Clinical Dermatology

Editors

DANIEL O. MORRIS
ROBERT A. KENNIS

VETERINARY CLINICS OF NORTH AMERICA: SMALL ANIMAL PRACTICE

www.vetsmall.theclinics.com

January 2013 • Volume 43 • Number 1

ELSEVIER

1600 John F. Kennedy Blvd. • Suite 1800 • Philadelphia, PA 19103-2899
http://www.vetsmall.theclinics.com

VETERINARY CLINICS OF NORTH AMERICA: SMALL ANIMAL PRACTICE Volume 43, Number 1
January 2013 ISSN 0195-5616, ISBN-13: 978-1-4557-7350-3

Editor: John Vassallo; j.vassallo@elsevier.com
Developmental Editor: Teia Stone

Veterinary Clinics of North America: Small Animal Practice (ISSN 0195-5616) is published bimonthly (For Post Office use only: volume 42 issue 1 of 6) by Elsevier Inc., 360 Park Avenue South, New York, NY 10010-1710. Months of issue are January, March, May, July, September, and November. Business and Editorial Offices: 1600 John F. Kennedy Blvd., Ste. 1800, Philadelphia, PA 19103-2899. Customer Service Office: 3251 Riverport Lane, Maryland Heights, MO 63043. Periodicals postage paid at New York, NY and additional mailing offices. Subscription prices are $283.00 per year (domestic individuals), $455.00 per year (domestic institutions), $138.00 per year (domestic students/residents), $375.00 per year (Canadian individuals), $559.00 per year (Canadian institutions), $416.00 per year (international individuals), $559.00 per year (international institutions), and $201.00 per year (international and Canadian students/residents). To receive student/resident rate, orders must be accompanied by name of affiliated institution, date of term, and the *signature* of program/residency coordinator on institution letterhead. Orders will be billed at individual rate until proof of status is received. Foreign air speed delivery is included in all *Clinics* subscription prices. All prices are subject to change without notice. **POSTMASTER:** Send address changes to *Veterinary Clinics of North America: Small Animal Practice*, Elsevier Health Sciences Division, Subscription Customer Service, 3251 Riverport Lane, Maryland Heights, MO 63043. Customer Service (orders, claims, online, change of address): Elsevier Periodicals Customer Service, Elsevier Health Sciences Division Subscription Customer Service 3251 Riverport Lane Maryland Heights, MO 63043. Tel: 1-800-654-2452 (U.S. and Canada); 314-447-8871 (outside U.S. and Canada). Fax: 314-447-8029. E-mail: journalscustomerservice-usa@elsevier.com (for print support); journalsonlinesupport-usa@elsevier.com (for online support).

Reprints. For copies of 100 or more of articles in this publication, please contact the Commercial Reprints Department, Elsevier Inc., 360 Park Avenue South, New York, NY 10010-1710. Tel.: 212-633-3812; Fax: 212-462-1935; E-mail: reprints@elsevier.com.

Veterinary Clinics of North America: Small Animal Practice is also published in Japanese by Inter Zoo Publishing Co., Ltd., Aoyama Crystal-Bldg 5F, 3-5-12 Kitaaoyama, Minato-ku, Tokyo 107-0061, Japan.

Veterinary Clinics of North America: Small Animal Practice is covered in *Current Contents/Agriculture, Biology and Environmental Sciences, Science Citation Index, ASCA, MEDLINE/PubMed (Index Medicus), Excerpta Medica, and BIOSIS.*

Printed in the United States of America.

Contributors

GUEST EDITORS

DANIEL O. MORRIS, DVM, MPH
Diplomate, American College of Veterinary Dermatology; Professor and Chief of
Dermatology and Allergy, School of Veterinary Medicine, University of Pennsylvania,
Philadelphia, Pennsylvania

ROBERT A. KENNIS, DVM, MS
Diplomate, American College of Veterinary Dermatology; Associate Professor,
Department of Clinical Sciences, College of Veterinary Medicine, Auburn University,
Auburn, Alabama

AUTHORS

PAUL BLOOM, DVM
Diplomate, American College of Veterinary Dermatology; Diplomate, American Board of
Veterinary Practitioners (Canine and Feline Speciality); Owner, Allergy, Skin and Ear Clinic
for Pets, Livonia; Assistant Adjunct Professor, Small Animal Clinical Sciences, Department
of Dermatology, College of Veterinary Medicine, Michigan State University, East Lansing,
Michigan

JEANNE B. BUDGIN, DVM
Diplomate, American College of Veterinary Dermatology; Staff Dermatologist, Department
of Dermatology and Allergy, Animal Specialty Center, Yonkers, New York

CHRISTINE L. CAIN, DVM
Diplomate, American College of Veterinary Dermatology; Assistant Professor of
Dermatology, Department of Clinical Studies-Philadelphia, School of Veterinary Medicine,
University of Pennsylvania, Philadelphia, Pennsylvania

DAVID DUCLOS, DVM
Diplomate, American College of Veterinary Dermatology; Clinical Veterinary Dermatology
Specialist, Animal Skin and Allergy Clinic, Lynnwood, Washington

MOLLY J. FLAHERTY, DVM
Associate Veterinarian, Integrative Pet Care, Chicago, Illinois

KINGA GORTEL, DVM, MS
Diplomate, American College of Veterinary Dermatology; Lake Country Veterinary
Specialist Hospital, British Columbia, Canada

MARIE INNERÅ, Dr med Vet
Finnsnes Dyreklinikk, Finnsnes, Norway

JAMES G. JEFFERS, VMD
Diplomate, American College of Veterinary Dermatology; Staff Dermatologist, Animal
Dermatology and Behavior Clinics, Inc., Gaithersburg, Maryland

ROBERT A. KENNIS, DVM, MS
Diplomate, American College of Veterinary Dermatology; Associate Professor,
Department of Clinical Sciences, College of Veterinary Medicine, Auburn University,
Auburn, Alabama

ELIZABETH A. MAULDIN, DVM
Diplomate, American College of Veterinary Pathologists; Diplomate, American College of
Veterinary Dermatology; Associate Professor of Dermatopathology, School of Veterinary
Medicine, University of Pennsylvania, Philadelphia, Pennsylvania

DANIEL O. MORRIS, DVM, MPH
Diplomate, American College of Veterinary Dermatology; Professor and Chief of
Dermatology and Allergy, School of Veterinary Medicine, University of Pennsylvania,
Philadelphia, Pennsylvania

CATHERINE A. OUTERBRIDGE, DVM, MVSc
Diplomate, American College of Veterinary Internal Medicine; Diplomate, American
College of Veterinary Dermatology; Associate Professor of Clinical Dermatology,
Department of Veterinary Medicine and Epidemiology, William Pritchard Veterinary
Medical Teaching Hospital, University of California Davis, California

BRIAN S. PALMEIRO, VMD
Diplomate, American College of Veterinary Dermatology; Fish Hospital, Lehigh Valley
Veterinary Dermatology, Allentown, Pennsylvania

Contents

> Although bacterial pyoderma is among the most commonly encountered dermatologic conditions in dogs, some cases present diagnostic challenges even to experienced clinicians. This article presents several unusual manifestations of pyoderma, including bullous impetigo, superficial spreading pyoderma, mucocutaneous pyoderma, and post-grooming furunculosis. Conditions mimicking pyoderma, including juvenile cellulitis, immunomodulatory-responsive lymphocytic-plasmacytic pododermatitis, and pemphigus foliaceus are also described. Diagnostic techniques used for diagnosing and characterizing pyoderma are also discussed.

> Staphylococcal antimicrobial resistance presents an emerging challenge for both human and veterinary medical professionals. Infections associated with methicillin- and multidrug-resistant staphylococci are increasingly encountered by veterinarians and are frequently associated with empiric therapeutic failures and limited systemic antimicrobial options. This article addresses mechanisms of antimicrobial resistance in common staphylococcal pathogens and implications for clinical practice, including indications for culture and susceptibility testing, rational antimicrobial selection, and potential for zoonotic transmission.

> The appearance and increasing prevalence of methicillin-resistant and multidrug-resistant staphylococcal skin infections has necessitated a change in how those infections are treated. Topical antibacterial treatments have evolved from elective adjunctive therapy to a more essential part of the treatment plan. This article reviews the ingredients and vehicles available for aggressive topical antibacterial treatment and prevention of *Staphylococcus* skin infections. Additionally, the basic tenets of improving client compliance and product efficacy are outlined.

> Feline otitis is reviewed by evaluating the predisposing, primary, and secondary causes. Diagnostic and treatment options are summarized. Emphasis is placed on comparing feline and canine otitis.

One of the best-recognized cutaneous manifestations of internal disease includes the skin changes seen in endocrine diseases. Cutaneous manifestations of internal disease can also be seen with certain neoplastic processes. Metabolic disturbances in zinc, lipid metabolism, or increased amino acid catabolism can result in zinc-responsive dermatosis, cutaneous xanthomas, and superficial necrolytic dermatitis, respectively. Certain infectious diseases can result in skin lesions that may provide visual clues but also critical diagnostic information if the skin is biopsied and cultured. Recognizing those skin changes that are clinical markers for internal disease can expedite the diagnosis and timely management of several systemic diseases.

Cyclosporine is an immunomodulatory medication that is efficacious and approved for atopic dermatitis in dogs and allergic dermatitis in cats; it has also been used to successfully manage a variety of immune-mediated dermatoses in dogs and cats. This article reviews the use of cyclosporine in veterinary dermatology including its mechanism of action, pharmacokinetics, drug interactions, side effects, and relevant clinical updates. Dermatologic indications including atopic/allergic dermatitis, perianal fistulas, sebaceous adenitis, and other immune-mediated skin diseases are discussed.

Pruritus, or itch, is defined as "a sensation that, if sufficiently strong, will provoke scratching or the desire to scratch." Pruritus is a symptom associated with a wide variety of causes and treatment options. Topical therapy is becoming the new target for the treatment of pruritus. The treatment of pruritus in the dog must be approached in a systematic manner and should include the search and resolution of the primary causes. Identifying and treating the primary cause of pruritus greatly increases the success rate of any therapy for pruritus.

This article presents an overview of alternative therapies for skin disorders including traditional Chinese medicine (acupuncture and Chinese herbs), homeopathy, and Western herbs and plant extracts. The medical and veterinary literature on the aforementioned modalities will be reviewed with a focus on reduction of inflammation and pruritus of the skin and ear canal in the canine species. Clinical application and potential adverse effects will also be included when available.

VETERINARY CLINICS OF NORTH AMERICA: SMALL ANIMAL PRACTICE

FORTHCOMING ISSUES

March 2013
Feline Diabetes
Jacquie Rand, BVSc, DVSc, *Guest Editor*

May 2013
Clinical Veterinary Dentistry
Steven Holmstrom, DVM, *Guest Editor*

July 2013
Emergency Medicine
Justine Lee, DVM, and Lisa Powell, DVM,
Guest Editors

RECENT ISSUES

November 2012
Otology and Otic Disease
Bradley L. Njaa, DVM, MVSc and
Lynette K. Cole, DVM, MS
Guest Editors

September 2012
Minimally Invasive Fracture Repair
Brian S. Beale, DVM and
Antonio Pozzi, DMV, MS, *Guest Editors*

July 2012
Geriatrics
William D. Fortney, DVM, *Guest Editor*

RELATED INTEREST

Veterinary Clinics of North America: Exotic Animal Practice
September 2012 (Vol. 14, No. 3)
Zoonoses, Public Health and the Exotic Animal Practitioner
Marcy J. Souza, DVM, MPH, Dipl. ABVP-Avian, Dipl. ACVPM, *Guest Editor*

Preface

Clinical Dermatology

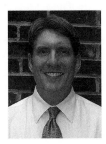 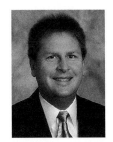

Daniel O. Morris, DVM, MPH, DACVD   Robert A. Kennis, DVM, MS, DACVD
Guest Editors

Over the past 10 years, our profession has witnessed a veritable explosion in research within the sciences of cutaneous biology and medicine. As such, it has become ever more difficult for veterinarians to stay abreast of advances in the specialties of dermatology and allergy. Our hope in presenting this issue of *Veterinary Clinics of North America: Small Animal Practice* is to provide updates and roadmaps that might assist our colleagues in navigating these ever-changing and exciting avenues of clinical medicine. With this goal in mind, we have organized the articles into 3 general topic areas:

1. The emerging challenges of recognizing and treating staphylococcal pyoderma: One of the hottest topics in veterinary dermatology (and indeed, in the broad field of infectious diseases) is the emergence of multiple-drug resistance in bacterial pathogens. In the first 3 articles, our authors review the disturbing trends in antimicrobial resistance of staphylococci that have occurred over the past decade and suggest strategies to overcome these formidable pathogens on behalf of our patients.
2. Cutaneous reaction patterns: Of the many challenges encountered in dermatologic practice, perhaps the most frustrating is the fact that the skin can react in only a limited number of ways to a seemingly endless variety of insults. As students just learning about dermatology so often lament, "everything looks the same!" In articles 4 to 9, our authors suggest diagnostic and therapeutic strategies to help us recognize and cope with some of the most common (and even a few uncommon) reaction patterns faced by practitioners in their daily work.
3. Dermatologic therapies: Veterinarians continue to search for less toxic compounds and minimally invasive interventions by which to treat a wide array of skin diseases. In the final 3 articles, our authors address various advances in cutaneous therapeutics. These include alternative therapies (such as acupuncture and nutraceuticals),

Vet Clin Small Anim 43 (2013) ix–x
http://dx.doi.org/10.1016/j.cvsm.2012.09.013   **vetsmall.theclinics.com**

options for the nonsteroidal treatment of pruritus, and an entire article dedicated to what many would consider to be the preeminent drug of the past decade: cyclosporine A.

Daniel O. Morris, DVM, MPH, DACVD
School of Veterinary Medicine
University of Pennsylvania
3900 Delancey Street
Philadelphia, PA 19104, USA

Robert A. Kennis, DVM, MS, DACVD
College of Veterinary Medicine
Auburn University
Auburn, AL 36849, USA

E-mail addresses:
domorris@vet.upenn.edu (D.O. Morris)
kennira@auburn.edu (R.A. Kennis)

Recognizing Pyoderma
More Difficult than it May Seem

Kinga Gortel, DVM, MS

KEYWORDS

- Canine pyoderma • Impetigo • Furunculosis • Mucocutaneous
- Bacterial overgrowth • Staphylococcus • Cytology • Bacterial culture

KEY POINTS

- Bacterial pyoderma is common in canine dermatology, but unusual manifestations including bullous impetigo, exfoliative superficial pyoderma (superficial spreading pyoderma), mucocutaneous pyoderma, and post-grooming furunculosis, can create diagnostic difficulty.
- Although it involves the same etiologic agents, the recently described bacterial overgrowth syndrome is distinct from pyoderma.
- Conditions such as juvenile cellulitis, immunomodulatory-responsive lymphocytic-plasmacytic pododermatitis, and pemphigus foliaceus can closely mimic pyoderma.
- Cutaneous cytology is among the most valuable, rapid, and inexpensive tools in veterinary dermatology, and is particularly useful in the diagnosis and characterization of pyoderma.
- Bacterial culture and susceptibility testing has become particularly useful with the increased incidence of resistant staphylococci as etiologic agents in canine pyoderma.

INTRODUCTION
Relevance

Bacterial pyoderma, a pyogenic bacterial infection of the skin, is among the most commonly encountered dermatologic conditions in dogs. Despite its prevalence and often typical clinical appearance, some cases present diagnostic challenges even to experienced clinicians. These difficulties can be posed by the development of unique clinical lesions, the presence of an unexpected etiologic agent, or by a close resemblance to another disease.

Bacteria and Canine Skin

The skin surface in animals and humans is colonized by bacteria that reside in the superficial epidermis and the infundibulum of the hair follicles.[1] The most common etiologic agent of pyoderma, *Staphylococcus pseudintermedius*, can frequently be

Lake Country Veterinary Specialist Hospital, 10564 Powley Court, Unit A, Lake Country, British Columbia V4V 1V5, Canada
E-mail address: dermvet@gmail.com

Vet Clin Small Anim 43 (2013) 1–18
http://dx.doi.org/10.1016/j.cvsm.2012.09.004
0195-5616/13/$ – see front matter © 2013 Elsevier Inc. All rights reserved.

isolated from oral, nasal, genital, and anal mucocutaneous sites. These sites are likely reservoirs for cutaneous colonization.[2] The organisms can be seeded onto the skin and hair by licking or grooming.[3] Pyoderma is very common in dogs compared with other domestic animals and humans. Reasons for their susceptibility to pyoderma are not fully characterized, but may include both physiologic and anatomic factors. The canine stratum corneum, the key physical barrier preventing the entry of bacteria into deeper parts of the skin, is thinner and more compact that that of other species studied. It also exhibits a paucity of intercellular lipids, a lack of a lipid follicular plug, and a higher pH.[1]

IS THIS PYODERMA?

Canine bacterial pyoderma assumes myriad clinical manifestations and is classified in various ways based on its appearance, depth of infection, and anatomic location. Pyoderma in dogs is often easy to identify by its typical clinical appearance. There are, however, manifestations of bacterial infection that are easily mistaken for other conditions, or in which a bacterial etiology is sometimes not suspected. For example, the very commonly encountered superficial bacterial folliculitis can sometimes lack obvious inflammatory lesions, manifesting with patchy alopecia and a "moth-eaten" appearance in short coated dogs such as Boxers. In silky coated dogs such as Yorkshire terriers, a patchy thinning of the hair coat can be the predominant abnormality[4] English Bulldogs uniquely often develop patches of alopecia with marked hyperkeratosis.[1] In these cases, lesions resolve with systemic anti-staphylococcal therapy. There also exist several conditions that can closely mimic pyoderma, but are distinctly different. The conditions most likely to create diagnostic difficulties are listed in **Box 1**, and several are discussed.

Box 1
Diagnostic challenges

Unusual manifestations of pyoderma or bacterial overgrowth

- Bullous impetigo
- Exfoliative superficial pyoderma (superficial spreading pyoderma)
- Mucocutaneous pyoderma
- Post-grooming furunculosis
- Acral lick dermatitis
- Nasal folliculitis and furunculosis
- Bacterial overgrowth syndrome

Conditions easily mistaken for pyoderma

- Juvenile cellulitis
- Imunomodulatory-responsive lymphocytic-plasmacytic pododermatitis
- Pemphigus foliaceus (and other pemphigus complex diseases)
- Subcorneal pustular dermatosis
- Superficial pustular drug reactions
- Sterile eosinophilic pustulosis
- Nasal eosinophilic folliculitis and furunculosis

UNUSUAL MANIFESTATIONS OF PYODERMA OR BACTERIAL OVERGROWTH
Bullous Impetigo

Bullous impetigo is a distinctive infectious pustular dermatosis of dogs characterized by the development of enlarging non-follicular pustules (**Fig. 1**). Bullous impetigo is reported to preferentially affect puppies or immunosuppressed adult dogs. It is seen most often with spontaneous or iatrogenic hyperadrenocorticism, but can also accompany other immunosuppressive diseases.[5] The condition is not pruritic.[6] Lesions appear most often in the glabrous areas of the groin and axillae, but can become generalized.[5]

The lesions of bullous impetigo are flaccid large pustules (bullae) typically ranging from 5 to 15 mm in diameter. The lesions are visually distinctive because they are much larger than the typical transient pustules seen with superficial folliculitis. Their contents can appear white, yellow, or even light green.[5] A margin of erythema is common. The pustules or bullae rupture easily and become overlain with yellow crust, often forming expanding epidermal collarettes.

Histopathology shows discrete subcorneal or intragranular pustules composed primarily of neutrophils. They can span several hair follicles. There can be mild separation of keratinocytes (acantholysis), but in some cases acantholysis is profound.[5] In the latter case, microscopic characteristics can be very similar to those seen in pemphigus foliaceus.[5,6] Two novel exfoliative toxins that digest canine desmoglein 1 and induce superficial epidermal acantholysis have been identified in *S pseudintermedius*. This finding highlights the likely importance of exfoliative toxin-induced acantholysis in dogs.[6–9]

Exfoliative Superficial Pyodermas

In dogs, exfoliative superficial pyodermas exist in 2 often-overlapping subtypes. The more common subtype is also called superficial spreading pyoderma.[6] Superficial spreading pyoderma is a common type of superficial bacterial skin disease in dogs that often accompanies superficial bacterial folliculitis.[5] In its less florid form, superficial spreading pyoderma is easy to recognize as a pyoderma lesion owing to the hallmark lesion of a rapidly expanding, and often erythematous and pruritic epidermal collarette, often affecting the axillae and groin (**Figs. 2 and 3**).[5]

In its more florid form, superficial spreading pyoderma can have an unusual and dramatic clinical appearance owing to the extent and severity of the lesions (**Fig. 4**). This form is seen most commonly in the Shetland Sheepdog, a breed in which it is

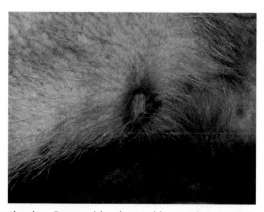

Fig. 1. Bullous impetigo in a Boxer with advanced hyperadrenocorticism.

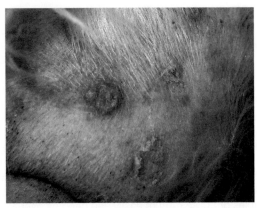

Fig. 2. Superficial folliculitis and superficial spreading pyoderma in the inguinal skin of a dog.

usually idiopathic. Border Collies, Australian Shepherds, and Collies are also predisposed to very severe lesions. A breed predisposition to colonization by exfoliative toxin-producing staphylococci has been suggested.[5] An initial pustular stage can be present, but is transient; the clinical signs are dominated by centrifugal peeling of the stratum corneum forming distinctive collarettes with erythematous borders and alopecia.[5,6] Individual coalescing collarettes can reach several centimeters in diameter, leading to extensive alopecia.[5] Treatment with an appropriate antibiotic usually results in rapid resolution of pruritus and inflammation, but relapses are frequent and often severe.[4]

The less common subtype of exfoliative superficial pyoderma closely resembles staphylococcal scalded skin syndrome in humans. The clinical signs are characterized by an acute onset of regionalized or generalized erythema with overlying scaling composed of large sheets of stratum corneum.

Mucocutaneous Pyoderma

Mucocutaneous pyoderma is a relapsing dermatosis of unknown etiology most commonly affecting the lips and perioral skin (**Fig. 5**).[1,4] The nasal planum and nares can also be affected. Less commonly, the eyelids, vulva, prepuce, and anus are involved.[10] The clinical appearance of the disease is variable and includes erythema

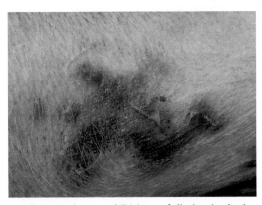

Fig. 3. Superficial spreading pyoderma exhibiting exfoliation in the inguinal skin of a dog.

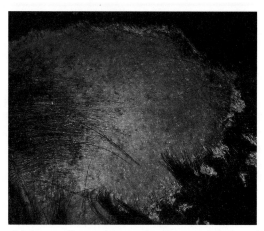

Fig. 4. Severe superficial spreading pyoderma leading to extensive alopecia in a Border Collie.

and swelling that progresses to crusting, fissuring, erosion, ulceration, and focal depigmentation.[10] German shepherds and their crosses are at increased risk of developing mucocutaneous pyoderma. The condition is easily confused with lip fold intertrigo, because it affects the same area, but the latter does not cause ulceration and is most common in spaniels.[5,10] Mucocutaneous pyoderma can be secondary to causes that typically cause bacterial infections, such as atopic dermatitis.[10]

When mucocutaneous pyoderma affects the nasal planum, it closely resembles discoid lupus erythematosus both clinically and histolopathogically. In many cases of nasal dermatitis, histopathologic changes cannot predict the response to treatment and distinguish an autoimmune from an infectious process.[4,11] Clinically, mucocutaneous pyoderma resolves with oral antibiotics. The response can be slow and relapses are common.[5] Treatment directed at staphylococci (based on culture if possible) should be attempted before immunomodulatory therapy whenever mucocutaneous pyoderma is suspected.[4]

Post-Grooming Furunculosis

Post-grooming furunculosis, an uncommon and distinctive subgroup of deep pyoderma, has a unique and severe clinical presentation. The onset is dramatically

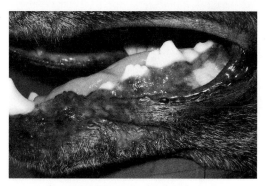

Fig. 5. Mucocutaneous pyoderma in a German shepherd.

acute, occurring 24 to 48 hours after bathing, hand stripping, or traumatic brushing.[4,5] The dorsal trunk is most commonly affected and lesions consist of pustules, hemorrhagic bullae, and fistulae typical of deep pyoderma (**Fig. 6**).[12] The affected skin is painful, even before the appearance of lesions.[12] Systemic symptoms of illness and fever often precede the onset of cutaneous lesions. The condition commonly affects dogs with thick hair shafts, such as dogs with wired haircoats and large-breed dogs. Minor trauma to the hair follicles combined with contaminated bathing products likely initiates the infection. Bacterial contamination of shampoo or cream rinse seems to be pivotal in the development of the condition.[5,12] In particular, self-serve dog washing facilities and grooming parlors using large communal containers of bathing products have been implicated.[5]

The diagnosis is based on the unique and rapidly appearing clinical signs and history. Bacterial culture is indicated because of the unpredictable susceptibility profiles of *Pseudomonas aeruginosa* and other gram-negative bacteria, which are often implicated. Cutaneous cytology and skin biopsies are useful adjunctive tests. Recommendations for avoiding post-grooming furunculosis include diluting shampoo or cream rinse on the day it is used, sterilizing all community containers (including pump nozzles) on a daily basis, encouraging sterilization of grooming tools (especially stripping combs), and postponing bathing for at least 2 weeks after hand stripping.[12] Instituting systemic therapy with an antibiotic targeted at gram-negative bacteria, such as a fluoroquinolone, is appropriate while culture/susceptibility is pending.[4]

Bacterial Overgrowth Syndrome

Bacterial overgrowth syndrome is not considered to be a form of pyoderma because it lacks neutrophilic inflammation or typical pyoderma lesions. It is included in this summary because like pyoderma, the condition is owing to bacteria, usually staphylococci. Bacterial overgrowth syndrome is a superficial cutaneous disorder characterized by marked pruritus, greasy seborrhea, offensive odor, erythema, lichenification, hyperpigmentation, excoriations, and alopecia (**Fig. 7**).[13] It most commonly affects that ventral aspect of the body, particularly the axillae and inguinal regions. Papules, pustules, epidermal collarettes, and crusts are absent in the syndrome, because the bacteria are present only on the skin surface. Its clinical appearance can closely resemble *Malassezia* dermatitis. As with *Malassezia* dermatitis, the condition is

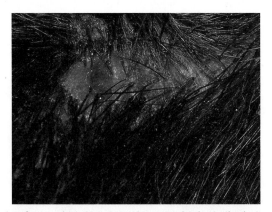

Fig. 6. Post-grooming furunculosis in a Great Dane. Multiple similar lesions were present on the dorsal trunk.

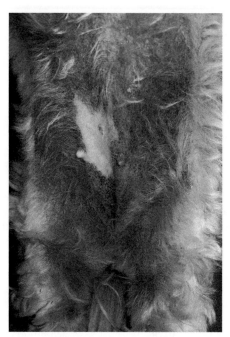

Fig. 7. Bacterial overgrowth syndrome in a mixed-breed dog. Note the clinical similarity to *Malassezia* dermatitis.

secondary to underlying allergic skin disease in some dogs. Cutaneous cytology in affected dogs shows significantly higher numbers of extracellular cocci on the lesional skin compared with normal dogs. Affected dogs show a reduction in pruritus and odor after treatment with antibiotics but can relapse upon discontinuation of treatment.[13] Topical antimicrobial therapy is important in the treatment of this condition because of the very superficial location of the organisms.

CONDITIONS EASILY MISTAKEN FOR PYODERMA
Juvenile Cellulitis

Juvenile cellulitis, also called juvenile pyoderma or puppy strangles, is a visually distinctive and often severe sterile inflammatory condition affecting puppies between 3 weeks and 4 months of age. The initial symptom of acute facial swelling is followed by the rapid development of papules and pustules that progress to draining tracts and crusts within 48 hours. The lesions are most prevalent on the lips, muzzle, chin, periocular area, and bridge of nose.[1] Juvenile cellulitis responds to corticosteroids. The condition can be diagnostically challenging for practitioners facing their first case of this uncommon dermatosis. Although it is distinguished by the age of onset, the clinical findings closely resemble what would be expected from severe deep pyoderma and cellulitis of bacterial etiology. Several cases have been reported in older puppies and adult dogs, which can also present significant diagnostic uncertainty.[14–16] Because corticosteroids are generally contraindicated in similarly presenting infectious conditions, the diagnosis relies on coupling the typical signalment, history, and clinical appearance with cytologic, parasitologic, and bacteriologic evidence of a sterile process. Histopathology is sometimes used to confirm the diagnosis.

Imunomodulatory-Responsive Lymphocytic-Plasmacytic Pododermatitis

The term lymphocytic-plasmacytic pododermatitis has been used to describe an idiopathic condition that closely resembles interdigital pyoderma. Affected dogs most commonly have chronic inflammatory lesions in all 4 feet. There are no age, gender, or seasonal predilections. The affected feet exhibit erythema, swelling, pain, alopecia, and occasionally sinous tracts. Despite a methodical search for an underlying infectious etiology, none is found in these cases. Histopathologically, the condition is characterized by epidermal hyperplasia, hyperkeratosis, spongiosis, dermal edema, and perivascular aggregates of lymphocytes and plasma cells. Affected dogs do not respond to appropriate antimicrobial therapy, but do improve with oral corticosteroids or cyclosporine.[17] Because it is an uncommon condition,[18] dogs presenting with pododermatitis must be subjected to diagnostic tests appropriate to rule out more common causes of pedal inflammation including interdigital pyoderma and pododemodicosis before this differential diagnosis is considered (see article by Duclos elsewhere in this issue). Histopathology and response to therapy can be used to support the diagnosis of imunomodulatory-responsive lymphocytic-plasmacytic pododermatitis.

Pemphigus Foliaceus

Pemphigus foliaceus, with its primary lesions of erythematous papules and pustules (**Fig. 8**), and secondary lesions of crusts, can be strikingly similar to superficial folliculitis, superficial spreading pyoderma, or bullous impetigo. This is particularly true when pemphigus affects the trunk. In most cases, pemphigus foliaceus involves areas that are rare for staphylococcal infections, such as the nasal planum, face, inner pinnae, and footpads. When it spares these sites, however, its presence can be overlooked. The appearance of the lesions can subtly different, with epidermal collarettes and centrifugal spreading typical of bacterial lesions being less common in pemphigus foliaceus.[9] Cytologic and histopathologic findings are usually helpful in determining the diagnosis, because pemphigus foliaceus lesions are characterized by sterile neutrophilic pustules with significant acantholysis (**Fig. 9**). In cases of bullous impetigo with significant acantholysis, however, histologic and cytologic features closely mimic those of pemphigus foliaceus and differentiating the 2 conditions can be difficult. In such cases, antimicrobial therapy based on culture/susceptibility testing of exudate from one or more of the pustules is an appropriate diagnostic and therapeutic step.

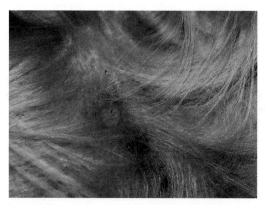

Fig. 8. Canine pemphigus foliaceus pustule bearing close resemblance to bacterial pyoderma.

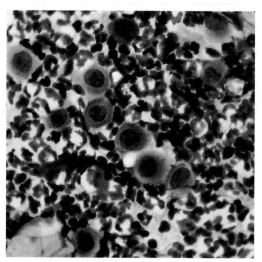

Fig. 9. Abundant acantholytic cells in a background of neutrophils found on cytologic examination of a canine pemphigus foliaceus pustule.

Diagnostic testing in pyoderma

The diagnosis of pyoderma is made based on history, physical examination, and additional diagnostic tests. Several tests are used in canine pyoderma, either to confirm the diagnosis, rule out similar conditions, or to guide therapy. The following tests are used most commonly:

- Cutaneous cytology;
- Bacterial culture and sensitivity;
- Histopathology; and
- Response to therapy.

CUTANEOUS CYTOLOGY
Indications

Cutaneous cytology is among the most valuable, rapid, and inexpensive tools in veterinary dermatology. It is recommended in nearly all cases of inflammatory skin and ear disease, and as an adjunct test in all samples submitted for bacterial culture. Although cytology can be collected and examined in various ways, in all cases the aim is to examine the lesions for pathogenic organisms (cocci, bacilli, yeast, or others) and to evaluate the cellular response or infiltrate.

Sample Collection and Processing

Many techniques exist for collecting cutaneous cytology, and the preferred technique varies between clinicians. A simple technique is the examination of exudate applied directly to a microscope slide and stained with a cytologic stain. A modified Wright's stain (Diff-Quik) is commonly used. With a few exceptions, the more time-consuming Gram stain is not a useful adjunctive step.[19] Acid-fast staining can be requested from a commercial laboratory when certain types of pathogens, particularly mycobacteria, are suspected. Collected material is allowed to air dry before fixation and staining. An alternative technique utilizing clear tape can also be very useful and is preferred by some clinicians. For the direct collection of cytologic specimens, material can be transferred to the microscope slide in various ways depending on the type of lesion examined. These techniques are listed in **Box 2**.

Interpretation

The interpretation of cutaneous cytology requires practice for proficiency. Because it is such a useful adjunct to clinical examination, it should be collected in nearly all cases with skin lesions. Stained slides are usually examined using the oil immersion lens (1000× magnification) using bright illumination with the light condenser up. The slide is first scanned at lower magnification to find areas containing a thin layer of material. A number of fields should then be scanned under oil immersion; the findings can vary substantially in various portions of the slide. Among the many things that can be gained by collecting cytology, the following are the most important.

- Microbiologic examination
    - Bacteria

Box 2
Techniques for collecting cytology specimens from various dermatologic lesions

- Pustule
    - Usually the most informative lesions
    - Open pustules with the edge of a microscope slide or needle
    - Touch microscope slide several times to purulent material
- Papule
    - Abrade with the edge of slide
    - Touch slide to abraded skin
- Epidermal collarette or crust
    - Undermine edge of the collarette with the edge of slide, or remove crust
    - Touch slide to skin under advancing edge of collarette or under crust
- Moist dermatitis, greasy skin, lichenified skin, dry seborrhea, patchy alopecia
    - Press slide several times to the affected skin to collect corneocytes
    - Heat fix to help dry or greasy debris adhere to the slide[19]
    - Tape technique or adhesive slides preferable for dry skin lacking surface exudate
- Draining tracts, fistulae, hemorrhagic bullae
    - Contamination with surface flora is likely in draining lesions
    - Pick intact lesions such as hemorrhagic bullae and furuncles
    - Aspirate by needle or squeeze lesion to extrude contents to the skin surface
- Skin folds
    - Swab with cotton-tipped applicator and roll
    - Sample small claw folds with the end of a broken cotton tipped applicator
- Unusual lesions
    - If biopsies are collected, touch the cut side surface of the biopsy onto 2 or 3 sterile glass slides
    - Stain with Diff-Quik and additional stains if needed

- *Cocci* (**Figs. 10** and **11**). These are the most common organisms found on cutaneous cytology, and usually represent *S pseudintermedius.* They are often found in pairs or tetrads.
- *Bacilli.* Rod-shaped bacteria are much less common as a cause of superficial pyoderma, but more common in surface infections or deep pyoderma.[4] Their presence should be interpreted in light of lesions and the sampling technique. Finding rod-shaped bacteria from an intact pustule, within neutrophils, or as the sole bacteria in a cytology preparation is suggestive of their role in the infection. When they are found in mixed populations, or from open lesions, the possibility of surface contamination must be considered (**Fig. 12**).
- Approximate numbers of bacteria should be recorded. Cytologic examination of the skin of normal dogs yields fewer than 2 bacteria per oil immersion field.[1] Because bacteria are generally difficult to count, some clinicians rely on a rating scale for bacterial numbers, such as a 0 (none) to 4+ (too numerous to count) scale. Although serial examination of bacterial counts can be useful to follow the progress of an infection, it is difficult to ascribe significance purely to their numbers. For example, the number of bacteria tends to be very high in surface infections, lower in superficial pyoderma, and very low in deep pyoderma. A pitfall of cytologic examination is that in some cases of deep pyoderma, bacteria cannot be found despite extensive examination (**Fig. 13**). Finally, because both Gram-positive and Gram-negative bacteria stain a dark blue using Diff-Quik stain, this staining should not be used to classify them as Gram positive.
- Melanin granules are oval- to rod-shaped and similar in size to bacteria. They are easily mistaken for bacteria on cytologic examination (see **Figs. 10** and **14**). The key difference is color: Unlike bacteria, melanin granules are refractory to stain but retain their brown to black color. The color difference is best appreciated when the fine focus is manipulated.[19]

○ Yeast
- The most common cutaneous yeast is the visually distinctive *Malassezia* sp. Its numbers are generally quantitated as the approximate number per oil immersion field.

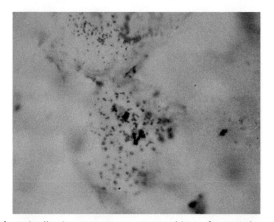

Fig. 10. Clusters of cocci adhering to a corneocyte on skin surface cytology from the trunk of a dog. The corneocyte is visible as a faint outline of a flat, angular cell. No inflammatory cells are present to suggest infection; bacterial overgrowth is likely. Note the numerous melanin granules associated with the corneocytes.

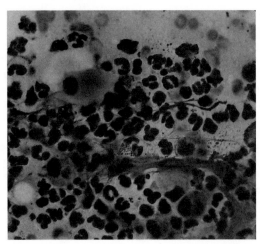

Fig. 11. Cytologic examination of a pustule in a dog with superficial folliculitis showing intracellular and extracellular cocci with neutrophils.

○ Rarely, other organisms are seen. These include positively staining fungal hyphae, yeast, and filamentous bacteria. Mycobacteria do not stain using Diff-Quik, but can be visible as "negative images" within macrophages. *Simonsiella* sp., a harmless very large bacterial saprophyte of the oral cavity can be found in areas subjected to licking (see **Fig. 14**).[19] Non-staining *Demodex* mites can sometimes be collected on a cytologic preparation, but this method is not recommended for their detection. Cutaneous cytology can also show a wide variety of pollens and mold spores that are sometimes be mistaken for pathogens.

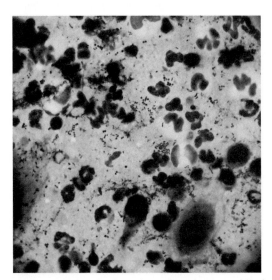

Fig. 12. Mixed bacterial population (rods and cocci) and neutrophils from the surface of a severely ulcerated deep pyoderma lesion. Because of the collection site, the status of the bacteria as primary etiologic agents or surface contaminants is difficult to ascertain.

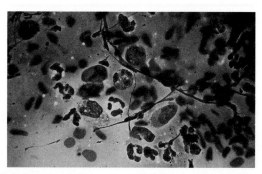

Fig. 13. Neutrophils, erythrocytes, macrophages, and an eosinophil from an intact lesion of deep pyoderma in a dog. Etiologic agents can be elusive in these cases. Nuclear streaming from neutrophil lysis is likely an artifact of the collection technique.

- Cellular examination
  - Neutrophilic inflammation is a hallmark of pyoderma lesions. In its absence, pyoderma is unlikely and the presence of bacteria can be associated with surface colonization, as seen with bacterial overgrowth syndrome (see **Fig. 10**). Even in these cases, the bacteria can still be clinically relevant. Conversely, the finding of intracellular bacteria is highly suggestive of infection rather than colonization (see **Fig. 11**). Neutrophils associated with infection can show degenerative or "toxic" changes, including karyolysis, swollen nuclei that tend to lose their lobate appearance.[20] The presence of degenerate neutrophils should prompt the close examination for microbial organisms. In some cases of bullous impetigo in immunosuppressed dogs, the number of bacteria is very high and neutrophils exhibit profound degenerative changes, sometimes making recognition of nuclear lobes difficult. A common artifact encountered with neutrophilic inflammation is that cellular destruction releases nuclear streaks that are sometimes mistaken for fungal hyphae (see **Fig. 13**).[20]
  - Neutrophilic inflammation with an absence or relative paucity of bacteria and with well-preserved neutrophils lacking degenerative changes warrants

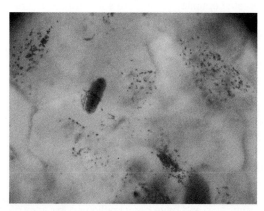

Fig. 14. Skin surface cytology showing the large *Simonsiella sp.* bacterium, a normal inhabitant of the canine oral cavity whose presence on the skin is associated with licking. Note several rod-shaped bacteria are also present, as well as abundant melanin granules associated with corneocytes.

consideration of a sterile inflammatory condition. The most common of these is pemphigus foliaceus. Cytologic examination of pustules in this disease typically shows large numbers of acantholytic keratinocytes, large round cells with a central nucleus, and basophilic cytoplasm (see **Fig. 9**).[19,20] These can uncommonly be mistaken for macrophages, which have an eccentric, oval, and sometimes indented nucleus and often marked vacuolation (see **Fig. 13**).[20] Although finding acantholytic cells in abundance is suggestive of pemphigus, a pitfall is that some infectious conditions, including certain subtypes of dermatophytes and bullous impetigo, can also show marked acantholysis.

o Other inflammatory cells can be found in pyoderma lesions concurrently with neutrophils. Macrophages are often abundant in deep pyoderma and eosinophils are common when furunculosis is present (see **Fig. 13**).

BACTERIAL CULTURE AND SENSITIVITY
Indications

Bacterial culture and susceptibility testing are a useful adjunctive test in canine pyoderma and has become particularly useful with the increasing incidence of resistant staphylococcal pyoderma. Because bacterial growth can be expected from any area of lesional skin even if bacteria are playing a minor role, culture is not used to confirm the diagnosis of pyoderma unless an unusual organism is suspected. Instead, it is most often used to choose an appropriate systemic antibiotic for treatment or to investigate treatment failures. Some of the indications for collecting bacterial cultures include the following.

o Infections responding poorly to empiric therapy;
o Suspected gram-negative bacteria (rod-shaped bacteria on cytology);
o Suspected atypical bacterial infection (*Mycobacterium*, *Actinomyces*, *Nocardia*, and others);
o Deep pyoderma;
o Severe or life-threatening infections; and
o Frequently relapsing pyoderma.

Sample Collection and Submission

Bacterial culture and susceptibility testing are submitted to reference laboratories. In all cases, cytology should be collected concurrently to ensure concordance between the 2 tests. Cytologic findings should be reported to the microbiology laboratory at the time of submission. In cases requiring immediate treatment, therapy is initiated based on cytology results and adjusted as needed based on culture.

The techniques used for collection of bacterial cultures vary with the type of lesion present. Except for certain cases of deep pyoderma, aseptic preparation of the skin is not recommended. Dogs with multiple pustules usually, but not always, exhibit the same strain of bacteria from several pustules.[21] When multiple lesions are present, more than one can be sampled with the material combined on one swab. The techniques used to collect culture samples are summarized in **Box 3**.

Samples should be submitted to laboratories capable of identifying staphylococci to their species level. In particular, the coagulase-variable organism *S schleiferi* must be accurately reported. Both the coagulase-positive and coagulase-negative subtypes of this organism are pathogenic and have been implicated in cases of pyoderma.[25] They are associated with recurrent infections and show a high rate of methicillin resistance.[25–27] The coagulase-positive subtype, *S schleiferi coagulans*, has likely been underreported by automated staphylococcal identification systems because it is

---

Box 3
Techniques for collecting cytology specimens from various dermatologic lesions

- *Pustules* are the most desirable lesions to sample for culture so a close examination should be performed to find intact pustules, particularly in the more sparsely haired skin of the ventral abdomen. They are punctured with a needle and swabbed.

- *Papules* are superficially punctured using a needle or scalpel blade, with purulent or serous material collected by swab.

- *Epidermal collarettes* are sampled by rolling a dry sterile swab across the lesion several times (this technique showed a sensitivity of 81.8% in 1 study).[22]

- *Crusts* are removed to swab the underlying skin.

- If suspecting *bacterial colonization and overgrowth*, a representative area of affected skin is swabbed.

- *Deep pyoderma* lesions should be sampled by aspirate or expression before they ulcerate or rupture (hemorrhagic bullae or furuncles are ideal); aspirated material is transferred to a swab. Alternatively, skin punch biopsy can be collected after disinfection of the skin surface.[1] Acral lick dermatitis should be sampled by biopsy, because deep cultures do not correlate well with superficial cultures and often show resistance to empiric drugs.[23] Care should be taken to rinse the skin well with non-preserved saline solution or water, to prevent the disinfectant solution from inhibiting the growth of bacteria in vitro.[4,24] Tissue samples are submitted in a culturette or sterile glass vial for minced tissue culture.[1,4]

- *Folliculitis* lesions lacking surface pathology can also be sampled by skin punch biopsy.

- *Unusual lesions* in which atypical organisms (eg, *Mycobacteria*, anaerobes) are suspected are also usually sampled by biopsy, but may require special handling and transport media; consult with the laboratory before sample collection

---

phenotypically similar to other coagulase-positive staphylococci.[2] The importance of the coagulase-negative subtype, *S schleiferi schleiferi*, as an emerging pathogen underlines the necessity for microbiology laboratories to also fully speciate the coagulase negative staphylococci.[4] It is likely that this coagulase negative subspecies, previously considered nonpathogenic, has been previously underreported.[2]

Interpretation

The results of the culture should always be interpreted in light of the cytology findings. Agreement between the 2 tests is expected. The most common species isolated in canine pyoderma is *S pseudintermedius*. Finding other staphylococci is not uncommon, but their significance varies depending on species. The other coagulase-positive staphylococci, *S aureus* and *S schleiferi coagulans*, should be considered pathogenic. Coagulase-negative staphylococci have previously been considered nonpathogenic, but this has changed with the characterization of *S schleiferi schleiferi* as a significant (and often resistant) pathogen in canine pyoderma. *S schleiferi schleiferi* should always be considered pathogenic. Other species of coagulase-negative staphylococci, despite frequently exhibiting multiple drug resistance, are much less likely to be pathogenic. Thus, if the culture has been collected from a contaminated site such as a skin surface swab, the result must be interpreted with caution. However, if they are isolated from an intact primary lesion such as a pustule they are much more likely to be significant. The culture can be repeated in cases where their significance seems unclear.[4]

Gram-negative bacteria such as *P aeruginosa* are uncommon agents in superficial pyoderma, but are more common in deep pyoderma[28] and surface infections such as intertrigo either as the sole pathogens or in combination with staphylococci. Resistance to empiric antimicrobials is common, particularly with *Pseudomonas* sp.,[28] so systemic antimicrobial therapy should be guided by susceptibility results.

Increasingly common and problematic isolates from cases of canine pyoderma are methicillin-resistant staphylococci, discussed in greater detail in article by Cain elsewhere in this issue. Although the term methicillin-resistant is commonly used, most veterinary diagnostic laboratories use oxacillin or cefoxitin as a surrogate for methicillin.[29] Isolates exhibiting methicillin resistance can appear susceptible to some β-lactam antibiotics in vitro, but are actually resistant to this entire class of drugs in vivo. This is important to realize; some veterinary diagnostic laboratories incorrectly report susceptibility to various β-lactam antibiotics in methicillin-resistant strains.[2] Therapeutic options can be limited by resistance to various classes of commonly used antimicrobial drugs. Veterinarians should also be aware of inducible clindamycin resistance, which has been reported in canine staphylococci and complicates with interpretation of susceptibility reports.[30,31] This phenomenon causes isolates to seem to be clindamycin-susceptible but erythromycin-resistant in vitro. Treatment failure can be expected when clindamycin is used for these strains.[30,31]

The zoonotic and reverse-zoonotic potential of methicillin-resistant *S aureus*, and less so the other staphylococci, should be considered and discussed with clients when these organisms are isolated.[32,33]

HISTOPATHOLOGY

Because most cases of pyoderma are straightforward to diagnose, histopathology is rarely used to confirm the diagnosis. In fact, pyoderma is usually treated before collecting skin biopsies because the infection can obscure subtle lesions of underlying diseases. However, histopathology is essential to securing a diagnosis in certain cases. These include infections with more unusual etiologic agents that can be difficult or slow to culture. A variety of histologic stains are available to highlight suspected etiologic agents. Histopathology is also useful in differentiating infection from immune-mediated pustular or crusting lesions.

RESPONSE TO THERAPY

Evaluating the response to therapy, usually to antimicrobial drugs, is a helpful diagnostic step when other tests have not yielded a definitive diagnosis or cannot be performed. A response to therapy can help to differentiate conditions such as mucocutaneous pyoderma from discoid lupus erythematosus, juvenile cellulitis from infectious cellulitis, and bullous impetigo from pemphigus foliaceus.

SUMMARY

Although canine pyoderma is common, certain cases present significant diagnostic challenges. Cytologic examination is among the most useful and rapid diagnostic tests used to investigate patients with suspected pyoderma. Bacterial culture and susceptibility testing is an increasingly important tool used to choose therapy for this condition owing to the emergence of resistant etiologic agents.

REFERENCES

1. Scott DW, Miller WH, Griffin CE. Muller & Kirk's small animal dermatology. Philadelphia: W.B. Saunders Company; 2001.

2. May ER. Bacterial skin diseases: current thoughts on pathogenesis and management. Vet Clin North Am Small Anim Pract 2006;36(1):185–202.
3. Saijonmaa-Koulumies LE, Lloyd DH. Colonization of the canine skin with bacteria. Vet Dermatol 1996;7(3):153–62.
4. Morris DO. Unusual pyoderma. 25th Annual Congress of the ESVD-ECVD Brussels (Belgium), September 7-10, 2011.
5. Gross TL, Ihrke PJ, Walder EJ, et al. Skin diseases of the dog and cat: clinical and histopathologic diagnosis. 2nd edition. Oxford (United Kingdom): Blackwell Science Ltd; 2005.
6. Olivry T, Linder KE. Dermatoses affecting desmosomes in animals: a mechanistic review of acantholytic blistering skin diseases. Vet Dermatol 2009;20(5–6): 313–26.
7. Iyori K, Hisatsune J, Kawakami T, et al. Identification of a novel Staphylococcus pseudintermedius exfoliative toxin gene and its prevalence in isolates from canines with pyoderma and healthy dogs. FEMS Microbiol Lett 2010;312(2): 169–75.
8. Iyori K, Futagawa-Saito K, Hisatsune J, et al. Staphylococcus pseudintermedius exfoliative toxin EXI selectively digests canine desmoglein 1 and causes subcorneal clefts in canine epidermis. Vet Dermatol 2011;22(4):319–26.
9. Olivry T. Update on canine autoimmune skin diseases: selected topics. North American Veterinary Dermatology Forum Galveston (TX), April 2011;26(1):41–7.
10. Bassett RJ, Burton GG, Robson DC. Antibiotic responsive ulcerative dermatoses in German shepherd dogs with mucocutaneous pyoderma. Aust Vet J 2004;82(8): 485–9.
11. Wiemelt SP, Goldschmidt MH, Greek JS, et al. A retrospective study comparing the histopathological features and response to treatment in two canine nasal dermatoses, DLE and MCP. Vet Dermatol 2004;15(6):341–8.
12. Ihrke PJ, Gross TL. Warning about postgrooming furunculosis. J Am Vet Med Assoc 2006;229(7):1081–2.
13. Pin D, Carlotti DN, Jasmin P, et al. Prospective study of bacterial overgrowth syndrome in eight dogs. Vet Rec 2006;158(13):437–41.
14. Bassett RJ, Burton GG, Robson DC. Juvenile cellulitis in an 8-month-old dog. Aust Vet J 2005;83(5):280–2.
15. Neuber AE, van den Broek AH, Brownstein D, et al. Dermatitis and lymphadenitis resembling juvenile cellulitis in a four-year-old dog. J Small Anim Pract 2004; 45(5):254–8.
16. Jeffers JG, Duclos DD, Goldschmidt MH. A dermatosis resembling juvenile cellulitis in an adult dog. J Am Anim Hosp Assoc 1995;31(3):204–8.
17. Breathnach RM, Baker KP, Quinn PJ, et al. Clinical, immunological and histopathological findings in a subpopulation of dogs with pododermatitis. Vet Dermatol 2005;16(6):364–72.
18. Breathnach RM, Fanning S, Mulcahy G, et al. Canine pododermatitis and idiopathic disease. Vet J 2008;176(2):146–57.
19. Mendelsohn C, Rosenkrantz W, Griffin CE. Practical cytology for inflammatory skin diseases. Clin Tech Small Anim Pract 2006;21(3):117–27.
20. Albanese F. Atlas of dermatological cytology of dogs and cats. Milan (Italy): Merial Italia; 2010.
21. Pinchbeck LR, Cole LK, Hillier A, et al. Pulsed-field gel electrophoresis patterns and antimicrobial susceptibility phenotypes for coagulase-positive staphylococcal isolates from pustules and carriage sites in dogs with superficial bacterial folliculitis. Am J Vet Res 2007;68(5):535–42.

22. White SD, Brown AE, Chapman PL, et al. Evaluation of aerobic bacteriologic culture of epidermal collarette specimens in dogs with superficial pyoderma. J Am Vet Med Assoc 2005;226(6):904–8.
23. Shumaker AK, Angus JC, Coyner KS, et al. Microbiological and histopathological features of canine acral lick dermatitis. Vet Dermatol 2008;19(5):288–9.
24. Hnilica KA. Small animal dermatology: a color atlas and therapeutic guide. St Louis: Elsevier Saunders; 2011.
25. Frank LA, Kania SA, Hnilica KA, et al. Isolation of Staphylococcus schleiferi from dogs with pyoderma. J Am Vet Med Assoc 2003;222(4):451–4.
26. Kania SA, Williamson NL, Frank LA, et al. Methicillin resistance of staphylococci isolated from the skin of dogs with pyoderma. Am J Vet Res 2004;65(9):1265–8.
27. Morris DO, Rook KA, Shofer FS, et al. Screening of Staphylococcus aureus, Staphylococcus intermedius, and Staphylococcus schleiferi isolates obtained from small companion animals for antimicrobial resistance: a retrospective review of 749 isolates (2003-04). Vet Dermatol 2006;17(5):332–7.
28. Hillier A, Alcorn JR, Cole LK, et al. Pyoderma caused by Pseudomonas aeruginosa infection in dogs: 20 cases. Vet Dermatol 2006;17(6):432–9.
29. van Duijkeren E, Catry B, Greko C, et al. Review on methicillin-resistant Staphylococcus pseudintermedius. J Antimicrob Chemother 2011;66(12):2705–14.
30. Faires MC, Gard S, Aucoin D, et al. Inducible clindamycin-resistance in methicillin-resistant Staphylococcus aureus and methicillin-resistant Staphylococcus pseudintermedius isolates from dogs and cats. Vet Microbiol 2009; 139(3–4):419–20.
31. Rubin JE, Ball KR, Chirino-Trejo M. Antimicrobial susceptibility of Staphylococcus aureus and Staphylococcus pseudintermedius isolated from various animals. Can Vet J 2011;52(2):153–7.
32. Faires MC, Tater KC, Weese JS. An investigation of methicillin-resistant Staphylococcus aureus colonization in people and pets in the same household with an infected person or infected pet. J Am Vet Med Assoc 2009;235(5):540–3.
33. Weese JS, Dick H, Willey BM, et al. Suspected transmission of methicillin-resistant Staphylococcus aureus between domestic pets and humans in veterinary clinics and in the household. Vet Microbiol 2006;115(1–3):148–55.

Antimicrobial Resistance in Staphylococci in Small Animals

Christine L. Cain, DVM

KEYWORDS

- *Staphylococcus* • Methicillin resistance • Multidrug resistance • Pyoderma
- Antimicrobial therapy

KEY POINTS

- Methicillin resistance is the most important mechanism of antimicrobial resistance in staphylococci and conveys resistance to all β-lactam derivatives.
- Methicillin-resistant staphylococci are frequently multidrug resistant by additional genetic mechanisms, making empiric antimicrobial selection difficult.
- Culture and susceptibility testing are often overlooked, but are increasingly indicated, in the clinical management of staphylococcal pyoderma.
- Systemic antimicrobial options for resistant staphylococcal pyoderma are often limited; potential adverse drug effects and drug interactions should be considered in treatment decisions.
- The medical literature suggests that transmission of methicillin-resistant staphylococci between humans and animals can occur; strict hygiene practices should be observed when handling infected patients.

INTRODUCTION

During the past several decades, the prevalence of staphylococcal antimicrobial resistance, particularly methicillin resistance, has risen substantially in both the human and the veterinary health care arenas. Infections associated with antimicrobial resistant *Staphylococcus* spp are increasingly encountered by veterinary practitioners. Staphylococcal resistance, in turn, presents significant challenges for successful empiric therapy, limits antimicrobial treatment options, and raises concerns of potential zoonotic transmission. This article will review common mechanisms of antimicrobial resistance in *Staphylococcus pseudintermedius*, *Staphylococcus aureus*, *Staphylococcus schleiferi*, and coagulase-negative staphylococci (CoNS). Implications of staphylococcal antimicrobial resistance for clinical practice, including rational antimicrobial selection and indications for culture and susceptibility testing, will be highlighted.

The author has no disclosures.
Department of Clinical Studies - Philadelphia, School of Veterinary Medicine, University of Pennsylvania, 3900 Delancey Street, Philadelphia, PA 19104, USA
E-mail address: ccain@vet.upenn.edu

Vet Clin Small Anim 43 (2013) 19–40
http://dx.doi.org/10.1016/j.cvsm.2012.09.003
0195-5616/13/$ – see front matter © 2013 Elsevier Inc. All rights reserved.
vetsmall.theclinics.com

METHICILLIN RESISTANCE

Methicillin resistance is the most important antimicrobial resistance mechanism in staphylococci. Methicillin resistance is conveyed by the *mecA* gene, carried on the mobile genetic element staphylococcal chromosome cassette *mec* (SCCmec), which encodes for an altered penicillin binding protein (PBP2a). Production of this altered penicillin binding protein renders resistance to all β-lactam derivatives, including penicillins, potentiated penicillins, cephalosporins, and carbapenems.[1] In veterinary staphylococcal isolates, the source of the *mecA* gene is unknown, although there is evidence in human medicine that the *mecA* gene likely originated in *Staphylococcus sciuri* (a CoNS) with possible horizontal transfer to *S aureus*.[2] Although references to methicillin resistance are pervasive in the medical literature, oxacillin is commonly used in veterinary microbiology laboratories as the correlate for testing antimicrobial resistance. Both drugs are semisynthetic penicillinase-resistant penicillins, but oxacillin possesses greater in vitro stability.[3,4] In keeping with the common vernacular, "methicillin resistance" will be used throughout this article.

METHICILLIN-RESISTANT STAPHYLOCOCCI OF VETERINARY IMPORTANCE
Methicillin-Resistant S pseudintermedius

S pseudintermedius is the most common cause of pyoderma in dogs and also normally colonizes the skin and mucosal sites.[5] This species was previously known as *S intermedius*. Recently, investigators used molecular techniques to more correctly classify 3 closely related staphylococcal species (*Staphylococcus intermedius*, *S pseudintermedius*, and *Staphylococcus delphini*) as the *S intermedius* group. Furthermore, it now seems that all previously classified *S. intermedius* isolates from dogs, cats, and humans were actually *S pseudintermedius* isolates.[5–7] For simplification purposes, isolates from these species will be referred to as *S pseudintermedius* throughout this article, even in referencing results of studies published before the reclassification of the *S. intermedius* group.

The prevalence of methicillin-resistant *S pseudintermedius* (MRSP) infections in veterinary patients has increased substantially during the past decade. Two reports of antimicrobial susceptibility of veterinary *S pseudintermedius* isolates in the mid-1980s failed to identify any methicillin-resistant isolates.[8,9] Following sporadic reports of MRSP isolates in the 1990s,[10,11] reports of MRSP infections are now commonplace in the veterinary literature. MRSP is a potential pathogen of dogs, cats, and horses; infection has been associated with pyoderma, otitis, urinary tract infections, wounds, surgical site infections, and septicemia.[12–17] In the United States, 2 large retrospective studies of clinical submissions to veterinary microbiology laboratories documented an overall MRSP prevalence of 15.6% (Jones and colleagues; 2001–2005) and 17% (Morris and colleagues[13]; 2003–2004), respectively.[18] Since that time, clinical isolation of MRSP seems to have increased; in 2008, nearly 30% of *S pseudintermedius* isolates from the University of Tennessee veterinary bacteriology laboratory were methicillin resistant.[3] Reported frequency of MRSP isolation from canine pyoderma varies with geographic location. For example, one recent Japanese study reported an MRSP prevalence of 66.7% from dogs with pyoderma,[19] whereas MRSP has only been more recently documented in Europe and isolation rates from clinical samples are low, but they may be increasing.[12,14,20]

MRSP has also been isolated from carriage sites of healthy dogs and cats. Multiple recent studies have investigated MRSP carriage in healthy dogs and/or cats in different geographic areas; sampled sites vary but include the nares, oral mucosa, skin, and rectal mucosa.[21–33] Reported prevalence of MRSP carriage in healthy dogs ranges from 0% to 30%, although several studies support a carriage rate in healthy dogs of 1.5% to 3%.[21,22,24–33] One study by Griffeth and colleagues[24] also investigated MRSP carriage in dogs with inflammatory skin disease; an overall prevalence of 7% was found, compared with 2% prevalence in healthy dogs. Far fewer investigators have examined MRSP carriage in cats. Abraham and colleagues[23] demonstrated a prevalence of MRSP carriage of 4% in healthy cats, but MRSP was not isolated from cats with inflammatory skin disease. Couto and colleagues[26] failed to isolate MRSP from the carriage sites of healthy cats. In a study of veterinary dermatology staff and their household pets, Morris and colleagues[33] found relatively high rates of MRSP carriage in dogs (6.2%) and cats (3.1%), suggesting that the pets of veterinary dermatology staff may be at increased risk for colonization by MRSP. Taken together, the literature suggests that reported prevalence of MRSP in clinical specimens may significantly exceed the prevalence of MRSP colonization in healthy animals, although there may be variation by geographic region and the sampled population.

As is the case for methicillin-resistant *S aureus* (MRSA), several closely related (clonal) MRSP lineages have been identified.[6,12,15,34–36] Furthermore, epidemic clonal strain types may differ by geographic region, suggesting that multiple methicillin-susceptible *S pseudintermedius* (MSSP) strains have acquired the *mecA* gene and successfully proliferated among the canine population.[6,34,36] For example, by the molecular technique of multilocus sequence typing, most MRSP isolates from North America have been classified as the clonal lineage ST68, whereas most European MRSP isolates are ST71.[6,12,15,34,36]

Although methicillin-resistant staphylococci are not necessarily more virulent than methicillin-susceptible staphylococci,[37] treatment of MRSP infections may present a major clinical challenge because of the multidrug resistance of isolates. High rates of resistance to non–β-lactam antimicrobials, including macrolides, lincosamides, tetracyclines, fluoroquinolones, and potentiated sulfonamides, have been reported in the United States, Europe, and Asia.[3,12–15,18–20,26,29,30,34,38–40] Resistance to these additional antimicrobials is mediated by genetic mechanisms other than the *mecA* gene. Antimicrobials to which MRSP isolates often exhibit susceptibility include fusidic acid, mupirocin, amikacin, rifampin, vancomycin, linezolid, and teicoplanin.[12,14,20,29,39,40] Susceptibility to chloramphenicol is variable; many European isolates are resistant to chloramphenicol,[15,39] whereas good susceptibility has been reported in MRSP isolates in the United States.[3,13] In the author's experience, chloramphenicol resistance seems to be increasing in the United States and is dependent on the region of practice. In a study of 103 MRSP isolates from various countries in Europe, various regions of the United States, and Canada, Perreten and colleagues[34] showed that 57.3% of isolates showed resistance to chloramphenicol, whereas only 1.9% of isolates showed resistance to rifampin. Options for antimicrobial treatment of MRSP infections will be further discussed later in the article.

Risk factors for MRSP acquisition have been investigated in only a few veterinary studies. In a recent retrospective study by Bryan and colleagues,[41] dogs with pyoderma caused by MRSP were no more likely to have a concurrent endocrinopathy, neoplasia, or to be receiving immunosuppressive drug therapy than dogs with MSSP isolated on skin culture. In a 2011 study by Huerta and colleagues,[42] dogs with methicillin-resistant staphylococci isolated on skin culture, mainly belonging to the *S intermedius* group, were more likely to be housed in an urban setting and to have received systemic antimicrobial treatment within the year before culture. Prior antimicrobial therapy may play a significant role in the acquisition of MRSP. As shown by Beck and colleagues,[43] subsequent MRSP isolation from the skin and mucosal sites of dogs with previous MSSP pyoderma following antimicrobial therapy is common. In this study, no association was found between prior antimicrobial exposure and MRSP isolation from infection or carriage sites, but treatment of pyoderma with clindamycin was associated with MRSP isolation on follow-up culture. Taken together, these results suggest that systemic antimicrobial therapy may alter the patient's commensal staphylococcal flora and thus allow for colonization by methicillin-resistant strains. This concept is supported by work in horses showing an increase in commensal staphylococci harboring drug-resistance genes, including *mecA*, following hospitalization and prophylactic penicillin treatment.[44]

Given the increase in MRSP infections, as well as the frequent multidrug resistance of isolates, the risk of MRSP transmission to other in-contact pets and humans, and of environmental contamination, has been a topic of concern. MRSP colonization of dogs and cats residing in the same household as a dog with a clinical MRSP infection has been demonstrated. For the most part, risk of MRSP colonization for healthy in-contact pets seems to correspond with active clinical lesions in dogs with diagnosed MRSP infections and to decrease after clearance of the infection.[45,46] Rare MRSP infections in humans have been reported; in most cases, dog-to-human transmission is suspected.[47–49] Nasal colonization of humans with MSSP and MRSP has also been shown, particularly in veterinarians, veterinary personnel, and persons residing in households with dogs with *S pseudintermedius* infections.[30,33,45,46,50–56] In several cases, MRSP isolates obtained from pets and from humans have been found to be identical on pulsed-field gel electrophoresis (PFGE), further supporting pet-to-human transmission.[33,45,54,56] In one study, lack of handwashing after the handling of pets was found to be a risk factor for nasal MRSP isolation.[50] Human colonization with MRSP is likely transient and seems to clear after clinical resolution of the pet's infection.[46,54,55] Environmental contamination of households and veterinary hospital with MRSP has also been demonstrated.[45,46,52] Environmental isolation of MRSP also seems to be associated with active lesions in patients with MRSP infections, although the organism has been isolated from environmental samples even in the absence of MRSP isolation from household humans or pets.[46]

MRSA

In humans, *S aureus* is a major cause of skin and soft tissue infections and colonizes approximately 30% of the human population worldwide.[57] Although *S aureus* colonization of healthy dogs has been reported,[58] the prevalence seems to be much lower than that of *S pseudintermedius* colonization.[59] In cats, there is conflicting evidence as to whether *S pseudintermedius* or *S aureus* is the primary colonizing coagulase-positive staphylococcal species.[60–63]

There has been a dramatic increase in the number of infections caused by MRSA in human medicine since the 1960s.[64] Although human MRSA infections were once regarded as primarily hospital-associated and nosocomial in origin, community-associated MRSA infections of healthy individuals have rapidly emerged during the past decade.[64,65] Both hospital-associated and community-associated MRSA infections are now recognized as major causes of human morbidity, mortality, and health care expenditures.[64,66] With the increasing importance of MRSA in the human health care arena, there has been a great deal of interest in MRSA infections in animals. Prevalence of methicillin resistance in clinical veterinary *S aureus* isolates has been reported to approximate 25% to 35%.[13,18] MRSA infections have been reported in a variety of companion and exotic animal species, including dogs, cats, horses, parrots, rabbits, guinea pigs, turtles, bats, elephants, and marine mammals.[13,16,67–94] Most infections involve wounds, both postsurgical and traumatic, but MRSA has also been isolated from cases of pyoderma, otitis, respiratory disease, cystitis, prostatitis, joint infections, and septicemia.[13,16,67,69–94] MRSA infections in companion and exotic animals are most often associated with predominant hospital-acquired or community-acquired clonal strains in the surrounding human population; this supports, but does not prove, human-to-animal transmission.[68–71,73–77,82–88,90–94]

Risk factors for MRSA infection in dogs and cats may include recent administration of antimicrobials, particularly β-lactams or fluoroquinolones; multiple antimicrobial courses; multiple-day hospitalization; surgical implants; intravenous catheterization; or contact with an ill or hospitalized human.[78,95] As with MRSP infections, empiric therapy can be challenging because of potential drug resistance; MRSA isolates are often resistant to non–β-lactam antibiotics, particularly fluoroquinolones, macrolides, and lincosamides.[13]

Healthy dogs and cats may be colonized by MRSA, although this colonization may be transient, particularly in dogs, and the organism may not be isolated on repeated sampling.[81,96,97] Reported prevalence of MRSA colonization in healthy dogs or on admission to veterinary hospitals ranges from 0% to approximately 3%, whereas reported prevalence in cats ranges from 0% to 4%.[21–26,33,50,77,98] In one study, animals presenting for veterinary care were significant more likely to carry MRSA than were healthy animals.[98] Several studies have suggested the possibility of MRSA transmission from colonized or infected humans to animals, or vice versa, often via demonstration of genotypically identical strains.[33,52,69,72,73,86,90,96,97,99–112] The true direction of transmission often cannot be proved, however. Although human-to-animal transmission is usually assumed, the epidemiologic relationships may be complex; even in households with infected or colonized humans, that person may not be identified as the MRSA source for the pet.[96,113] The risk of direct pet-to-pet transmission seems to be low, especially among healthy colonized dogs.[81]

MRSA is an emerging pathogen in horses and farm animals, particularly pigs. In North America, horses may be colonized by or infected with a clonal MRSA strain known as USA500 (or Canadian epidemic MRSA-5).[114–120] Although this strain was initially associated with nosocomial infections in humans, it has now become well adapted to horses, but it may colonize or cause infection in humans with close horse contact.[115–118] Pigs may harbor a clonal MRSA strain known as ST398; this strain seems to have arisen in swine and may colonize large numbers of pigs in some herds, particularly in Europe.[121,122] MRSA ST398 has been isolated from infections in dogs and humans,[121,123] from commercial pork products in the United States and Canada,[124,125] and from carriage sites of humans with pig contact.[126,127]

Colonization by MRSA may be an occupational risk for veterinarians and veterinary staff. In 2001 through 2004, the prevalence of human nasal MRSA colonization in the United States was 1.5%.[128] By contrast, nasal colonization prevalence rates in veterinarians and veterinary staff of 3.5% to 21.4% have been reported in screening studies in North America, Europe, and Australia.[33,129–132] Although some studies have reported a much higher prevalence of nasal colonization in large animal (including equine) practitioners,[129,133] others have reported equal isolation from the nares of small and large animal practitioners.[130] MRSA may also be isolated from environmental sites in veterinary hospitals, although the role of the environment in MRSA transmission is not entirely clear.[134–137]

Methicillin Resistant S schleiferi

S schleiferi is a unique staphylococcal species in that 2 variants have been described based on coagulase production: *S schleiferi* subsp *schleiferi* (coagulase negative) and *S schleiferi* subsp *coagulans* (coagulase positive). Recent work suggests that the 2 subspecies are not genotypically distinct and do not differ in clinical behavior.[138,139] Coagulase-positive and coagulase-negative S schleiferi have been reported to cause infections in dogs and are mainly associated with pyoderma and otitis in dogs with allergic dermatitis.[138–144] When isolated from dogs with pyoderma, there may be an association with recurrent pyoderma and prior or concurrent antimicrobial therapy.[139,142]

Methicillin resistance seems to be particularly prevalent in clinical isolates of S schleiferi with rates of methicillin resistance exceeding 50% in several reports.[1,138,139,142,145] Despite frequent methicillin resistance, S schleiferi isolates may maintain favorable susceptibility to non–β-lactam antimicrobials, especially to potentiated sulfonamides.[13,138,139] Fluoroquinolone resistance is common in methicillin-resistant S schleiferi (MRSS) isolates.[13,19,138,139,146,147] Risk factors for clinical isolation of MRSS identified in one retrospective study of 225 infections in dogs included recent (30 days to 6 months before culture) treatment with penicillins, potentiated penicillins, or first- and second-generation cephalosporins or treatment with third-generation cephalosporins within 30 days of culture.[139] These results suggest that alteration of the patients' methicillin-susceptible flora may have predisposed to colonization by MRSS, as has been found with S pseudintermedius after antimicrobial therapy.[43]

S schleiferi colonization of companion animals has been infrequently investigated in the veterinary literature. Coagulase-positive S schleiferi has been isolated from carriage sites of cats and dogs[21,23,24,33] and may be found together with S pseudintermedius.[148] Prevalence of colonization with coagulase-positive MRSS has been reported to be 0.5% in a convenience sampled population of dogs entering a veterinary teaching hospital[21]; 2% in healthy dogs and dogs with inflammatory skin disease[24]; and 0.4% in dogs belonging to veterinary dermatologists or staff.[33] Coagulase-positive MRSS was not isolated from healthy cats or cats with inflammatory skin disease in the study by Abraham and colleagues.[23] Coagulase-negative S schleiferi has been less frequently documented as a normal inhabitant of dogs and cats. This variant has been isolated from the ears of healthy dogs.[143] Coagulase-negative MRSS has been isolated from carriage sites of cats[23] and dogs[24] with inflammatory skin disease, with a 2% prevalence in both species, and from 1 of 258 dogs (0.4%) belonging to veterinary dermatology practice staff.[33] MRSS may also be isolated from carriage sites of dogs with pyoderma caused by MRSS, as well as dogs with other staphylococci isolated from skin lesions.[43]

In humans, coagulase-negative S schleiferi is well documented as a normal component of preaxillary flora, although it has been associated with nosocomial infections, including surgical and pacemaker implantation site infections.[149–151] By contrast, coagulase-positive S schleiferi is an infrequent cause of human infections; only 2 infections have been documented in the medical literature to date.[152,153] In the second reported infection, a case of endocarditis in a human liver transplant recipient, a family dog with recurrent otitis was suspected as the source, but molecular characterization was not done to show identical strains from the person and the dog.[153] In the 2010 study by Morris and colleagues[33] of methicillin-resistant staphylococcal colonization in veterinary dermatology staff and pets, a higher prevalence of MRSS colonization, with a predominance of coagulase-positive isolates, was demonstrated in humans compared with dogs and cats. This finding suggests that MRSS colonization, particularly by the coagulase-positive variant, may be an occupational risk for veterinarians and veterinary staff.

Methicillin-Resistant CoNS

Both coagulase-negative and coagulase-positive S schleiferi are important pathogens in veterinary medicine. The clinical importance of other CoNS, which have historically been considered to be commensal organisms or contaminants with limited pathogenic potential, is less well established. In human medicine, CoNS represent an emerging cause of opportunistic infections, particularly nosocomial infections. Isolates may produce a variety of different virulence factors and exhibit high levels of methicillin resistance.[154–156] In veterinary medicine, CoNS may be isolated from the skin and mucosal sites of healthy animals,[157–162] as well as from cultures of infection sites[75,163–165] and from environmental sites in veterinary hospitals.[158,166] Methicillin resistance in veterinary isolates of CoNS has been reported,[75,157,158,160,161,167,168] highlighting their potential importance as both reservoirs of drug resistance and opportunistic pathogens.

OTHER MECHANISMS OF STAPHYLOCOCCAL ANTIMICROBIAL RESISTANCE

As discussed previously, methicillin-resistant staphylococci frequently exhibit coresistance to non–β-lactam antimicrobials by mechanisms unrelated to acquisition of the *mecA* gene. Clindamycin resistance, resistance to tetracyclines, and fluoroquinolone resistance will be specifically discussed.

Clindamycin Resistance

Resistance to the related macrolides and lincosamides, including clindamycin, may be conveyed by the staphylococcal *msrA* gene, which encodes for antimicrobial efflux, or the *erm* genes, which encode for changes to the ribosomal antimicrobial target site. Clindamycin resistance encoded by the *erm* genes may be either constitutive, in which resistance is shown to all drugs in these related classes (ie, both erythromycin and clindamycin), or inducible, in which the presence of an inducing agent (eg, erythromycin) promotes expression of a resistant phenotype. Use of clindamycin in infections caused by isolates exhibiting inducible resistance may result in treatment failure.[169,170] Inducible clindamycin resistance has been well documented in MRSA isolates from humans and animals and has been reported in some MRSP isolates as well.[34,169–171] Microbiology laboratories can test for inducible clindamycin resistance using a double disc diffusion test (D-test) with adjacent erythromycin and clindamycin discs (**Fig. 1**).[169] In the absence of this test, clinicians may predict inducible resistance based on susceptibility reports indicating erythromycin resistance and clindamycin susceptibility. In these cases, clindamycin use should be avoided.[169,171]

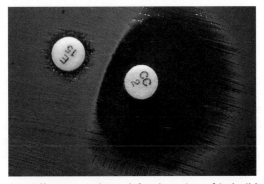

Fig. 1. The double disc diffusion test (D-test) for detection of inducible clindamycin resistance illustrating the D-shaped zone around the clindamycin disc ("CC") when in close proximity to the erythromycin disc ("E"). (*Courtesy of* Dr David A. Bemis and the University of Tennessee Veterinary Bacteriology Laboratory.)

Tetracycline Resistance

Staphylococcal resistance to tetracyclines may be mediated by plasmid-situated genes (tetK or tetL) encoding for antimicrobial efflux, or by the chromosomal or transposon-situated tetM or tetO genes, which encode for alteration of the ribosomal antimicrobial target site.[172] The tetK and tetM genes seem to be the most important mediators of resistance in MRSP isolates.[34] Isolates possessing the tetM gene are considered to be resistant to all tetracylines, including doxycycline and minocycline.[172] Tetracycline-resistant isolates belonging to the ST68 lineage, the predominant MRSP clone in North America, have been found to carry the tetM gene.[34] Staphylococcal isolates possessing the tetK gene, by contrast, are considered to be resistant to tetracycline and susceptible to minocycline. Doxycycline resistance in both tetM- and tetK-positive MRSA isolates may be induced by incubation with subinhibitory concentrations of tetracyclines,[172] suggesting that doxycycline may be a poor choice for any staphylococcal isolate exhibiting resistance to tetracycline by susceptibility testing. Tetracycline-resistant isolates belonging to the ST71 lineage, the predominant European MRSP clone, have been found to carry the tetK gene, indicating the minocycline may be an appropriate therapeutic option for MRSP infections in Europe if supported by susceptibility test results.[34]

Fluoroquinolone Resistance

Fluoroquinolones exhibit rapid bactericidal activity via inhibition of bacterial topoisomerase (TP) II, also known as DNA gyrase, and TP-IV, thus preventing bacterial DNA synthesis.[89,173,174] Staphylococcal resistance to fluoroquinolones may be mediated by chromosomal mutations in the genes encoding DNA gyrase and TP-IV. Both of these enzymes contain 2 subunits: DNA gyrase is made up of GyrA and GyrB (encoded by the gyrA and gyrB genes, respectively) and TP-IV is made up of GrlA and GrlB (encoded by the grlA and grlB genes, respectively). In S aureus, mutations encoding for amino acid substitutions in GyrA and GrlA, and subsequent fluoroquinolone resistance, occur most often in the well-conserved quinolone resistance determining regions of the gyrA and grlA genes.[89,147] Mutations in genes encoding for DNA gyrase and topoisomerase IV have been demonstrated in veterinary isolates of fluoroquinolone-resistant MRSA, MRSP, and MRSS.[29,38,89,147] Other potential mechanisms of staphylococcal fluoroquinolone resistance include drug efflux pumps and reduced intracellular accumulation caused by altered membrane diffusion channels.[147,175] One study demonstrated that fluoroquinolone resistance may be induced in vitro by subinhibitory drug concentrations, although the molecular mechanism was not investigated.[175]

IMPLICATIONS OF STAPHYLOCOCCAL ANTIMICROBIAL RESISTANCE

The increase in methicillin resistance in veterinary staphylococcal isolates presents significant challenges in clinical management of infections, particularly staphylococcal pyoderma, by limiting therapeutic options. Many methicillin-resistant isolates are also multidrug resistant, making successful empiric therapy difficult. The remainder of the article will discuss the changing face of clinical practice in the age of antimicrobial resistance, including indications for culture and susceptibility testing, rational empiric therapy for staphylococcal pyoderma, and potential treatment options for resistant staphylococcal infections.

Indications for Culture and Susceptibility Testing

The importance of bacterial culture and susceptibility testing is often overlooked in the management of staphylococcal pyoderma. Given the increasing prevalence of methicillin resistance, as well as the unpredictable antimicrobial susceptibility of MRSP, MRSA, and MRSS isolates, culture and susceptibility testing are likely indicated much more than are routinely performed by practitioners. Indications for culture and susceptibility testing include:

- Infections that have failed to respond to appropriate empiric therapy[176]
- Clinical lesions (nodules, hemorrhagic bullae, draining tracts, furuncles) consistent with deep pyoderma
- Cytologic evidence of mixed infection (such as intracellular rods and cocci)[176]
- Recurrent or relapsing pyoderma[42,95]
- Recent antimicrobial administration, which may predispose to colonization, and subsequent infection, by methicillin-resistant strains[42,43,78,139]
- Prior methicillin-resistant staphylococcal infection, because colonization, particularly with MRSP, may persist for extended periods of time[177]

Rational Empiric Therapy

Despite the increasing importance of culture and susceptibility testing in management of staphylococcal pyoderma, empiric therapy may be appropriate in selected cases, particularly first-time or treatment-naïve infections. β-Lactam derivatives, especially cephalosporins, are frequently considered to be first-line choices in the treatment of pyoderma because of their good tissue penetration, low risk of adverse effects, and bactericidal activity against methicillin-susceptible staphylococci.[178] Concerns about selection for colonization by methicillin-resistant strains may support the empiric choice of other antimicrobials, such as macrolides, lincosamides, or potentiated sulfonamides, instead of cephalosporins or potentiated penicillins, for treatment-naïve infections.[139] In the study by Beck and colleagues,[43] however, administration of clindamycin was associated with subsequent MRSP isolation from dogs with pyoderma. With recognition of the role of systemic antimicrobial therapy in the acquisition of methicillin-resistant strains, there may be a paradigm shift to increased reliance on topical antimicrobial therapy in the treatment of canine pyoderma, especially first-time, mild, or localized infections.[43]

Systemic fluoroquinolone therapy may be indicated in selected instances, such as treatment of mixed infections according to culture and susceptibility results,[176] but their empiric use for canine pyoderma is not recommended. As discussed previously, many methicillin-resistant staphylococcal isolates exhibit coresistance to fluoroquinolones, often leading to therapeutic failure with empiric administration. Fluoroquinolone exposure is also a potential risk factor for MRSA isolation in humans[179] and in dogs,[78] possibly by increasing susceptibility to colonization by highly fluoroquinolones-resistant strains,[179] as well as by promoting adhesion of MRSA to host cells.[180]

Treatment of Methicillin-Resistant Staphylococcal Infections

Potential antimicrobial options for methicillin-resistant staphylococcal pyoderma, as based on susceptibility test results, are listed in **Table 1**. Treatment duration, as for methicillin-susceptible staphylococcal pyoderma, should be a minimum of 3 to 4 weeks, with 1 week past clinical resolution, for superficial infections; and a minimum of 6 to 8 weeks, with 2 weeks past clinical resolution, for deep infections.[176] Clinical resolution of MRSP-associated pyoderma may take longer than clinical resolution of MSSP-associated pyoderma.[41] This may be a result of infection chronicity and secondary pathologic changes to the skin, instead of an indication that methicillin resistant strains are more virulent than methicillin-susceptible strains.[41,80]

Table 1
Potential systemic antimicrobial options for methicillin resistant staphylococcal infections in dogs (as based on culture and susceptibility data)

Drug (Brand Name)	Dose, mg/kg	Dosing Interval	Typical Route
Erythromycin	10–15	q8 h	PO
Lincomycin (Lincocin)	22	q12 h	PO
Clindamycin (Antirobe)	10	q12 h	PO
	11	q24 h	
Trimethoprim-sulfa (Tribrissen, Bactrim, Septra)	15–30	q12 h	PO
Ormetoprim-sulfadimethoxine (Primor)	55 (d 1) 27.5 (subsequent d)	q24 h	PO
Doxycycline (Vibramycin)	5–12	q12 h	PO
Minocycline (Minocin)	5–12	q12 h	PO
Enrofloxacin (Baytril)	5–20	q24 h	PO
Marbofloxacin (Zeniquin)	2.75–5.5	q24 h	PO
Chloramphenicol (Viceton)	50	q8 h	PO
Rifampin (Rifadin, Rimactane)	5–10	q12–24 h	PO
Amikacin (Amiglyde-V)	15–20	q24 h	IV, SC

Antimicrobial options for treatment of pyoderma associated with multidrug-resistant staphylococci are often severely limited. Chloramphenicol, rifampin, and aminoglycosides, particularly amikacin, may be the only remaining effective systemic antimicrobial agents indicated by susceptibility tests.[3,12–14] Despite good in vitro susceptibility,[12] use of antimicrobial agents that are more common for serious MRSA infections in humans, such as linezolid and vancomycin,[181] should be avoided in veterinary patients because of ethical concerns.[34,39] These drugs are also often prohibitively expensive in veterinary patients.[182]

When prescribing chloramphenicol, rifampin, or amikacin, practitioners should be aware of potential adverse effects in treated patients. Chloramphenicol has the potential for dose-dependent bone marrow suppression, with cats more susceptible to this effect than dogs.[183] In humans, chloramphenicol may rarely cause idiosyncratic and irreversible pancytopenia[182,183]; clients should be warned to take precautions when handling this medication. The most common side effects of chloramphenicol administration in dogs seem to be gastrointestinal upset, inappetence, and weight loss; these adverse effects may be severe enough to warrant drug discontinuation.[41] Chloramphenicol may also interact with other drugs via inhibition of hepatic cytochrome P450 microenzymes.[182,183] This effect must be kept in mind when prescribing chloramphenicol in combination with other cytochrome P450 substrates, particularly anticonvulsants.[183]

Rifampin is most often administered in combination with other antimicrobials for treatment of mycobacterial and rhodococcal infections,[182,183] although it also exhibits antistaphylococcal activity.[184,185] Resistance to rifampin is rare, even among methicillin-resistant strains.[34] Resistance may arise quickly, however, when rifampin is used as a monotherapy by mutations within the rifampin resistance-determining region of the staphylococcal *rpoB* gene.[186] Adverse effects of rifampin include hepatic enzyme induction and increase in hepatic enzyme activity, particularly alkaline phosphatase.[187] In some dogs, serious, and potentially fatal, hepatotoxicity may occur, with corresponding increases in hepatic enzyme activity indicting hepatocellular damage and hyperbilirubinemia.[183,187] Other potential effects include gastrointestinal upset, hemolytic anemia, thrombocytopenia, and orange discoloration of bodily fluids.[182,183,187] To decrease the risk of adverse effects, it is recommended not to exceed a total daily dose of 10 mg/kg in dogs.[187] Rifampin is also a potent inducer of hepatic cytochrome P450 microenzymes and may, thus, reduce serum levels and activity of other cytochrome P450 substrates.[182,183]

Like other aminoglycosides, amikacin must be administered parenterally.[183] When used for treatment of pyoderma, it may be administered subcutaneously by the client at home. The primary adverse effect of concern is nephrotoxicity, specifically renal proximal tubular necrosis.[182,183] Amikacin may be less nephrotoxic than other amino-glycosides, particularly gentamicin.[183] Urinalyses should be frequently monitored for signs of nephrotoxicity; decreased specific gravity, casts, proteinuria, or glucosuria should precede azotemia.[183] When using amikacin, the author advises twice-weekly urinalyses. At the first sign of nephrotoxicity, amikacin administration should be discontinued; renal toxicity is generally reversible with early drug withdrawal.[188] Amino-glycosides also have the potential to cause ototoxicity via induction of inner ear hair cell apoptosis and may result in permanent deafness.[189]

With the increase in staphylococcal multidrug resistance, limited options for systemic therapy, and potential for adverse drug effects, interest in the role of topical antimicrobial therapy for resistant staphylococcal infections has increased. Topical therapy alone has been found to be effective for treatment of pyoderma associated with methicillin-resistant staphylococci.[14,41,190] Readers are referred to the article by Jeffers elsewhere in this issue for further exploration of topical therapy for drug-resistant pyoderma.

Infection Prevention and Decolonization

Standardized guidelines for preventing the spread of methicillin-resistant staphylo-cocci have not been established in veterinary medicine. Strict hygiene practices seem to be of the utmost importance in limiting transmission of methicillin-resistant staphylococci from pets to pets, from pets to humans (or from infected humans to pets), and from pets to the environment. Recommended hygiene practices include regular handwashing, particularly after handling infected patients and between patients; covering open or draining wounds; preventing pets from licking human care-takers; restricting infected pets from sleeping in the bed with human caretakers (or vice versa); frequent environmental disinfection, washing of pet bedding, and cleaning of pet dishes; and barrier precautions within veterinary hospitals when working with infected patients (disposable gloves, etc).[37,39,50,96,112,191,192]

Several case reports in the medical literature have discussed decolonization of pets by use of topical or systemic antimicrobials as a strategy for management of MRSA transmission in households.[101,104,107,109] Fusidic acid application has also been reported to reduce *S pseudintermedius* colonization of mucosal sites in dogs.[193] Neither the efficacy nor the optimal types of decolonization strategies for methicillin resistant staphylococci have been well established in veterinary patients. Moreover, staphylo-coccal colonization seems to be widespread over the skin and mucosal sites,[24] making targeted decolonization difficult to impossible.

SUMMARY

In conclusion, methicillin- and multi-drug resistant staphylococci are increasingly iso-lated from veterinary patients, particularly from dogs with pyoderma and otitis. Prac-titioners should be aware of the most common mechanisms of staphylococcal antimicrobial resistance and the implications for successful clinical management of resistant infections. Judicious antimicrobial usage, including basing treatment decisions on culture and susceptibility data when appropriate, should be encouraged.

REFERENCES

1. Kania SA, Williamson NL, Frank LA, et al. Methicillin resistance of staphylococci isolated from the skin of dogs with pyoderma. Am J Vet Res 2004;65:1265–8.
2. Wu S, Piscitelli C, de Lencastre H, et al. Tracking the evolutionary origin of the methicillin resistance gene: cloning and sequencing of a homologue of *mecA* from a methicillin susceptible strain of Staphylococcus sciuri. Microb Drug Resist 1996;2:435–41.
3. Bemis DA, Jones RD, Frank LA, et al. Evaluation of susceptibility test breakpoints used to predict *mecA*-mediated resistance in *Staphylococcus pseudintermedius* isolated from dogs. J Vet Diagn Invest 2009;21:53–8.
4. Cole LK, Kwochka KW, Hillier A, et al. Identification of oxacillin-resistant staphylococci in dogs with end-stage otitis. Vet Rec 2006;159:418–9.
5. Sasaki T, Kikucki K, Tanaka Y, et al. Reclassification of phenotypically identified *Staphylococcus intermedius* strains. J Clin Microbiol 2007;45:2770–8.
6. Bannoehr J, Ben Zakour NL, Waller AS, et al. Population genetic structure of the *Staphylococcus intermedius* group: insights into *agr* diversification and the emergence of methicillin-resistant strains. J Bacteriol 2007;189: 8685–92.
7. Fitzgerald JR. The *Staphylococcus intermedius* group of bacterial pathogens: species re-classification, pathogenesis and the emergence of methicillin resistance. Vet Dermatol 2009;20:490–5.
8. Phillips WE, Williams BJ. Antimicrobial susceptibility patterns of canine *Staphylococcus intermedius* isolates from veterinary clinical specimens. Am J Vet Res 1984;45:2376–9.
9. Medleau L, Long RE, Brown J. Frequency and antimicrobial susceptibility of *Staphylococcus* species isolated from canine pyodermas. Am J Vet Res 1986;47:229–31.
10. Piriz S, Valle J, Mateos EM, et al. In vitro activity of fifteen antimicrobial agents against methicillin-resistant and methicillin-susceptible Staphylococcus intermedius. J Vet Pharmacol Ther 1996;19:118–23.
11. Gortel K, Campbell KL, Kakoma I, et al. Methicillin resistance among staphylococci isolated from dogs. Am J Vet Res 1999;60:1526–30.
12. Ruscher C, Lubke-Becker A, Semmler T, et al. Widespread rapid emergence of a distinct methicillin- and multidrug-resistant *Staphylococcus pseudintermedius* (MRSP) genetic lineage in Europe. Vet Microbiol 2010;144:340–6.
13. Morris DO, Rook KA, Shofer FS. Screening of *Staphylococcus aureus, Staphylococcus intermedius*, and *Staphylococcus schle*iferi isolates obtained from small companion animals for antimicrobial resistance: a retrospective review of 749 isolates (2003-04). Vet Dermatol 2006;17:332–7.
14. Loeffler A, Linek M, Moodley A, et al. First report of multiresistant, *mecA*-positive *Staphylococcus intermedius* in Europe: 12 cases from a veterinary dermatology referral clinic in Germany. Vet Dermatol 2007;18:412–21.
15. Kadlec K, Schwarz S, Perreten V, et al. Molecular analysis of methicillin-resistant *Staphylococcus pseudintermedius* of feline origin from different European countries and North America. J Antimicrob Chemother 2010;65:1826–37.
16. Penna B, Varges R, Martins R, et al. In vitro antimicrobial resistance of staphylococci isolated from canine urinary tract infection. Can Vet J 2010;51:738–42.

17. Weese JS. A review of multidrug resistant surgical site infections. Vet Comp Orthop Traumatol 2008;21:1–7.
18. Jones RD, Kania SA, Rohrbach BW, et al. Prevalence of oxacillin- and multidrug-resistant staphylococci in clinical samples from dogs: 1,772 samples (2001-2005). J Am Vet Med Assoc 2007;230:221–7.
19. Kawakami T, Shibata S, Murayama N, et al. Antimicrobial susceptibility and methicillin resistance in *Staphylococcus pseudintermedius* and *Staphylococcus schleiferi* subsp. *coagulans* isolated from dogs with pyoderma in Japan. J Vet Med Sci 2010;72:1615–9.
20. Ruscher C, Lubke-Becker A, Wleklinski CG, et al. Prevalence of methicillin-resistant *Staphylococcus pseudintermedius* isolated from clinical samples of companion animals and equidaes. Vet Microbiol 2009;136:197–201.
21. Hanselman BA, Kruth S, Weese JS. Methicillin-resistant staphylococcal colonization in dogs entering a veterinary teaching hospital. Vet Microbiol 2008;126: 277–81.
22. Gingrich EN, Kurt T, Hyatt DR, et al. Prevalence of methicillin-resistant staphylococci in northern Colorado shelter animals. J Vet Diagn Invest 2011;23:947–50.
23. Abraham JL, Morris DO, Griffeth GC, et al. Surveillance of healthy cats and cats with inflammatory skin disease for colonization of the skin by methicillin-resistant coagulase-positive staphylococci and *Staphylococcus schleiferi* ssp. schleiferi. Vet Dermatol 2007;18:252–9.
24. Griffeth GC, Morris DO, Abraham JL, et al. Screening for skin carriage of methicillin-resistant coagulase-positive staphylococci and *Staphylococcus schleiferi* in dogs with healthy and inflamed skin. Vet Dermatol 2008;19:142–9.
25. Vanderhaeghen W, Van De Velde E, Crombe F, et al. Screening for methicillin-resistant staphylococci in dogs admitted to a veterinary teaching hospital. Res Vet Sci 2011;93(1):133–6.
26. Couto N, Pomba C, Moodley A, et al. Prevalence of methicillin-resistant staphylococci among dogs and cats at a veterinary teaching hospital in Portugal. Vet Rec 2011;169:72.
27. Vengust M, Anderson ME, Rousseau J, et al. Methicillin-resistant staphylococcal colonization in clinically normal dogs and horses in the community. Lett Appl Microbiol 2006;43:602–6.
28. Epstein CR, Yam WC, Peiris JS, et al. Methicillin-resistant commensal staphylococci in healthy dogs as a potential zoonotic reservoir for community-acquired antibiotic resistance. Infect Genet Evol 2009;9:283–5.
29. Onuma K, Tanabe T, Sato H. Antimicrobial resistance of *Staphylococcus pseudintermedius* isolates from healthy dogs and dogs affected with pyoderma in Japan. Vet Dermatol 2011;23:17–22.e5.
30. Sasaki T, Kikuchi K, Tanaka Y, et al. Methicillin-resistant *Staphylococcus pseudintermedius* in a veterinary teaching hospital. J Clin Microbiol 2007;45: 1118–25.
31. Rubin JE, Chirino-Trejo M. Prevalence, sites of colonization, and antimicrobial resistance among *Staphylococcus pseudintermedius* isolates from healthy dogs in Saskatoon, Canada. J Vet Diagn Invest 2011;23:351–4.
32. Gomez-Sanz E, Torres C, Lozano C, et al. Detection and characterization of methicillin-resistant *Staphylococcus pseudintermedius* in healthy dogs in La Rioja, Spain. Comp Immunol Microbiol Infect Dis 2011;34:447–53.
33. Morris DO, Boston RC, O'Shea K, et al. The prevalence of carriage of methicillin-resistant staphylococci by veterinary dermatology practice staff and their respective pets. Vet Dermatol 2010;21:400–7.

34. Perreten V, Kadlec K, Schwarz S, et al. Clonal spread of methicillin-resistant *Staphylococcus pseudintermedius* in Europe and North America: an international multicentre study. J Antimicrob Chemother 2010;65:1145–54.
35. Osland AM, Vestby LK, Fanuelson H, et al. Clonal diversity and biofilm-forming ability of methicillin-resistant Staphylococcus pseudintermedius. J Antimicrob Chemother 2012;67:841–8.
36. Black CC, Solyman SM, Eberlein LC, et al. Identification of a predominant multilocus sequence type, pulsed-field gel electrophoresis cluster, and novel staphylococcal chromosomal cassette in clinical isolates of *mecA*-containing, methicillin-resistant Staphylococcus pseudintermedius. Vet Microbiol 2009; 139:333–8.
37. Cohn LA, Middleton JR. A veterinary perspective on methicillin-resistant staphylococci. J Vet Emerg Crit Care (San Antonio) 2010;20:31–45.
38. Descloux S, Rossano A, Perreten V. Characterization of new staphylococcal cassette chromosome *mec* (SCC*mec*) and topoisomerase genes in fluoroquinolone- and methicillin-resistant Staphylococcus pseudintermedius. J Clin Microbiol 2008;46:1818–23.
39. Bond R, Loeffler A. What's happened to *Staphylococcus intermedius*? Taxonomic revision and emergence of multi-drug resistance. J Small Anim Pract 2012;53(3):147–54.
40. Wang Y, Yang J, Logue CM, et al. Methicillin-resistant *Staphylococcus pseudintermedius* isolated from canine pyoderma in North China. J Appl Microbiol 2012; 112:623–30.
41. Bryan J, Frank LA, Rohrbach BW, et al. Treatment outcome of dogs with methicillin-resistant and methicillin-susceptible *Staphylococcus pseudintermedius* pyoderma. Vet Dermatol 2012;23(4):361–8.e65.
42. Huerta B, Maldonado A, Ginel PJ, et al. Risk factors associated with the antimicrobial resistance of staphylococci in canine pyoderma. Vet Microbiol 2011;150: 302–8.
43. Beck KM, Waisglass SE, Dick HL, et al. Prevalence of methicillin-resistant *Staphylococcus pseudintermedius* (MRSP) from skin and carriage sites of dogs after treatment of their methicillin-resistant or methicillin-sensitive staphylococcal pyoderma. Vet Dermatol 2012;23(4):369–75.e67.
44. Schnellmann C, Gerber V, Rossano A, et al. Presence of new *mecA* and *mph(C)* variants conferring antibiotic resistance in *Staphylococcus* spp. isolated from the skin of horses before and after clinic admission. J Clin Microbiol 2006;44: 4444–54.
45. van Duijkeren E, Kamphuis M, van der Mije IC, et al. Transmission of methicillin-resistant *Staphylococcus pseudintermedius* between infected dogs and cats and contact pets, humans and the environment in households and veterinary clinics. Vet Microbiol 2011;150:338–43.
46. Laarhoven LM, de Heus P, van Luijn J, et al. Longitudinal study on methicillin-resistant *Staphylococcus pseudintermedius* in households. PLoS One 2011;6: e27788.
47. Lee J. *Staphylococcus intermedius* isolated from dog-bite wounds. J Infect 1994;29:105.
48. Tanner MA, Everett L, Youvan DC. Molecular phylogenetic evidence for noninvasive zoonotic transmission of *Staphylococcus intermedius* from a canine pet to a human. J Clin Microbiol 2000;38:1628–31.
49. Kempker R, Mangalat D, Kongphet-Tran T, et al. Beware of the pet dog: a case of *Staphylococcus intermedius* infection. Am J Med Sci 2009;338:425–7.

50. Hanselman BA, Kruth SA, Rousseau J, et al. Coagulase positive staphylococcal colonization of humans and their household pets. Can Vet J 2009;50:954–8.
51. Boost MV, So SY, Perreten V. Low rate of methicillin-resistant coagulase positive staphylococcal colonization of veterinary personnel in Hong Kong. Zoonoses Public Health 2011;58:36–40.
52. Ishihara K, Shimokubo N, Sakagami A, et al. Occurrence of molecular characteristics of methicillin-resistant *Staphylococcus aureus* and methicillin-resistant *Staphylococcus pseudintermedius* in an academic veterinary hospital. Appl Environ Microbiol 2010;76:5165–74.
53. Paul NC, Moodley A, Ghibaudo G, et al. Carriage of methicillin-resistant *Staphylococcus pseudintermedius* in small animal veterinarians: indirect evidence of zoonotic transmission. Zoonoses Public Health 2011;58:533–9.
54. Guardabassi L, Loeber ME, Jacobson A. Transmission of multiple antimicrobial-resistant *Staphylococcus intermedius* between dogs affected by deep pyoderma and their owners. Vet Microbiol 2004;98:23–7.
55. Frank LA, Kania SA, Kirzeder EM. Risk of colonization or gene transfer to owners of dogs with methicillin-resistant Staphylococcus pseudintermedius. Vet Dermatol 2009;20:496–501.
56. van Duijkeren E, Houwers DJ, Schoormans A, et al. Transmission of methicillin-resistant *Staphylococcus intermedius* between humans and animals [letter to the editor]. Vet Microbiol 2008;128:213–5.
57. Tang YW, Stratton CW. *Staphylococcus aureus*: an old pathogen with new weapons. Clin Lab Med 2010;30:179–208.
58. Rubin JE, Chirino-Trejo M. Pharyngeal, rectal and nasal colonization of clinically healthy dogs with *Staphylococcus aureus* [letter to the editor]. Vet Microbiol 2010;143:440–1.
59. Fazakerley J, Nuttall T, Sales D, et al. Staphylococcal colonization of mucosal and lesional skin sites in atopic and healthy dogs. Vet Dermatol 2009;20: 179–84.
60. Cox HU, Hoskins JD, Newman SS, et al. Distribution of staphylococcal species on clinical normal cats. Am J Vet Res 1985;46:1824–8.
61. Igimi S, Atobe H, Tohya Y, et al. Characterization of the most frequently encountered *Staphylococcus* sp. in cats. Vet Microbiol 1994;39:255–60.
62. Lilenbaum W, Nunes EL, Azeredo MA. Prevalence and antimicrobial susceptibility of staphylococci isolated from the skin surface of clinically normal cats. Lett Appl Microbiol 1998;27:224–8.
63. Lilenbaum W, Esteves AL, Souza GN. Prevalence and antimicrobial susceptibility of staphylococci isolated from saliva of clinically normal cats. Lett Appl Microbiol 1998;28:448–52.
64. Ippolito G, Leone S, Lauria FN, et al. Methicillin-resistant *Staphylococcus aureus*: the superbug. Int J Infect Dis 2010;14(Suppl 4):S7–11.
65. Duquette RA, Nuttall TJ. Methicillin-resistant *Staphylococcus aureus* in dogs and cats: an emerging problem? J Small Anim Pract 2004;45:591–7.
66. Cosgrove SE, Qi Y, Kaye KS, et al. The impact of methicillin resistance in *Staphylococcus aureus* bacteremia on patient outcomes: mortality, length of stay, and hospital charges. Infect Control Hosp Epidemiol 2005;26:166–74.
67. Middleton JR, Fales WH, Luby CD, et al. Surveillance of *Staphylococcus aureus* in veterinary teaching hospitals. J Clin Microbiol 2005;43:2916–9.
68. Rubin JE, Chirino-Trejo M. Antimicrobial susceptibility of canine and human *Staphylococcus aureus* collected in Saskatoon, Canada. Zoonoses Public Health 2011;58:454–62.

69. Leonard FC, Abbott Y, Rossney A. Methicillin-resistant *Staphylococcus aureus* isolated from a veterinary surgeon and five dogs in one practice. Vet Rec 2006;158:155–9.
70. Abbott Y, Leonard FC, Markey BK. Detection of three distinct genetic lineages in methicillin-resistant *Staphylococcus aureus* (MRSA) isolates from animals and veterinary personnel. Epidemiol Infect 2010;138:764–71.
71. Abdel-moein KA, El-Hariri M, Samir A. Methicillin-resistant *Staphylococcus aureus*: an emerging pathogen of pets in Egypt with a public health burden. Transbound Emerg Dis 2011;59(4):331–5.
72. McLean CL, Ness MG. Methicillin-resistant *Staphylococcus aureus* in a veterinary orthopaedic referral hospital: staff nasal colonization and incidence of clinical cases. J Small Anim Pract 2008;49:170–7.
73. Vitale CB, Gross TL, Weese JS. Methicillin-resistant *Staphylococcus aureus* in cat and owner [letter to editor]. Emerg Infect Dis 2006;12:1998–9.
74. Grinberg A, Kingsbury DD, Gibson IR, et al. Clinically overt infections with methicillin-resistant *Staphylococcus aureus* in animals in New Zealand: a pilot study. N Z Vet J 2008;56:237–42.
75. Malik S, Coombs GW, O'Brien FG, et al. Molecular typing of methicillin-resistant staphylococci isolated from cats and dogs. J Antimicrob Chemother 2006;58: 428–31.
76. Strommenger B, Kehrenberg C, Kettlitz C, et al. Molecular characterization of methicillin-resistant *Staphylococcus aureus* strains from pet animals and their relationship to human isolates. J Antimicrob Chemother 2006;57:461–5.
77. Abbott Y, Leggett B, Rossney S, et al. Isolation rates of methicillin-resistant *Staphylococcus aureus* in dogs, cats and horses in Ireland. Vet Rec 2010; 166:451–5.
78. Faires MC, Traverse M, Tater KC, et al. Methicillin-resistant and -susceptible *Staphylococcus aureus* infections in dogs. Emerg Infect Dis 2010;16:69–75.
79. Tomlin J, Pead MJ, Lloyd DH, et al. Methicillin-resistant *Staphylococcus aureus* infections in 11 dogs. Vet Rec 1999;144:60–4.
80. Pak SI, Han HR, Shimizu A. Characterization of methicillin-resistant *Staphylococcus aureus* isolated from dogs in Korea. J Vet Med Sci 1999;61:1013–8.
81. Loeffler A, Pfeiffer DU, Lindsay JA, et al. Lack of transmission of methicillin-resistant *Staphylococcus aureus* (MRSA) between apparently healthy dogs in a rescue kennel. Vet Microbiol 2010;141:178–81.
82. Baptiste KE, Williams K, Williams NJ, et al. Methicillin-resistant staphylococci in companion animals. Emerg Infect Dis 2005;11:1942–4.
83. O'Mahony R, Abbott Y, Leonard FC, et al. Methicillin-resistant *Staphylococcus aureus* (MRSA) isolated from animals and veterinary personnel in Ireland. Vet Microbiol 2005;109:285–96.
84. Rankin S, Roberts S, O'Shea K, et al. Panton valentine leukocidin (PVL) toxin positive MRSA strains isolated from companion animals. Vet Microbiol 2005; 108:145–8.
85. Bender JB, Torres SM, Gilbert SM, et al. Isolation of methicillin-resistant *Staphylococcus aureus* from a non-healing abscess in a cat. Vet Rec 2005;157:388–9.
86. Weese JS, Dick H, Willey BM, et al. Suspected transmission of methicillin-resistant *Staphylococcus aureus* between domestic pets and humans in veterinary clinics and in the household. Vet Microbiol 2006;115:148–55.
87. Walther B, Wieler LH, Friedrich AW, et al. Methicillin-resistant *Staphylococcus aureus* (MRSA) isolated from small and exotic animals at a university hospital during routine microbiological examinations. Vet Microbiol 2008;127:171–8.

88. Lin Y, Barker E, Kislow J, et al. Evidence of multiple virulence subtypes in nosocomial and community-associated MRSA genotypes in companion animals from the Upper Midwestern and Northeastern United States. Clin Med Res 2011;9:7–16.

89. Lin AE, Davies JE. Occurrence of highly fluoroquinolone-resistant and methicillin-resistant *Staphylococcus aureus* in domestic animals. Can J Microbiol 2007;53:925–9.

90. Faires MC, Tater KC, Weese JS. An investigation of methicillin-resistant *Staphylococcus aureus* colonization in people and pets in the same household with an infected person or infected pet. J Am Vet Med Assoc 2009;235:540–3.

91. Morris DO, Mauldin EA, O'Shea K, et al. Clinical, microbiological, and molecular characterization of methicillin-resistant *Staphylococcus aureus* infections of cats. Am J Vet Res 2006;67:1421–5.

92. Briscoe JA, Morris DO, Rankin SC, et al. Methicillin-resistant *Staphylococcus aureus*-associated dermatitis in a Congo African Grey Parrot. J Avian Med Surg 2008;22:336–43.

93. Centers for Disease Control and Prevention. Methicillin-resistant *Staphylococcus aureus* skin infections from an elephant calf—San Diego, California, 2008. Morb Mortal Wkly Rep 2009;58:194–8.

94. Faires MC, Gehring E, Mergl J, et al. Methicillin-resistant *Staphylococcus aureus* in marine mammals [letter to the editor]. Emerg Infect Dis 2009;15:2071–2.

95. Magalhaes RJ, Loeffler A, Lindsay J, et al. Risk factors for methicillin-resistant *Staphylococcus aureus* (MRSA) infection in dogs and cats: a case-control study. Vet Res 2010;41:55.

96. Morris DO, Lautenbach E, Zaoutis T, et al. Potential for pet animals to harbour methicillin-resistant *Staphylococcus aureus* when residing with human MRSA patients. Zoonoses Public Health 2012;59:286–93.

97. Bender JB, Waters KC, Nerby J, et al. Methicillin-resistant *Staphylococcus aureus* (MRSA) isolated from pets living in households with MRSA-infected children [letter to the editor]. Clin Infect Dis 2012;54:449–50.

98. Loeffler A, Pfeiffer DU, Lindsay JA, et al. Prevalence of and risk factors for MRSA carriage in companion animals: a survey of dogs, cats and horses. Epidemiol Infect 2011;139:1019–28.

99. Zhang W, Hao Z, Wang Y, et al. Molecular characterization of methicillin-resistant *Staphylococcus aureus* strains from pet animals and veterinary staff in China. Vet J 2011;190:e125–9.

100. Loeffler A, Pfeiffer DU, Lloyd DH, et al. Methicillin-resistant *Staphylococcus aureus* carriage in UK veterinary staff and owners of infected pets: new risk groups. J Hosp Infect 2010;74:282–8.

101. Manian FA. Asymptomatic nasal carriage of mupirocin-resistant, methicillin-resistant *Staphylococcus aureus* (MRSA) in a pet dog associated with MRSA infection in household contacts. Clin Infect Dis 2003;36:e26–8.

102. Boost MV, O'Donoghue MM, James A. Prevalence of *Staphylococcus aureus* carriage among dogs and their owners. Epidemiol Infect 2008;136:953–64.

103. Loeffler A, Boag AK, Sung J, et al. Prevalence of methicillin-resistant *Staphylococcus aureus* among staff and pets in a small animal referral hospital in the UK. J Antimicrob Chemother 2005;56:692–7.

104. van Duijkeren E, Wolfhagen MJ, Box AT, et al. Human-to-dog transmission of methicillin-resistant Staphylococcus aureus. Emerg Infect Dis 2004;10:2235–7.

105. Rutland BE, Weese JS, Bolin C, et al. Human-to-dog transmission of methicillin-resistant *Staphylococcus aureus* [letter to editor]. Emerg Infect Dis 2009;15:1328–30.

106. Ferreira JP, Anderson KL, Correa MT, et al. Transmission of MRSA between companion animals and infected human patients presenting to outpatient medical care facilities. PLoS One 2011;6:e26978.

107. Sing A, Tuschak C, Hormansdorfer S. Methicillin-resistant *Staphylococcus aureus* in a family and its pet cat [letter to the editor]. N Engl J Med 2008; 358:1200–1.

108. Coughlan K, Olsen KE, Boxrud D, et al. Methicillin-resistant *Staphylococcus aureus* in resident animals of a long-term care facility. Zoonoses Public Health 2010;57:220–6.

109. van Duijkeren E, Wolfhagen MJ, Heck ME, et al. Transmission of a panton- valentine leucocidin-positive, methicillin-resistant *Staphylococcus aureus* strain between humans and a dog. J Clin Microbiol 2005;43:6209–11.

110. Ferreira JP, Fowler VG, Correa MT, et al. Transmission of methicillin-resistant *Staphylococcus aureus* between human and hamster. J Clin Microbiol 2011; 49:1679–80.

111. Walther B, Wieler LH, Friedrich AW, et al. *Staphylococcus aureus* and MRSA colonization rates among personnel and dogs in a small animal hospital: association with nosocomial infections. Berl Munch Tierarztl Wochenschr 2009;122:178–85.

112. Lefebvre SL, Reid-Smith RJ, Waltner-Toews D, et al. Incidence of acquisition of methicillin-resistant *Staphylococcus aureus, Clostridium difficile*, and other health-care- associated pathogens by dogs that participate in animal-assisted interventions. J Am Vet Med Assoc 2009;234:1404–17.

113. Kottler S, Middleton JR, Perry J, et al. Prevalence of *Staphylococcus aureus* and methicillin-resistant *Staphylococcus aureus* carriage in three populations. J Vet Intern Med 2010;24:132–9.

114. Burton S, Reid-Smith R, McClure JT, et al. *Staphylococcus aureus* colonization in healthy horses in Atlantic Canada. Can Vet J 2008;49:797–9.

115. Weese JS, Rousseau J, Traub-Dargatz JL, et al. Community-associated methicillin- resistant *Staphylococcus aureus* in horses and humans who work with horses. J Am Vet Med Assoc 2005;226:580–3.

116. Weese JS, Caldwell F, Willey BM, et al. An outbreak of methicillin-resistant *Staphylococcus aureus* skin infections resulting from horse to human transmission in a veterinary hospital. Vet Microbiol 2006;114:160–4.

117. Anderson ME, Lefebvre SL, Rankin SC, et al. Retrospective multicentre study of methicillin-resistant *Staphylococcus aureus* infections in 115 horses. Equine Vet J 2009;41:401–5.

118. Weese JS, van Duijkeren E. Methicillin-resistant *Staphylococcus aureus* and *Staphylococcus pseudintermedius* in veterinary medicine. Vet Microbiol 2010; 140:418–29.

119. Maddox TW, Clegg PD, Diggle PJ, et al. Cross-sectional study of antimicrobial-resistant bacteria in horses. Part 1: prevalence of antimicrobial-resistant escherichia coli and methicillin-resistant staphylococcus aureus. Equine Vet J 2012;44: 289–96.

120. Tokateloff N, Manning ST, Weese JS, et al. Prevalence of methicillin-resistant *Staphylococcus aureus* colonization of horses in Saskatchewan, Alberta, and British Columbia. Can Vet J 2009;50:1177–80.

121. Smith TC, Pearson N. The emergence of *Staphylococcus aureus* ST398. Vector Borne Zoonotic Dis 2011;11:327–39.

122. Guardabassi L, Stegger M, Skov R. Retrospective detection of methicillin resistant and susceptible *Staphylococcus aureus* ST398 in Danish slaughter pigs. Vet Microbiol 2007;122:384–6.

123. Floras A, Lawn K, Slavic D, et al. Sequence type 398 methicillin-resistant *Staphylococcus aureus* infection and colonisation in dogs. Vet Rec 2010;166:826–7.
124. O'Brien AM, Hanson BM, Farina SA, et al. MRSA in conventional and alternative retail pork products. PLoS One 2012;7:e30092.
125. Weese JS, Reid-Smith R, Rousseau J, et al. Methicillin-resistant *Staphylococcus aureus* (MRSA) contamination of retail pork. Can Vet J 2010;51:749–52.
126. van Loo I, Huijsdens X, Tiemersma E, et al. Emergence of methicillin-resistant *Staphylococcus aureus* of animal origin in humans. Emerg Infect Dis 2007;13: 1834–9.
127. Garcia-Graells C, Antoine J, Larsen J, et al. Livestock veterinarians at high risk of acquiring methicillin-resistant *Staphylococcus aureus* ST398. Epidemiol Infect 2012;140:383–9.
128. Gorwitz RJ, Kruszon-Moran D, McAllister SK, et al. Changes in the prevalence of nasal colonization with *Staphylococcus aureus* in the United States, 2001-2004. J Infect Dis 2008;197:226–34.
129. Jordan D, Simon J, Fury S, et al. Carriage of methicillin-resistant *Staphylococcus aureus* by veterinarians in Australia. Aust Vet J 2011;89:152–9.
130. Burstiner LC, Faires M, Weese JS. Methicillin-resistant *Staphylococcus aureus* colonization in personnel attending a veterinary surgery conference. Vet Surg 2010;39:150–7.
131. Moodley A, Nightingale EC, Stegger M, et al. High risk for nasal carriage of methicillin- resistant *Staphylococcus aureus* among Danish veterinary practitioners. Scand J Work Environ Health 2008;34:151–7.
132. Anderson ME, Lefebvre SL, Weese JS. Evaluation of prevalence and risk factors for methicillin-resistant *Staphylococcus aureus* colonization in veterinary personnel attending an international equine veterinary conference. Vet Microbiol 2008;129:410–7.
133. Hanselman BA, Kruth SA, Rousseau J, et al. Methicillin-resistant *Staphylococcus aureus* colonization in veterinary personnel. Emerg Infect Dis 2006;12:1933–8.
134. Heller J, Armstrong SK, Girvan EK, et al. Prevalence and distribution of methicillin- resistant *Staphylococcus aureus* within the environment and staff of a university veterinary clinic. J Small Anim Pract 2009;50:168–73.
135. Hoet AE, Johnson A, Nava-Hoet RC, et al. Environmental methicillin-resistant *Staphylococcus aureus* in a veterinary teaching hospital during a nonoutbreak period. Vector Borne Zoonotic Dis 2011;11:609–15.
136. Weese JS, DaCosta T, Button L, et al. Isolation of methicillin-resistant *Staphylococcus aureus* from the environmentl in a veterinary teaching hospital. J Vet Intern Med 2004;18:468–70.
137. Murphy CP, Reid-Smith RJ, Boerlin P, et al. *Escherichia coli* and selected veterinary and zoonotic pathogens isolated from environmental sites in companion animal veterinary hospitals in southern Ontario. Can Vet J 2010;51:963–72.
138. Cain CL, Morris DO, O'Shea K, et al. Genotypic relatedness and phenotypic characterization of *Staphylococcus schleiferi* subspecies in clinical samples from dogs. Am J Vet Res 2011;72:96–102.
139. Cain CL, Morris DO, Rankin SC. Clinical characterization of Staphylococcus schleiferi infections and identification of risk factors for acquisition of oxacillin-resistant strains in dogs: 225 cases (2003-2009). J Am Vet Med Assoc 2011; 239:1566–73.
140. Igimi S, Takahashi E, Mitsuoka T. *Staphylococcus schleiferi* subsp. *coagulans* subsp. nov., isolated from the external auditory meatus of dogs with external ear otitis. Int J Syst Bacteriol 1990;40:409–11.

141. Bes M, Guerin-Faublee V, Freney J, et al. Isolation of *Staphylococcus schleiferi* subspecies *coagulans* from two cases of canine pyoderma. Vet Rec 2002;150: 487–8.

142. Frank LA, Kania SA, Hnilica KA, et al. Isolation of *Staphylococcus schleiferi* from dogs with pyoderma. J Am Vet Med Assoc 2003;222:451–4.

143. May ER, Hnilica KA, Frank LA, et al. Isolation of *Staphylococcus schleiferi* from healthy dogs and dogs with otitis, pyoderma, or both. J Am Vet Med Assoc 2005;227:928–31.

144. Yamashita K, Shimizu A, Kawano J, et al. Isolation of characterization of staphylococci from external auditory meatus of dogs with or without otitis externa with special reference to *Staphylococcus schleiferi* subsp. *coagulans* isolates. J Vet Med Sci 2005;67:263–8.

145. Bemis DA, Jones RD, Hiatt LE, et al. Comparison of tests to detect oxacillin resistance in *Staphylococcus intermedius, Staphylococcus schleiferi*, and *Staphylococcus aureus* isolates from canine hosts. J Clin Microbiol 2006;44: 3374–6.

146. Vanni M, Tognetti R, Pretti C, et al. Antimicrobial susceptibility of *Staphylococcus intermedius* and *Staphylococcus schleiferi* isolated from dogs. Res Vet Sci 2009;87:192–5.

147. Intorre L, Vanni M, Di Bello D, et al. Antimicrobial susceptibility and mechanism of resistance to fluoroquinolones in *Staphylococcus intermedius* and Staphylococcus schleiferi. J Vet Pharmacol Ther 2007;30:464–9.

148. Chanchaithong P, Prapasarakul N. Biochemical markers and protein pattern analysis for canine coagulase-positive staphylococci and their distribution on dog skin. J Microbiol Methods 2011;86:175–81.

149. Hernandez JL, Calvo J, Sota R, et al. Clinical and microbiological characteristics of 28 patients with *Staphylococcus schleiferi* infection. Eur J Clin Microbiol Infect Dis 2001;20:153–8.

150. Da Costa A, Lelievre H, Kirkorian G, et al. Role of the preaxillary flora in pacemaker infections. Circulation 1998;97:1791–5.

151. Kluytmans J, Berg H, Steegh P, et al. Oubreak of *Staphylococcus schleiferi* wound infections: strain characterization by randomly amplified polymorphic DNA analysis, PCR ribotyping, conventional ribotyping, and pulsed-field gel electrophoresis. J Clin Microbiol 1998;36:2214–9.

152. Vandenesch F, Lebeau C, Bes M, et al. Clotting activity in *Staphylococcus schleiferi* subspecies from human patients. J Clin Microbiol 1994;32:388–92.

153. Kumar D, Cawley JJ, Irizarry-Alvarado JM, et al. Case of *Staphylococcus schleiferi* subspecies *coagulans* endocarditis and metastatic infection in an immune compromised host. Transpl Infect Dis 2007;9:336–8.

154. Piette A, Verschraegen G. Role of coagulase-negative staphylococci in human disease. Vet Microbiol 2009;134:45–54.

155. von Eiff C, Peters G, Heilmann C. Pathogenesis of infections due to coagulase-negative staphylococci. Lancet Infect Dis 2002;2:677–85.

156. Garza-Gonzalez E, Morfin-Otero R, Llaca-Diaz JM, et al. Staphylococcal cassette chromosome *mec* (SCC*mec*) in methicillin-resistant coagulase-negative staphylococci. A review and the experience in a tertiary-care setting. Epidemiol Infect 2010;138:645–54.

157. Bagcigil FA, Moodley A, Baptiste KE, et al. Occurrence, species distribution, antimicrobial resistance and clonality of methicillin- and erythromycin-resistant staphylococci in the nasal cavity of domestic animals. Vet Microbiol 2007;121: 307–15.

158. Moodley A, Guardabassi L. Clonal spread of methicillin-resistant coagulase-negative staphylococci among horses, personnel and environmental sites at equine facilities. Vet Microbiol 2009;137:397–401.

159. Briscoe JA, Morris DO, Rosenthal KL, et al. Evaluation of mucosal and seborrheic sites for staphylococci in two populations of captive psittacines. J Am Vet Med Assoc 2009;234:901–5.

160. Corrente M, D'Abramo M, Latronico F, et al. Methicillin-resistant coagulase negative staphylococci isolated from horses. New Microbiol 2009;32:311–4.

161. Yasuda R, Kawano J, Onda H, et al. Methicillin-resistant coagulase-negative staphylococci isolated from healthy horses in Japan. Am J Vet Res 2000;61:1451–5.

162. Stepanovic S, Dimitrijevic V, Vukovic D, et al. *Staphylococcus sciuri* as part of skin, nasal and oral flora in healthy dogs. Vet Microbiol 2001;82:177–85.

163. Lilenbaum W, Veras M, Blum E, et al. Antimicrobial susceptibility of staphylococci isolated from otitis externa in dogs. Lett Appl Microbiol 2000;31:42–5.

164. Lacasta D, Ferrer LM, Ramos JJ, et al. Unilateral scrotal pyocele in ram caused by Staphylococcus capitis. Aust Vet J 2009;87:484–6.

165. Griffin GM, Hold DE. Dog-bite wounds: bacteriology and treatment outcome in 37 cases. J Am Anim Hosp Assoc 2001;37:453–60.

166. Sidhu MS, Oppegaard H, Devor TP, et al. Persistence of multidrug-resistant *Staphylococcus haemolyticus* in an animal veterinary teaching hospital clinic. Microb Drug Resist 2007;13:271–80.

167. Moon BY, Youn JH, Shin S, et al. Genetic and phenotypic characterization of methicillin- resistant staphylococci isolated from veterinary hospitals in South Korea. J Vet Diagn Invest 2012;24:489–98.

168. Zhang Y, Wang X, LeJeune JT, et al. Comparison of phenotypic methods in predicting methicillin resistance in coagulase-negative *Staphylococcus* (CoNS) from animals. Res Vet Sci 2011;90:23–5.

169. Rich M, Deighton L, Roberts L. Clindamycin-resistance in methicillin-resistant *Staphylococcus aureus* isolated from animals. Vet Microbiol 2005;111:237–40.

170. Faires M, Gard S, Aucoin D, et al. Inducible clindamycin-resistance in methicillin- resistant *Staphylococcus aureus* and methicillin-resistant *Staphylococcus pseudintermedius* isolates from dogs and cats [letter to the editor]. Vet Microbiol 2009;139:419–20.

171. Rubin JE, Ball KR, Chirino-Trejo M. Antimicrobial susceptibility of *Staphylococcus aureus* and *Staphylococcus pseudintermedius* isolated from various animals. Can Vet J 2011;52:153–7.

172. Trzcinski K, Cooper BS, Hryniewicz W, et al. Expression of resistance to tetracyclines in strains of methicillin-resistant Staphylococcus aureus. J Antimicrob Chemother 2000;45:763–70.

173. Greene CE, Watson AD. Antibacterial chemotherapy. In: Greene CE, editor. Infectious diseases of the dog and cat. 3rd edition. St Louis (MO): Saunders Elsevier; 2006. p. 292.

174. Ihrke PJ, Papich MG, Demanuelle TC. The use of fluoroquinolones in veterinary dermatology. Vet Dermatol 1999;10:193–204.

175. Ganiere JP, Medaille C, Limet A, et al. Antimicrobial activity of enrofloxacin against *Staphylococcus intermedius* strains isolated from canine pyodermas. Vet Dermatol 2001;12:171–5.

176. Ihrke PJ. Bacterial infections of the skin. In: Greene CE, editor. Infectious diseases of the dog and cat. 3rd edition. St Louis (MO): Saunders Elsevier; 2006. p. 807–15.

177. Windahl U, Reimegard E, Holst BS, et al. Carriage of methicillin-resistant *Staphylococcus pseudintermedius* in dogs—a longitudinal study. BMC Vet Res 2012; 8:34.
178. Mason IS, Kietzmann M. Cephalosporins—pharmacological basis of clinical use in veterinary dermatology. Vet Dermatol 1999;10:187–92.
179. Weber SG, Gold HS, Hooper DC, et al. Fluoroquinolones and the risk for methicillin- resistant *Staphylococcus aureus* in hospitalized patients. Emerg Infect Dis 2003;9:1415–22.
180. Bisognano C, Vaudauz PE, Rohner P, et al. Induction of fibronectin-binding proteins and increased adhesion of quinolone-resistant *Staphylococcus aureus* by subinhibitory levels of ciprofloxacin. Antimicrob Agents Chemother 2000;44: 1428–37.
181. Liu C, Bayer A, Cosgrove SE, et al. Clinical practice guidelines by the infectious diseases society of America for the treatment of methicillin-resistant *Staphylococcus aureus* infections in adults and children: executive summary. Clin Infect Dis 2011;52:285–92.
182. Papich MG. Selection of antibiotics for methicillin-resistant *Staphylococcus pseudintermedius*: time to revisit some old drugs? Vet Dermatol 2012;23(4): 352–60.e64.
183. Greene CE, Hartmann K, Calpin J. Antimicrobial drug formulary. In: Greene CE, editor. Infectious diseases of the dog and cat. 3rd edition. St Louis (MO): Saunders Elsevier; 2006. p. 1197, 1226, 1259, 1310.
184. Arditi M, Yogev R. In vitro interaction between rifampin and clindamycin against pathogenic coagulase-negative staphylococci. Antimicrob Agents Chemother 1989;33:245–7.
185. Senturk S, Ozel E, Sen A. Clinical efficacy of rifampicin for treatment of canine pyoderma. Acta Vet Brno 2005;74:117–22.
186. Kadlec K, van Duijkeren E, Wagenaar JA, et al. Molecular basis of rifampicin resistance in methicillin-resistant *Staphylococcus pseudintermedius* isolates from dogs. J Antimicrob Chemother 2011;66:1236–42.
187. Frank LA. Clinical pharmacology of rifampin. J Am Vet Med Assoc 1990;197: 114–7.
188. Plumb DC. Amikacin sulfate. In: Plumb's veterinary drug handbook. 7th editon. Ames (IA): Wiley-Blackwell; 2011. p. 39–42.
189. Huth ME, Ricci AJ, Cheng AG. Mechanisms of aminoglycoside ototoxicity and targets of hair cell protection. Int J Otolaryngol 2011;2011:937861.
190. Murayama N, Nagata M, Terada Y, et al. Efficacy of a surgical scrub including 2% chlorhexidine acetate for canine superficial pyoderma. Vet Dermatol 2010; 21:586–92.
191. Weese JS, Faires M, Rousseau J, et al. Cluster of methicillin-resistant *Staphylococcus aureus* colonization in a small animal intensive care unit. J Am Vet Med Assoc 2007;231:1361–4.
192. Walther B, Hermes J, Cuny C, et al. Sharing more than friendship—nasal colonization with coagulase-positive staphylococci (CPS) and co-habitation aspects of dogs and their owners. PLoS One 2012;7:e35197.
193. Saijonmaa-Koulu L, Parsons E, Lloyd DH. Elimination of *Staphylococcus intermedius* in healthy dogs by topical treatment with fusidic acid. J Small Anim Pract 1998;39:341–7.

Topical Therapy for Drug-Resistant Pyoderma in Small Animals

James G. Jeffers, VMD

KEYWORDS

- Methicillin-resistant • Chlorhexidine • Benzoyl • Hypochlorous • Nisin • Mupirocin
- Liposomes • Barrier

KEY POINTS

- Methicillin- and multidrug-resistant staphylococcal skin infections are becoming more prevalent in small animal dermatology.
- Topical therapy is increasingly important for the treatment and prevention of bacterial skin infections.
- An expanding number of different topical antibacterial ingredients are available for use in small animal practice.
- Success in the topical treatment of bacterial skin infections hinges on choosing not only the correct ingredient but also the appropriate vehicle for application.
- Many of the topical antibacterial skin products contain ingredients that prolong the longevity of antimicrobial ingredients.

Topical treatment of bacterial skin infections has been an important part of veterinary dermatology since its inception. However, it was often relegated to elective adjunctive treatment with oral antibiotics positioned as primary therapy. The recent emergence of methicillin- and multidrug-resistant staphylococcal skin infections has necessitated a dramatic change in philosophy of oral antibiotic treatment (see articles by Gortel and Cain elsewhere in this issue). It has also heightened the need for a new approach to topical antibacterial treatment, not only as adjunctive treatment with empirically chosen or culture-based antibiotics, but also as primary therapy for multidrug-resistant strains. Topical antibacterial therapy also serves as the benchmark for prevention of future infections, especially because antibiotic resistance can occur after 1-pass antibiotic treatment.[1]

Strategies for effective topical antibacterial treatment include choosing both the ingredient as well as the vehicle used to deliver it. Ideally, the applied topical treatment

Disclosures and Conflicts of Interest: None.
Animal Dermatology and Behavior Clinics, Inc, 9039 Gaither Road, Gaithersburg, MD 20877, USA
E-mail address: 000927@comcast.net

Vet Clin Small Anim 43 (2013) 41–50
http://dx.doi.org/10.1016/j.cvsm.2012.09.006

has to be effective, adequate delivery vehicle, proper contact time, and residual activity. These 4 variables determine the success of treatment.

SHAMPOO/LEAVE-ON CONDITIONER THERAPY

There are many compounds or combination products that have antibacterial activity, such as iodine and triclosan, present in a shampoo vehicle. However, the most widely used and effective are benzoyl peroxide, chlorhexidine (also available in a leave-on conditioner, spray, or wipe), or ethyl lactate (in combination with other antibacterial ingredients propylene glycol, lactic acid, and benzalkonium chloride). Studies have been undertaken in dogs to prove the efficacy of each shampoo in killing *Staphylococcus* bacteria on the skin surface as sole therapy.[2–7] However, it is difficult to compare these studies to determine the best product and ideal protocol for use. The materials and methods of each were unique to that study, especially those involving chlorhexidine because the percentage tested ranged from 0.5% to 4%, with different chlorhexidine products (gluconate or acetate) used.[8] One study did directly compare the in vitro potencies of the 3 ingredients and found chlorhexidine to be superior in activity. However, in the skin, both benzoyl peroxide and ethyl lactate break down to a more effective state so that study may have underestimated their true in vivo potency.[9]

- Ethyl lactate (10%) is lipid soluble and penetrates all skin layers, including hair follicles and sebaceous glands. In the skin, ethyl lactate is hydrolyzed into ethanol and lactic acid, which exerts both its bacteriostatic and bacteriocidal action.[10,11] Its ability to diffuse through all skin layers contributes to its efficacy.
- Benzoyl peroxide (2.5%–3%) is an oxidizing agent that disrupts the bacterial cell wall membrane by increasing permeability or causing its rupture.[8] If used frequently, benzoyl peroxide shampoo can be drying and irritating to some animals. It also has a shorter shelf life and poor lathering compared with other shampoo ingredients.
- Chlorhexidine (0.5%–4%) kills bacteria by coagulating bacterial cytoplasmic proteins and deteriorating bacterial cell membranes.[10] An in vitro study[12] found that the concentration of chlorhexidine has a linear relationship with the degree of *Staphylococcus* bacteria kill; thus, higher concentration chlorhexidine products are recommended for treatment. An adequate dose of 2% chlorhexidine shampoo needed to kill *Staphylococcus* bacteria has been established as the amount of shampoo covering 1 US quarter coin on the area of a dog covered by 2 open adult hands.[13]

Shampoo therapy is best used for cases of generalized bacterial skin infections, particularly those affecting the torso and on patients with medium to long and/or thick coats. Ideally, bathing should be done as frequently as possible, even daily, if an infection is overtly present or to establish its efficacy as a preventative treatment. Afterward, the frequency of bathing can be decreased slowly and gradually over time but to no less often than every 7 to 14 days. To be most effective, dogs with thick or long coats should be clipped short. For larger dogs, inexpensive premedicated shampoo bathing removes grease, dirt, and debris for better contact time with the medicated product, with less product used and therefore less expense. It is ideal to have 10 to 15 minutes of contact time before rinsing.[14] In climates with temperate weather, it can be done outside, with dogs walked during the 10- to 15-minute contact time needed before rinsing. If undertaken inside in a shower or bathtub, a timer is needed and ideally some form of distraction for the patient. Peanut butter or squeeze cheese (aerosolized semisolid processed cheese product) can be spread around the tub or shower at the pet's head level to offer distraction. Once the contact time has elapsed, the patient should be rinsed thoroughly with tepid water. The patient should be allowed to air dry or use a hair dryer on the cool setting. Thorough rinsing, tepid bath water, and heat-free drying all minimize adverse reactions to the shampoo treatment that more often occur in dogs with irritated skin.

OINTMENT/CREAM/GEL/LIQUID THERAPY

There are a variety of topical ointments, creams, gels, or liquids that are available and effective for treating localized bacterial skin infections that can be used on both cats and dogs. For the treatment of methicillin and/or multidrug-resistant *Staphylococcus* infections, mupirocin, fusidic acid, and amikacin are most favored. The vehicle and packaging of these products limit their use to only focal areas of skin infection.

- Mupirocin (pseudomonic acid) is available in a 2% ointment in a polyethylene glycol base and is produced from *Pseudomonas fluorescens* bacteria. It is bacteriostatic at low concentrations and bacteriocidal at higher concentrations. It kills bacteria by selective inhibition of bacterial protein synthesis. Although staphylococcal bacterial resistance to mupirocin is rare in dogs and cats, it most frequently develops when used over a prolonged period of time and over large areas of the skin. It should be reserved for short-term treatment of acute infections because its chronic or recurring use may encourage resistance.[15] The ointment has been advocated for use in treating interdigital abscesses, callous pyoderma,[10] and acne in both dogs and cats.[10,16] However, its clinical use has expanded far beyond those applications with the increasing prevalence of resistant bacterial skin infections. If the treatment area of the skin exceeds the boundaries for ointment application, mupirocin ointment can be dissolved in water and sprayed onto infected skin. The author has found that 1 cup of water can be heated, not boiled, and a 30 g capped tube of mupirocin placed in the hot water (the ointment should stay within the tube). The ointment will liquefy inside the tube and then can be dissolved in 60 mL of water to make a 1% solution. The mupirocin stays in solution without precipitating and maintains its potency for at least 1 month.
- Fusidic acid, produced from *Fusidium* fungus, is available in an ointment, cream, or gel. Fusidic acid works by inhibiting bacterial protein synthesis and is bacteriocidal at all concentrations. It readily penetrates skin and there is almost no known staphylococcal bacterial resistance. Studies have shown fusidic acid to be as effective as mupirocin for killing *Staphylococcus* infections.[15] Fusidic acid is available for use in Canada but not in the United States.
- Topical amikacin use has been reported anecdotally in the treatment of multidrug-resistant *Staphylococcus* skin infections. It has already been widely and successfully used for the topical treatment of both gram-negative and gram-positive bacterial external ear canal infections with a low incidence of irritation to an area that is amenable to topical drug reactions.[17] The solution is prepared from the parenteral amikacin formulation and mixed with sterile water into a 1% (10 mg/mL) solution, with or without added parenteral-based corticosteroids (0.4–0.8 mg/mL dexamethasone). Although there is almost no *Staphylococcus* bacterial resistance to amikacin, its chronic use could promote conversion of a susceptible strain to a resistant one. The nephrotoxic potential of amikacin, used systemically for treatment of multidrug-resistant staphylococcal skin infections, is greatly minimized with its topical use.

Topical medications should be applied twice a day and ideally during times of distraction to allow adequate contact time. For dogs, that can be immediately before being walked or turned out into a fenced yard, or immediately before feeding. It has been established that a contact time of more than 10 minutes is required for topical mupirocin to exert its antibacterial benefit on infected skin.[18] Although other topical antibacterial ointments, gels, creams, or sprays have not been similarly tested for adequate contact time before removal, a similar minimum 10-minute contact time is recommended.

SPRAYS AND DIPS

- Chlorhexidine products
- Oxychlorine products: Hypochlorous acid and sodium hypochlorite
  - Both sodium hypochlorite, common household bleach, and its active ingredient hypochlorous acid are effective antibacterial agents.[19] Neutrophils contain hypochlorous acid as part of the normal mammalian host defense to kill invading micro-organisms. Hypochlorous acid causes oxidative unfolding of bacterial cell proteins in vitro and targets their thermolabile proteins for irreversible aggregation in vivo.[20]
    - If one half cup of common household bleach is added to a bathtub filled one quarter of the way, the resultant 2.5-μL/mL concentration of bleach kills 99.94% to 100% of methicillin-resistant *Staphylococcus aureus* organisms in vitro after 10 minutes of contact time. Both colonizing strains of methicillin-resistant *Staphylococcus aureus* and those methicillin-resistant *Staphylococcus aureus* bacteria associated with invasive infection are equally susceptible to bleach treatment[21]; thus, it can be used to both treat and potentially prevent bacterial skin infections by affecting the carrier state. To avoid bleaching household items, a children's plastic swimming pool can be used and the patient allowed to soak outdoors in the sodium hypochlorite-containing pool water. Otherwise, a bathtub is needed. Although most fabrics would not become bleached due to its dilute concentration, the pet should be thoroughly bathed with shampoo after the 10-minute sodium hypochlorite soaking to avoid potentially bleaching the coat or its surrounding environment. Although this treatment is economical, effective, and can be generally distributed throughout the skin with a low risk for skin irritation, it has the potential to ruin carpeting or furniture if the bleach is not thoroughly removed or if the patient escapes the bathroom during bathing.
    - Hypochlorous acid, the active ingredient found in bleach, is commercially available as a single-agent product, and offers several advantages over household bleach. Hypochlorous acid is more stable, nontoxic, pH neutral, and does not bleach. It is labeled for daily use as a wound care product, but also can be used at least once a day to treat superficial and deep bacterial skin infections as an adjunct to antibacterial shampoo or wipe therapy. It may also be used by itself in locations amenable to spray treatment. Hypochlorous acid is available as Vetericyn VF (veterinary), at a concentration of 150 parts per million of free active chlorine, or Dermacyn (human; Oculus Innovative Sciences, Inc. Petaluma, CA).[22]

WIPES

- Chlorhexidine products
- Lantibiotics: Nisin wipes

Lantibiotics (lanthionine-containing antibiotics) are a group of antimicrobial peptides that are produced by and primarily act on Gram-positive bacteria, of which nisin is a member.[23] Nisin is bacteriocidal and is derived from *Lactococcus* bacteria.[24] The primary but not exclusive[25] mechanism of action for nisin is targeting the *Staphylococcus* cytoplasmic membrane, which it disrupts, causing rapid efflux of cytoplasmic contents.[26] Nisin was first established as a preservative in processed cheese products and, since then, numerous other applications in foods and beverages have been developed. It is currently recognized as a safe food preservative in approximately 50 countries.[27] It is also used as an udder wipe to prevent mastitis in milking cows.[24] In a study on dogs with excessive surface bacterial colonization, 40% had a positive clinical and cytologic response to twice daily nisin wipe treatment. The improvement, however, was muted by the presence of *Pseudomonas* and/or *Malassezia* organisms, which in some cases eliminated the benefits of the nisin treatments.[24] The relatively large size of the nisin molecule prevents its penetration of the outer membrane of those organisms.[23] Nisin was also used in combination with culture-based oral antibiotics as adjunctive treatment for superficial *Staphylococcus* pyoderma cases. Fifty-six percent of treated dogs had more rapid clearing of bacterial infections in nisin treated areas when compared with their untreated sides.[24] The wipes can be purchased in approximately 8 × 8-inch impregnated squares in a 500-count pouch (Wipe Out, ImmuCell Corporation, Portland, ME) or in smaller sizes and quantities. The cost of nisin wipes are pennies per square, making them an extremely economical means of treating bacterial skin infections, even in giant breed dogs. Because the only clinical study in dogs was its adjunctive treatment to oral antibiotics in bacterially infected skin, it is difficult to extrapolate a frequency of treatment to prevent bacterial skin infections. However, twice daily use is reasonable because the wipes are easy to use and inexpensive. Clients can be instructed to leave the container of wipes by the door that serves as ingress from a walk or bathroom trip and use them in lieu of a towel that normally serves to wipe soiled body parts. Areas of the body that historically become infected with bacteria, regardless of location, are generously wiped. Ideally, the wipes are used in thinly haired areas (limbs, face, or glabrous torso skin) and in locations that are otherwise difficult to spray or shampoo. Because nisin is an edible protein, there is no chance for toxicity if the dog licks or chews the site of its application.

POTENTIATING INGREDIENTS

Some topical antimicrobial products have added molecules that extend the duration of treatment ingredients for several days after being applied to the skin. Chitosan, liposomes, and lipid barrier are the more commercially available ingredients incorporated into shampoo, leave-on conditioners, sprays, and wipes.

- Chitosan is produced commercially by deacetylation of chitin, the structural element in the exoskeleton of crustaceans (such as crabs and shrimp) and cell walls of fungi. It is the second most ubiquitous natural polysaccharide, with cellulose being the most common. Chitosan is water soluble, nontoxic, biocompatible, and biodegradable. The protonated amino groups contained in chitosan provide a positive charge in biologic environments; thus, it has a high affinity for normal negatively charged skin, hair, and nails. Chitosan readily adsorbs to skin and hair surfaces, providing a protective elastic film as its high molecular weight will not allow it to penetrate the skin. Additionally, it enhances the transport of polar drugs across epithelial surfaces and can trap non-polarized drugs on the skin surface.[28]

- Liposomes are artificially prepared phospholipid or surfactant vesicles and can be oligo- or multilamellar in construction, with as few as 2 or as many as 1000 layers. Liposomes have a hydrophilic head group attached to a hydrophobic tail. The fatty acid tails point into the membrane's interior and the polar head groups point out, form a bilayered membrane (**Fig. 1**). Both lipophilic and non-lipophilic ingredients can be incorporated into these vesicles and allow slow release of the ingredients contained within. Any water-soluble molecules present at the time of vesicle creation get incorporated into the aqueous spaces in between the multiple layers of the lipid bilayer membrane or in its core. Lipid-soluble molecules added at vesicle formation are trapped in the bilayer membrane between the polar heads in the tail region. The ingredients within the liposomes are released into the surrounding skin either by leaking through channels in the bilayer or are released progressively during membrane disruption. The surface of liposomes can be given different charges.[29,30] Cationic (positively charged) liposomes attach to negatively charged skin and hair to deliver ingredients to the surface, whereas non-ionic (neutral) liposomes are absorbed through the skin to deliver ingredients to deeper skin levels.[31]
- Lipid barrier treatments enhance the natural lipid film of the skin, produced by sebaceous and apocrine glands.[32] The lipid barrier offers physical, chemical, and microbial protection to the epidermis as well as waterproofing the skin and regulating its pH. The lipid film is made up of ceramides, cholesterol, and free fatty acids. Changes in the lipid barrier, created by certain skin diseases, can promote an environment more conducive to recurring bacterial skin infections.[32,33] Dogs with atopic disease, for example, have been shown to have decreased levels of cerumide 1 and 9, which may contribute to their tendencies to develop secondary bacterial skin infections.[34] There are commercially available sources of procerumides (phytosphingosine) in a shampoo, spray, wipe and ampule treatments, some of which contain chlorhexidine (Douxo, Sogeval Laboratories, Inc, Coppell, TX) as well as a composite product with cerumides and fatty acids in an ampule form (Allerderm Spot On, Virbac Animal Health, Fort Worth, TX).

When choosing topical therapy for treatment or prevention of bacterial skin infections, each case needs to be assessed independently for their needs, primarily based on the body location and length/thickness of hair coat. Just as important as the product choice for topical antibacterial therapy is the means by which it is delivered.

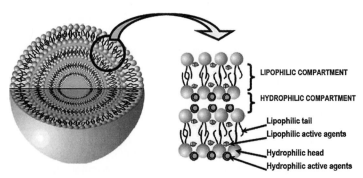

Fig. 1. The structure of a liposome. (*Courtesy of* Virbac Corporation, Fort Worth, TX; with permission.)

Shampoo, leave-on conditioners, sprays, wipes (big and small), and ointments/creams/gels/liquids are all available for use individually or in combination.

Shampoo/conditioner therapy is best used for cases of generalized torso skin infections, regardless of coat length and thickness. It is difficult to shampoo the face and distal extremities of dogs. If the coat is thick and/or long, shampoo therapy may be the only means by which one can deliver antimicrobial ingredients. Although shampoo therapy potentially offers the most effective mode of topical treatment, considering the majority of patients are haired and it is the most widely distributable vehicle, it is the mode with poorest client compliance. Depending on the size and length of hair coat of the dog as well as its temperament, the process can be physically difficult, time consuming, and stressful. There are few cats who will tolerate the process. Bathing is more commonly needed for generalized rather than localized or patterned infections, which can be addressed by more client-friendly products. The selection of the shampoo bottle size is important. Unless the dog is 5 kg of body weight or smaller, there is no value to small shampoo sizes. The 16-ounce bottle size is best suited for the majority of dogs, considering its generalized application and need for frequent and chronic use. To conserve on cost of the antibacterial shampoo, a bath can be first given with a lower cost non-medicated shampoo immediately followed by the medicated shampoo because there will be less medicated shampoo needed to cover the area once the scale, dead hair, and debris are first removed.

The presence of potentiating ingredient(s) in a shampoo is just as important as the shampoo ingredient choice itself. Whenever possible, the shampoo should contain some type of ingredient, such as chitosans, liposomes, or lipid barrier molecules that extend the life of the antibacterial agent being applied. Different antibacterial ingredients should be used, on a trial-and-error basis, until the most effective product is found for the patient being treated. Proper application, frequency of application and contact time must also be considered. The more often and thorough the application, the better the outcome.

If client compliance is an issue with shampoo therapy, an acceptable substitution may be a wipe. The treatment surface area dictates the choice of wipe treatment. If the infection covers a large area, nisin wipes are most appropriate because their large size and low cost allow for generous use and coverage area. Smaller areas are ideal for chlorhexidine-containing wipes, many of which also contain antifungal drugs and/or skin surface lipids. Just as with shampoo therapy, the actual act of wiping the skin with a moist cloth material has the added benefit of directly removing debris, adherent environmental allergens such as pollens or mold spores, and adherent bacteria, lessening the numbers of organisms needed to be killed on the skin surface. Wipes are ideal for thinly haired areas, the head, and extremity skin, areas otherwise more difficult to reach with shampoo therapy.

Spray treatments can be directly applied using the trigger sprayer or applied with a cotton ball or suitable substitute. A large (triple-sized) cotton ball is superior to regular sized cotton because the opening to most spray liquids, when the sprayer itself is removed, is too large for regular cotton balls. If the cotton ball is directly sprayed instead, the dispersion angle and volume of liquids propelled through the sprayer can easily exceed that which can be trapped by a regular sized cotton ball. Cotton ball application is best used in areas that require more careful targeted treatment (around the eyes, mouth, or feet) or for individuals who resent the direct spraying (especially cats). Sprays can be used by themselves or as adjunctive treatment to the wipes or shampoo treatments. Unlike the ointments or creams, which are typically used to treat skin infections, the sprays can both treat and prevent infections. They are better suited, however, for prevention.

Topical antibacterial treatment in cats represents a special challenge in veterinary medicine. Many of the topical products available to canine patients can be used in cats but there are practical limitations. Few cats allow themselves to be bathed with the frequency needed to be effective for treating or preventing bacterial skin infections. Fortunately, cats rarely develop generalized bacterial skin infections that would require whole-body antibacterial shampoo therapy. Leave-on conditioners are more attractive because they need only damp skin and can be applied in a manner acceptable to most cats who allow handling. Wipes are particularly attractive because cats are small and often have bacterial skin infections in localized regions. Generally, the smaller wipes are better than larger ones made for large surface area application. There is minimal residue left behind from wipe treatments, which is less likely to encourage a fastidious animal to lick off the applied product. Antibacterial sprays can accomplish the same objective. Most cats resent direct spray application and the contents within the spay bottle are better applied with the product soaked on a cotton ball. Ointments, creams, and gels are very helpful as treatment for localized infections. However, the vehicles often prompts cats to groom the treatment area and it can be difficult to distract the cat for the necessary contact time of more than 10 minutes. If topical therapy is needed, it is more practical to fit the cat with an Elizabethan collar before treatment and keep the collar in place for 15 to 20 minutes after the topical medication is applied.

Considering the current state of bacterial resistance and the ever-present pressure for recurring bacterial infections, it is critical that veterinarians incorporate aggressive topical antibacterial products into the regular treatment of bacterial skin infections. The client needs to be involved in the decision making process, so their willingness and ability to undertake the topical treatments can be assessed. Any physical limitations of the patient or pet owner, as well as the size and temperament of the patient, will play a role, along with the facilities and time needed to complete the topical treatment. Rather than relying on 1 individual product choice, a combination of products is ideal. This can entail regular shampoo therapy, with adjunctive spray or wipe treatment, or a combination of wipe and spray treatments. Topical ointments/creams/gels/liquids can also be prescribed for short-term treatment of localized infections. There also needs to be an assessment of the practice inventory, to carry at least a minimum of products than can serve the needs for effective and consistently administered topical treatment of bacterial skin infections.

REFERENCES

1. Beck KM, Waisglass SE, Dick HL, et al. Prevalence of methicillin-resistant Staphylococcus pseudintermedius (MRSP) from skin and carriage sites of dogs after treatment of their meticillin-resistant or meticillin-sensitive staphylococcal pyoderma. Vet Dermatol 2012;23(4):369–e67.
2. Kwochka KW, Kowalski JJ. Prophylactic efficacy of four antibacterial shampoos against Staphylococcus intermedius in dogs. Am J Vet Res 1991;52:115–8.
3. Nagata M, Murayama N, Shibata K. Efficacy of Nolvasan surgical scrub containing 2 chlorhexidine acetate in topical management of canine superficial pyoderma a randomized double-blinded controlled study. Jpn J Vet Dermatol 2006;12:1–6.
4. Ascher F, Maynard L, Laurent J, et al. Controlled trial of ethyl lactate and benzoyl peroxide shampoos in the management of canine surface pyoderma and superficial pyoderma. In: Von Tscharner C, Halliwell RE, editors. Advances in veterinary dermatology. London: Balliere Tindall; 1990. p. 375.

5. Murayama N, Nagata M, Terada Y, et al. Efficacy of a surgical scrub including 2% chlorhexidine acetate for canine superficial pyoderma. Vet Dermatol 2010;21: 586–92.

6. Loeffler A, Cobb MA, Bond R. Comparison of a chlorhexidine and a benzoyl peroxide shampoo as sole treatment in canine superficial pyodermas. Vet Rec 2011;169:249.

7. Scott DW, Miller WH, Cayette SM. A clinical study on the effect of two commercial veterinary benzoyl peroxide shampoos in dogs. Canine Practice 1994;19:7–10.

8. Murayama N, Nagata M, Terada Y, et al. Comparison of two formulations of chlorhexidine for treating canine superficial pyoderma. Vet Rec 2010;167:532–3.

9. Young R, Buckley L, McEwan N, et al. Comparative in vitro efficacy of antimicrobial shampoos: a pilot study. Vet Dermatol 2012;23:36–40.

10. Guaguere E. Topical treatment of canine and feline pyoderma. Vet Dermatol 1996;7:145–51.

11. Prottey C, George D, Leech RW, et al. The mode of action of ethyl lactate as a treatment for acne. Br J Dermatol 1984;110:475–85.

12. Abbott WH, Lemons CL, Gram WD. In vitro activity of chlorhexidine gluconate against Staphylococcus intermedius. In: Proceedings of the AAVD/ACVD 14th meeting. San Antonio (TX); 1998. p. 17.

13. Murayama N, Terada Y, Okuaki M, et al. Dose assessment of 2% chlorhexidine acetate for canine superficial pyoderma. Vet Dermatol 2011;22:449–53.

14. Scott DW, Miller WH, Griffin CE. Muller and Kirk's small animal dermatology. 6th edition. Philadelphia: WB Saunders; 2001. p. 221–4.

15. Werner AH, Russell AD. Mupirocin, fusidic acid and bacitracin: activity, action and clinical uses of three topical antibiotics. Vet Dermatol 1999;10:225–40.

16. White SD, Bordeau PB, Blumstein P, et al. Feline acne and results of treatment with mupirocin in an open clinical trial: 25 cases (1994–96). Vet Dermatol 1997; 8:157–64.

17. Dowling PM. Antimicrobial therapy of skin and ear infections. Can Vet J 1996;37: 695–9.

18. Burrows AK. Residual antimicrobial action of 2% mupirocin ointment. In: Proceedings of the AAVD/ACVD 10th meeting. Charleston (SC); 1994. p. 35.

19. Kaplan S. Implications of methicillin-resistant Staphylococcus aureus as a community-acquired pathogen in pediatric patients. Infect Dis Clin North Am 2005;19:747–57.

20. Winter J, Ilbert M, Graf PC, et al. Bleach activates a redox-regulated chaperone by oxidative protein unfolding. Cell 2008;135:691–701.

21. Fisher RG, Chain RL, Hair PS, et al. Hypochlorite killing of community- acquired methicillin-resistant Staphylococcus aureus. Pediatr Infect Dis J 2008;27:934–5.

22. Oculus Innovative Sciences, Inc. Vetericyn: one-step wound and infection care and animal wellness products. Available at: http://vetericyn.com/veterinarians/. Accessed May 31, 2012.

23. Brötzaand H, Sahl HG. New insights into the mechanism of action of lantibiotics— diverse biological effects by binding to the same molecular target. J Antimicrob Chemother 2000;46:1–6.

24. Frank LA, Kirzeder EM, Davis JA, et al. Nisin impregnated wipes for the treatment of canine pyoderma and surface bacterial colonization. In: Proceedings of the North American Veterinary Dermatology 24th Forum. Savannah (GA); 2009. p. 215.

25. Hasper HE, Kramer NE, Smith JL, et al. An alternative bactericidal mechanism of action for lantibiotic peptides that target lipid II. Science 2006;313:1636–7.

26. Ruhr E, Sahl HG. Mode of action of the peptide antibiotic nisin and influence on the membrane potential of whole cells and on cytoplasmic and artificial membrane vesicles. Antimicrobial Agents Chemother 1985;27:841–5.
27. Delves-Broughton J, Blackburn P, Evans RJ, et al. Applications of the bacteriocin, nisin. Antonie Van Leeuwenhoek 1996;69:193–202.
28. Dutta PK, Dutta J, Tripathi VS. Chitin and chitosan: chemistry, properties and applications. J Sci Ind Res 2004;63:20–31.
29. Singh A, Malviya R, Sharma PK. Novasome-a breakthrough in pharmaceutical technology a review article. Adv Biol Res 2011;5:184–9.
30. Quelch V. Exploring microvesicle technology: tiny structures lead to advances in dermatology therapy. Veterinary Product News May/June 1996;26–7.
31. Barthe N, Jasmin P, Brouillaud B, et al. Assessment of the distribution of radiolabelled non-ionic multilamellar surfactant microvesicles following topical application to canine skin biopsies: a preliminary study. J Drug Deliv Sci Technol 2005;15:183–5.
32. Piekutowska A, Pin D, Rème CA, et al. Effects of a topically applied preparation of epidermal lipids on the stratum corneum barrier of atopic dogs. J Comp Pathol 2008;138:197–203.
33. Coderch L, López O, Maza A, et al. Ceramides and skin function. Am J Clin Dermatol 2003;4:107–29.
34. Reiter LV, Torres SM, Wertz PW. Characterization and quantification of ceramides in the nonlesional skin of canine patients with atopic dermatitis compared with controls. Vet Dermatol 2009;20:260–6.

Feline Otitis: Diagnosis and Treatment

Robert A. Kennis, DVM, MS

KEYWORDS

- Feline • Otitis • Aural polyp • Atopy • Food allergy • Ear mites

KEY POINTS

- Cats may develop otitis media without overt otitis externa.
- Cats are less susceptible to secondary otic infections than dogs.
- Cats may be more susceptible to ototoxicity than dogs, and topical therapy should be used cautiously.

INTRODUCTION

Feline otitis can be a challenging clinical problem. The commonly used clinical approach to diagnosis and treatment of canine otitis rarely yields satisfactory results when applied to cats. Dr John August introduced the concept that otitis is a multifactorial problem in dogs, and his concepts are extrapolated to the cat in this article.

Otitis by definition is inflammation of the ear canal and/or the pinna. *Otitis externa* is a term used when only the external canal, outside of the tympanic membrane, is involved. When the tympanum and the tympanic bulla are involved, the term *otitis media* is used. *Otitis interna* implies damage to the hearing apparatus; neurologic symptoms and deafness are usually present.

Otitis in cats is usually a multifactorial problem. Predisposing factors are those that may allow inflammation to occur. Ear canal stenosis and pinnal deformity are far more common problems in dogs than in cats. There does not seem to be a breed predisposition for developing otitis in cats. Ear pinna conformation of the Scottish Fold is not associated with an increased risk of otitis. High-humidity environments or cats that are bathed frequently may be more at risk because of canal tissue maceration. One of the common predisposing causes of feline otitis is the use of a cotton swab to remove normal ear canal excretions. Trauma from cleaning may lead to inflammation and secondary infections. Some cats, especially Persians and older Siamese cats, have excessively ceruminous ears and should be left alone unless infection is identified.

Primary causes are those that induce otitis directly. Foreign bodies or ectoparasites are the most common causes. Although some allergic cats will have concurrent otitis, this occurs far less commonly than in the dog. Additional primary causes include autoimmune diseases, neoplasia, and fungal infections. A polyp is usually the result of

Department of Clinical Sciences, Auburn University, 612 Hoerlein Hall, Auburn, AL 36849, USA
E-mail address: kennira@auburn.edu

Vet Clin Small Anim 43 (2013) 51–56
http://dx.doi.org/10.1016/j.cvsm.2012.09.009
0195-5616/13/$ – see front matter © 2013 Elsevier Inc. All rights reserved.

chronic inflammation. However, in some cases, the presence of a polyp may lead to ear canal inflammation caused by obstruction.

The perpetuating factors, bacteria and yeast organisms that are the source of frustration in many canine otitis cases, are less frequently a problem for cats. An aural polyp is usually a perpetuating factor as a result of chronic inflammation or may be idiopathic. One of the most important, yet least discussed, risk factors is the allergic or irritant reaction that occurs after application of topical medications. Antiinflammatory corticosteroids may be the cause of the reaction. This reaction is counterintuitive considering that these should reduce the amount of inflammation and not be the source of the problem. Contact reactions may also occur with antibiotics or carrier agents.

DIFFERENTIAL DIAGNOSES

It is possible to limit the differential diagnoses based on the observation of a unilateral versus a bilateral problem. Unilateral causes are commonly associated with a foreign body, aural polyp, neoplasia, or trauma (aural hematoma). Bilateral otitis is usually associated with parasitic, metabolic (systemic illness), allergic, or autoimmune problems. Dermatophytosis, bacterial infections, or yeast infections may present as unilateral or bilateral problems.

Atopy and cutaneous adverse reactions to food should be considered for cases of recurrent otitis. These cases may be associated with either unilateral or bilateral otitis externa. Concurrent clinical signs of pruritus may be present in other regions of the body. Both of these allergic conditions may be very pruritic without overt secondary infection. Aural hematoma may be a consequence of excessive scratching.

Otitis media without overt otitis externa may occur more commonly in the cat than the dog. It is usually a unilateral problem but may be bilateral. Clinical signs may include head shaking or pawing at the ears. There may be no evidence of otitis externa. In dogs, otitis media is frequently associated with chronic otitis externa leading to damage of the tympanic membrane. The diagnosis of otitis media is usually made during otoscopic examination. The tympanic membrane may seem to be ballooning outward. Fluid and air bubbles may be seen behind the intact tympanum. Empiric treatment with a systemic antibiotic to cover a spectrum against *Staphylococcus*, *Streptococcus*, *Pasteurella*, and anaerobic bacteria should be considered. A myringotomy can be performed under general anesthesia to collect a sample for culture and susceptibility testing.

Ceruminous gland cysts (ceruminous cystomatosis) may occur in any aged cat. The clinical signs include single to multiple cystlike structures containing dark brown to dark bluish material (**Fig. 1**). In severe cases, the cysts may lead to a stenotic ear canal with secondary infection. When these lesions are present, it is usually recommended to perform a biopsy with histopathology to rule out neoplastic diseases. Treatment with topical or systemic medication is rarely helpful. Surgical excision or laser ablation can be considered for severe cases.

Some cats may develop an increase in cerumen production leading to a shiny-appearing inner pinna or waxy brown debris within the canal. This condition is sometimes referred to as idiopathic ceruminous otitis externa. Secondary infection may occur. Treatment of secondary infections should be considered; however, excessive topical treatment may lead to chronic clinical signs. It is usually best to treat these as conservatively as possible. Allergic diseases should be considered as a possible underlying cause of this condition. The use of topical or systemic glucocorticoid medications may be considered for short-term relief if excessive pruritus is present.

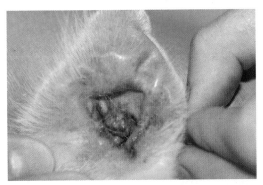

Fig. 1. Ceruminous gland cysts (ceruminous cystomatosis) in an aged cat. The clinical signs include single to multiple cystlike structures containing dark brown to dark bluish material.

Aural polyps are usually associated with unilateral otitis. Secondary infections may be present and may be the cause of clinical presentation. The cause of polyp formation is unknown but infectious causes have been investigated as a predisposing factor. The polyp may arise from anywhere within the mucosal lining of the ear canal and may originate in the pharynx and extend through the eustachian tube. They are most commonly seen in younger cats but can be identified at any age. The polyp itself is comprised of mixed inflammatory cells and has an epithelial layer. The clinical signs are variable and may include pruritus, head shaking, neurologic signs (Horner syndrome), and respiratory signs if the polyp extends to the oral pharynx. Infection or inflammatory to serous exudation may be evident on cytologic evaluation. The diagnosis may be made on otoscopic evaluation. A computed tomography (CT) scan is helpful to identify the extent and origination of the polyp and will aid in differentiating the mass from neoplastic causes. It will also help the surgeon determine the best method for removal because recurrence is a possibility if residual tissue remains. Middle ear polyps may require ventral bulla osteotomy for complete resection and removal. Secondary infection is a common consequence of aural polyps. Cytology will help with empiric therapy, but culture and susceptibility testing may be more appropriate to help achieve a complete remission.

Neoplasia is an uncommon cause of unilateral otitis in the cat. Squamous cell carcinoma or apocrine or sebaceous carcinomas may occur. These carcinomas tend to be highly malignant, so aggressive surgical and medical intervention is required. Some cats may present with recurrent infections caused by stenosis of the ear canal. Diagnosis is based on histopathology. The treatment options and the prognosis are variable.

Demodex cati may be identified when performing routine cytologic evaluation of debris mixed with mineral oil. Clinical signs may be minimal and confined only to the ear canals. If generalized demodicosis is present, then it is necessary to search for a disease process that may lead to immunosuppression. There are no standard protocols for treating localized aural demodex in the cat. Treatment options might include those suitable for the treatment of ear mites. Topical compounded ivermectin preparations can be considered. When generalized demodicosis caused by *Demodex cati* is diagnosed, the treatment should be aimed at the cause of the demodex rather than treatment of the demodex itself.

Ear mites caused by *Otodectes cynotis* is one of the most common causes of otitis externa in the cat. The diagnosis can usually be made with an otoscopic examination.

Alternatively, the waxy debris can be gently removed and mixed with mineral oil for microscopic examination. Treatment options are discussed later.

DIAGNOSTIC PROCEDURES

The proper treatment of feline otitis depends on an accurate identification of the predisposing primary and secondary problems. A thorough history is essential. Simple information regarding unilateral versus bilateral problems along with the treatments used are essential starting points. An otoscopic examination is also necessary. It is a way to determine if the tympanum and bulla are involved. It is also the easiest way to find otodectes ear mites and ear masses. Cytology is an important diagnostic tool to evaluate the perpetuating factors. However, care should be used in placing swabs into a cat's ear when only ceruminous debris and no exudation are present. Vigorous swabbing can be an inciting source of inflammation and further complications. A culture and susceptibility should be performed for refractory cases or those with highly exudative otitis.

Because many cats may have a metabolic cause for their otitis, additional laboratory work, including a complete blood count, serum chemistry profile, thyroid analysis, and feline immunodeficiency virus and feline leukemia virus testing, may be indicated. Routine radiograph imaging rarely yields useful information. A CT scan is better to analyze the extent of the problem when neoplasia or polyps are suspected. Biopsy of the ear canal tissue or pinnae is a commonly needed procedure when masses are present or when systemic/autoimmune disorders are suspected. Samples should be submitted in formalin for histopathologic analysis. The surgeon should be prepared for an extensive procedure, including bulla osteotomy, canal resection, or total ear canal ablation, depending on the extent of disease.

TREATMENT OPTIONS

Cats seem to be more susceptible to ototoxicity and Horner syndrome than dogs, which may be caused by differences in their tympanic bullae. General anesthesia is usually indicated for even minor ear cleaning procedures. Warmed sterile saline is recommended for cleaning a cat's ears, even when ear mites are present. Iodine has been shown to be ototoxic to cats. The aminoglycoside antibiotics can cause ototoxicity and should be avoided. Because chlorhexidine has been shown to be ototoxic to dogs, it is rational to also avoid this product in cats. There are currently no licensed veterinary products for the ear canal that contain chlorhexidine. Dioctyl sulfosuccinate and other ceruminolytic agents should be avoided, especially if the tympanic membrane is ruptured. A product containing Tris-EDTA or a commercially available ear cleaning product for dogs and cats may be considered. Sterile physiologic saline is probably the safest cleansing agent for cats.

One of the major differences in the approach to treating otitis in dogs from cats involves the usage of topical medications. Topical medications are the mainstay of therapy in canine otitis. It is the author's opinion that they should be mostly avoided in treating cats. Several cats have improved simply by discontinuing the use of topical medications. For undefined reasons, cats tend to develop irritant reactions and contact allergy reactions in the ear pinna and canal at a higher incidence than in dogs. Many cases of feline otitis can be successfully treated without the use of topical medications, which is rarely the case in dogs. Cats hate topical products. Their fastidious nature causes them to frantically remove any topical agent applied to the skin surface, including the ear canal and pinnae. Topical application is a potential source for aural hematoma formation and also for the clients to be wounded by a fractious cat. For these reasons, topical medications should be limited or avoided in the treatment of feline otitis.

There are exceptions to avoiding topical medications when it comes to treating feline ear mite infestations. Pyrethrin-based ear medications instilled into the ear canal for the treatment of ear mites are inexpensive compared with other products. They can be effective, but the precautions about topical medications should be considered. Also, ear mites may crawl out of the ear canal and avoid topical contact. Treatment can be prolonged and failure may occur. The spot-on topical application of selamectin (Revolution) is an excellent treatment option for resolving ear mites. This product is labeled for monthly treatment, but an accepted protocol is to use this product every 14 days for 3 treatments. A spot-on formulation containing imidacloprid and moxidectin (Advantage Multi for cats) is also highly effective in treating ear mites. Injectable or orally administered cattle ivermectin is not licensed or approved for use in the cat. It is commonly used off label for treating ear mites. Several off-label protocols are discussed in continuing education proceedings. Only licensed products are reviewed here. There is a topical otic suspension consisting of 0.01% ivermectin (Acarexx) that is licensed and approved and highly effective. This product is to be applied into each ear canal one time, but a second treatment is recommended. This product is licensed for application to kittens as young as 4 weeks of age. A 0.1% milbemycin containing otic product (Milbemite) is a topical preparation to be used as a single treatment. Few cases have needed a second treatment. This product can also be used on kittens 4 weeks of age or older. With the highly effective and licensed products available, there is no reason to use off-label ivermectin. Any untoward reaction from using cattle formulations of ivermectin will be the responsibility of the clinician.

There is no general agreement whether it is better to aggressively clean the canals and pinnae or to leave them alone when there is ear mite infestation. Systemic treatment will resolve the infestation either way. Topical medications may work better if the debris is removed, but package labeling states that efficacy is not altered regardless of whether the ears are cleaned or not. Cleaning usually requires at least sedation. The cats seem to be painful immediately after removing all of the debris. The argument to not clean them comes from the observation that much of this material may coalesce and form a ceruminolith leading to additional complications. A compromise might be to not clean them initially, and then address the cerumen accumulation later on if it becomes a problem.

When bacteria or *Malassezia* yeast (perpetuating factors) are present in the cat, systemic medications should be considered, even if the middle ear is not involved. This practice is absolutely contradictory to the common approach to treating canine otitis. Cats infrequently get bacteria or yeast infections except for iatrogenic causes, secondary to allergic causes, and those associated with ear masses. A good empiric selection of an antibiotic for the cat would include clindamycin, cefpodoxime (Simplicef), or amoxicillin with clavulanate (Clavamox) at the standard dosage. Although first-generation cephalosporin drugs are very useful in dogs, cats tend to vomit and become anorexic with these products. High dosages of enrofloxacin (Baytril) should be avoided because of retinal degeneration that has occurred in some cats. However, marbofloxacin (Zeniquin) may be indicated for usage only if based on culture and susceptibility testing. Many commercial topical antibacterial otic preparations contain aminoglycoside antibiotics and should generally be avoided in cats because of the increased risk of ototoxicity.

Itraconazole (Sporanox) is the recommended treatment of severe yeast otitis in the cat. The recommended dosage is 5 to 10 mg/kg every day until a remission is reached. This drug is not licensed for use in the cat and is relatively expensive. Anorexia and/or vomiting may occur. Ketoconazole should be avoided in cats because of hepatopathy. Fluconazole 5 to 10 mg/kg every day until remission is a reasonable option and is easier to dose than other azole medications. Cats rarely get primary yeast infections. Allergic causes should be sought for recurrent infections. Mild yeast otitis in the cat can be treated with topical 1% miconazole solution.

Surgery is indicated for any mass in the ear of a cat. The extent of the procedure is based on the problem. There are several surgical options for the removal of an inflammatory polyp and they are beyond the scope of this article. Appropriate diagnostic procedures, including a CT scan, will help to determine the extent of the disease and can aid the surgeon in giving the owner a reasonable prognosis. However, this depends on the histopathologic diagnosis. There are always potential postsurgical complications to consider. Head tilt or Horner syndrome caused by facial nerve damage may occur. Chronic draining tracts can also be a problem.

SUGGESTED READINGS

August JR. Otitis externa, a disease of multifactorial etiology. Vet Clin North Am Small Anim Pract 1988;18:731.

Bloom PB. Anatomy of the ear in health and disease. In: August JR, editor. Consultations in feline internal medicine, vol. 6. St Louis (MO): Saunders Elsevier; 2010. p. 319–30.

Moriello KA, Diesel A. Medical management of otitis. In: August JR, editor. Consultations in feline internal medicine, vol. 6. St Louis (MO): Saunders Elsevier; 2010. p. 347–57.

Donnelly K, Tillson D. Feline inflammatory polyps and ventral bulla osteotomy. Comp Cont Ed Vet 2004;29:446–54.

Gotthelf LN. Diagnosis and management of otitis media. In: Gotthelf LN, editor. Small animal ear diseases: an illustrated guide. 2nd edition. St Louis (MO): Mosby; 2005. p. 276.

Fan TM, de Lorimier LP. Inflammatory polyps and aural neoplasia. Vet Clin North Am Small Anim Pract 2004;34:489–509.

Canine Pododermatitis

David Duclos, DVM

KEYWORDS

- Pododermatitis • Dermatology • Veterinary • Dog diseases • Skin diseases

KEY POINTS

- Skin diseases that affect the canine paw cause changes that overlap and look very similar.
- The causes of pododermatitis can be grouped into the categories of infectious/parasitic, immunologic, metabolic, neoplastic, genetic/inherited, and foreign body/acquired.
- Demodicosis involving the feet in the adult dogs older than 4 years is one of the most commonly misdiagnosed skin diseases seen by dermatologists.
- Dermatophytosis can easily look like other conditions such as demodicosis, pyoderma, or atopic dermatitis.
- Deep pyoderma in the paws is one of the most frustrating conditions in the dog; dogs with this condition have nodules, fistula, and recurrent draining tracts.

INTRODUCTION

Skin diseases that affect the canine paw cause changes that overlap and look very similar. **Figs.1–5** show dogs with atopy, demodicosis, deep pyoderma, and dermatophytosis. In **Figs. 6–10**, changes caused by pemphigus, superficial necrolytic dermatitis, epitheliotropic lymphoma, and familial paw pad hyperkeratosis are represented. **Figs. 11–15** are of dogs with vasculitis, epitheliotropic lymphoma, deep pyoderma, demodicosis, and atopy. Could you tell the diagnosis of each by looking only at these pictures, and not the legend? The diagnosis for each figure is given and explained in the following paragraphs. The purpose of this article is to point out what information is necessary to make the right diagnosis for the different diseases that cause similar changes in the canine paw. To make a diagnosis, you will need to use key features from the signalment, history, and physical examination and to choose the right diagnostic tests.

A detailed discussion of treatment of these diseases is not the main goal of this article. Treatments will be briefly discussed, but it is assumed that the practicing veterinarian already knows most of the major details about treatment. Some of the conditions discussed here, such as neoplasia and autoimmune diseases, are not simple to treat and the veterinarian would need to have some advanced training for treatment and management. If the reader is has not taken this kind of advanced training or

Animal Skin & Allergy Clinic, 16429 7th Place West, Lynnwood, WA 98037, USA
E-mail address: david_duclos@msn.com

Vet Clin Small Anim 43 (2013) 57–87
http://dx.doi.org/10.1016/j.cvsm.2012.09.012
0195-5616/13/$ – see front matter © 2013 Elsevier Inc. All rights reserved.

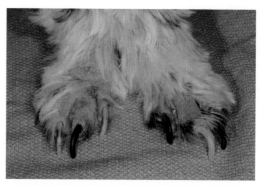

Fig. 1. Demodicosis.

does not have much experience in these types of treatment, referral to a specialist is recommended.

The causes of pododermatitis can be grouped into the categories of infectious/parasitic, immunologic, metabolic, neoplastic, genetic/inherited, and foreign body/acquired; see **Box 1**.

INFECTIOUS/PARASITIC DISEASES OF THE PAWS
Demodicosis

1. Demodicosis involving the feet in the adult dogs older than 4 years is one of the most commonly misdiagnosed skin diseases seen by dermatologists (see **Figs. 1**, **3**, and **15**; **Figs. 16–20**). Demodicosis can present with only paw lesions, however, most often other body parts are affected such as the perioral, periocular, and other areas on the trunk. All that is needed is the microscopic examination of a skin scraping, so why would so many of these be missed? Possibly it is because these dogs look very much like dogs with allergies or because they occur in dogs that have been seen by the veterinarian for chronic skin disease.[1,2] Veterinarians in general practice are not typically trained to notice the key subtle features that would alert them to something new going on in the dog's skin disease, so demodicosis is an easily missed, new condition in the skin of older dogs. Treating these dogs with corticosteroids or cyclosporine will worsen the condition, so it is

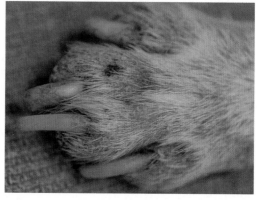

Fig. 2. Dermatophytosis.

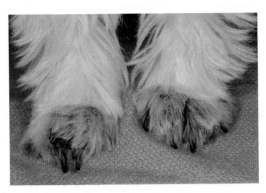

Fig. 3. Demodicosis.

important to pay attention to dogs with skin disease that are not responding to therapy. Most dogs with adult-onset demodicosis look very similar to dogs that have allergic skin disease, so it is easily missed. One should be aware that dogs with skin lesions on the face, feet, axillae, and groin are not always dogs with allergies. These signs are only part of the signs for allergy. In addition to these clinical signs, other historical and signalment information is needed. All of the signalment, history, and physical examination information needs to be put together to make a diagnosis of atopic dermatitis. One major tip is that dogs with demodicosis are really not very pruritic; they might have a recent history of licking at the more severely affected sites, but compared to dogs with allergies, they do not have a long-term history of pruritus. What is even more diagnostic is that most dogs with adult-onset demodicosis have no allergic signs and are not allergic.[1] The clinician needs to be careful to not turn all skin diseases into "allergy." There are numerous visible clinical signs that can alert the clinician to the possibility of demodicosis.

2. Key features for demodicosis
   a. Usually not pruritic (some are, but not common)
   b. Hyperpigmentation (see **Figs. 3** and **16**)
   c. Comedones—not easy to find; need to look closely for these but are usually present (see **Figs. 16** and **17**)
   d. Nodules, fistula, hemorrhagic draining lesions—especially on the paws (see **Figs. 15** and **17–19**)

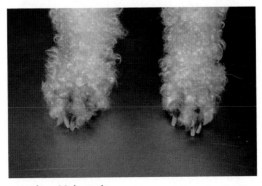

Fig. 4. Atopy with secondary *Malassezia.*

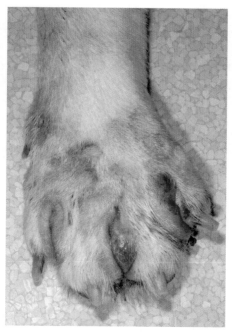

Fig. 5. Deep pyoderma/furunculosis.

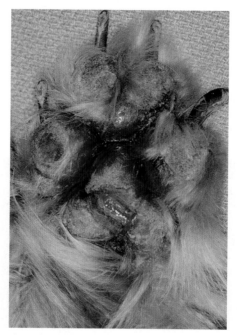

Fig. 6. Superficial necrolytic dermatitis.

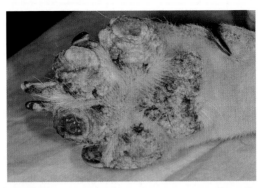

Fig. 7. Pemphigus foliaceus.

e. Alopecia—complete or thinning, with a white powder–like scale (see **Figs. 19** and **20**)
f. Skin is friable; bleeds very easily during skin scrapings
g. Body areas most often affected
   i. Paws (see **Figs. 1**, **3**, and **16–18**)
   ii. Muzzle and perioral (see **Fig. 20**)
   iii. Legs
   iv. Dorsal and lateral trunk
   v. Ventrum—comedones often present here
   vi. Pinnae—comedones often seen on concave surface
h. No skin scrapings have been performed; look like dogs with allergies
i. Do not take a biopsy sample before doing a skin scraping/hair plucking examination
j. Hair plucking works in the place of skin scraping in most cases; the mites are in the distal ends of the hairs[3]
k. When looking at the hairs on skin scraping, pay attention to the hairs; sometimes there will be dermatophyte arthrospores present
l. If treatment of demodicosis shows limited to no improvement, perform culture for dermatophytes; some of these dogs have both demodicosis and dermatophytosis
m. Look for underlying causes—hyperadrenocorticism, lymphoma, atopy, hypothyroidism[4]

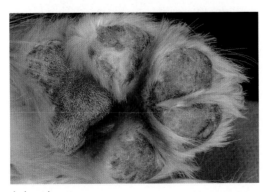

Fig. 8. Epitheliotropic lymphoma.

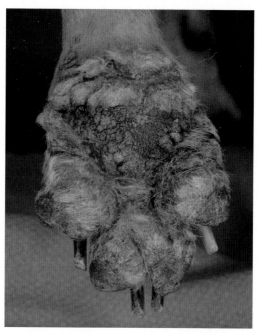

Fig. 9. Superficial necrolytic dermatitis.

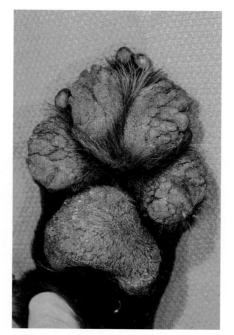

Fig. 10. Familial paw pad hyperkeratosis.

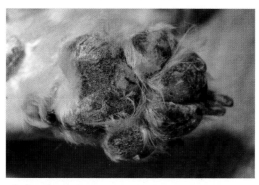

Fig. 11. Epitheliotropic lymphoma.

3. Treatment[2,5,6]

  a. Amitraz (Mitaban, Pfizer Animal Health, Exton, PA, USA) dips—the only approved treatment

  b. Ivermectin (400–600 μg/kg/d—not approved, potentially toxic but is effective[2,5,6]

  c. Milbemycin oxime (Interceptor, Novartis Animal Health, Greensboro, NC, USA) 1 to 2 mg/kg/d not approved, less toxic than ivermectin, expensive, also effective[7]

  d. Moxidectin/imidacloprid (Advantage Multi) spot on weekly[5,8–10]—not approved, efficacy looks good but not 100% effective; long-term follow-up studies have not been published

  e. Doramectin (Dectomax, Pfizer Animal Health, Exton, PA, USA)[11]—not approved, potentially toxic, is an ivermectin derivative but with longer action in the tissue so could use less frequently, possibly once per week, no long-term studies published

  f. Treat any pyoderma or underlying disease or both as needed.

Dermatophytosis

1. Dermatophytosis will affect the paws (see **Fig. 2**; **Figs. 21** and **22**) but affects other body sites as well. It can easily look like other conditions such as demodicosis, pyoderma, or atopic dermatitis. A major differentiating feature between dermatophytosis and demodicosis is the effects of where the disease organisms live in the skin. In demodicosis, the mites live deep within the hair follicle, so this disease will more likely cause hemorrhagic or follicular nodules and dilations and draining

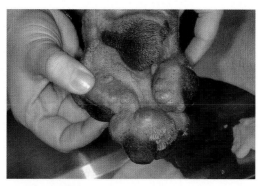

Fig. 12. Deep pyoderma/furunculosis.

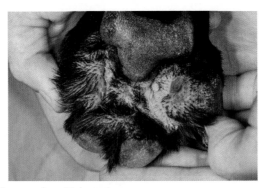

Fig. 13. Atopy with secondary *Malassezia.*

lesions. The dermatophytes live exclusively in keratin, so they are in the upper stratum corneum of the skin and in the keratinized upper portions of the hairs. Clinically, this means dermatophytosis is a disease with dry, scaly, and alopecic skin and broken hairs. There will be erythema and crusting because of the reactions to the infection. Hemorrhage can be seen but is not a common feature of dermatophytosis; nodular draining lesions are also not typical of dermatophytosis, whereas this is a common feature of demodicosis. Dermatophytes can affect any area of the body; in dogs, lesions are most commonly seen on the paws, bridge of the nose, and pinnae (see **Figs. 2**, **21**, and **22**). The other body parts can be affected, but when they are, the paws, pinna, and muzzle are also affected. The most common dermatophyte that affects the dog is *Trichophyton* spp, which do not produce fluorescence or arthrospores on hairs.[12,13] This means the Wood's lamp and skin scraping examination results in the dog with dermatophytosis are usually negative. In addition to the history, physical examination, and signalment, a fungal culture is the only way to make a diagnosis of dermatophytosis in these dogs. Histopathologic examination of biopsy specimens also can be an important diagnostic test to confirm a diagnosis for canine dermatophytosis. Some cases of dermatophytosis in the dog are very subtle and are first picked up by finding mycelia in the biopsy specimens; after this, a fungal culture will identify the dermatophyte.[12] The dog is not the normal host for *Trichophyton* spp, and because of this, there are fewer arthrospores and mycelia, which makes this dermatophyte

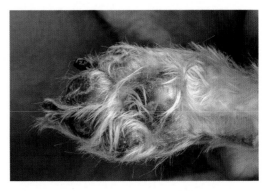

Fig. 14. Vasculitis.

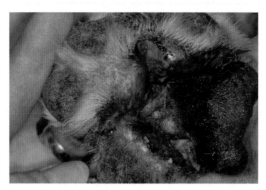

Fig. 15. Demodicosis.

difficult to find on histopathologic examination. Often, special stains are necessary. If a dermatophyte is suspected, special stains should be requested.[13]
2. Key features
   a. Dry scale, erythema, alopecia, broken hairs, some crusting with scale on the crusts
   b. Skin scraping and Wood's lamp negative
   c. Nonpruritic
   d. Misshapen nails—longstanding cases (see **Fig. 22**)

Box 1
Causes of pododermatitis in the dog
Infectious/Parasitic
1. Demodicosis
2. Dermatophytosis
3. Deep pyoderma/furunculosis
4. Malassezia
Immunologic
5. Pemphigus
6. Atopy
7. Vasculitis
Metabolic
8. Superficial necrolytic dermatitis
Neoplastic
9. Nailbed squamous cell carcinoma
10. Epitheliotropic lymphoma
Genetic/Inherited
11. Familial paw pad hyperkeratosis
Foreign body/acquired
12. Follicular cysts

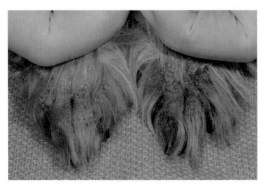

Fig. 16. Demodicosis.

  e. Fungal culture the only means of making a confirming diagnosis
  f. Most canine dermatophyte infections are caused by *Trichophyton; Microsporum canis* less frequently[12]
  g. Histopathology can reveal fungal hyphae in keratin structures of skin
  h. Body areas affected most commonly—paws, muzzle, and pinnae; other areas less often (see **Figs. 2, 21,** and **22**)
  i. *Trichophyton* infections in the canine are not highly contagious, because of the low numbers of arthrospores and mycelia, so other pets and humans are not usually affected[13]
  j. Typically only one dog in house is affected and can be affected for years while undiagnosed; the dog is not the normal host for this dermatophyte, so it does not act as a reliable source for contagion[12,13]
3. Treatments[12]
  a. Topical—only adjunctive in use
   i. Shampoo with miconazole-chlorhexidine or climbazole-chlorhexidine
   ii. Selenium sulfide shampoo
   iii. Rinses with lime sulfur
  b. Systemic—the primary therapy, can be used alone or with topicals
   i. Terbinafine (Lamisil, Pharma-US Novartis, East Hanover, NJ, USA)—25 to 30 mg/kg/d; very effective; some individuals have vomiting and gastrointestinal upset (diarrhea) with this drug and may need lower dose for a while or change to another drug

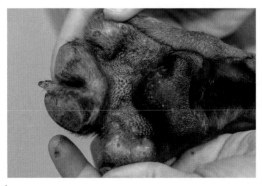

Fig. 17. Demodicosis.

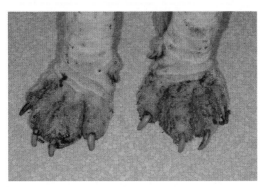

Fig. 18. Demodicosis.

   ii. Itraconazole (Sporanox, Ortho-McNeil-Janssen Pharmaceuticals, NJ, USA)— 10 mg/kg/d; expensive, few side effects

   iii. Fluconazole—10–20 mg/kg/d; may work but efficacy is not known; this drug is primarily for single-cell fungal (yeast) infections, not mycelial-type fungal (dermatophyte) infections. Studies of this drug for its efficacy against the common dermatophytes in the dog have not been done. In vitro studies suggest it may be effective.[14,15]

   iv. Griseofulvin—no longer used for dermatophyte infections in the dog

Deep Pyoderma/Furunculosis

1. Deep pyoderma in the paws is one of the most frustrating conditions in the dog (see **Figs. 5** and **12**). Dogs with this condition have nodules, fistula, and recurrent

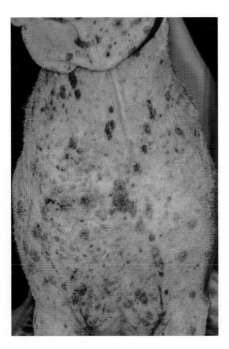

Fig. 19. Demodicosis.

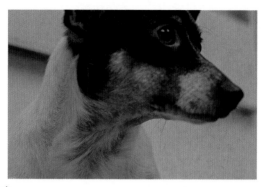

Fig. 20. Demodicosis.

draining tracts (see **Figs. 5** and **12**). Other diseases that have these signs are demodicosis and interdigital follicular cysts. Demodicosis can look exactly like the deep bacterial pododermatitis; in fact, demodicosis is complicated with a deep secondary pyoderma, so the 2 are often present together. Follicular cysts, on the other hand, usually only affect 1 interdigital space; see later discussion on follicular cysts. Any dog with deep draining lesions of the paws should have 2 diagnostic tests performed: skin scraping/hair plucking and bacterial culture and antibiotic sensitivity. The first test should be the skin scraping/hair plucking examination for *Demodex* mites. Because this is a very difficult area in which to obtain skin scrapings, hair plucking for microscopic examination for *Demodex* mites can be done first[3]; then, if this examination is negative for *Demodex* mites, a skin scraping is necessary. Sedation may be necessary in some dogs to perform adequate skin scrapings of the paws. If the tests for *Demodex* mites are negative, then a bacterial culture and antibiotic sensitivity should be done so that the correct antibiotic is used. Usually, dogs with a deep pyoderma have multiple paws and interdigital spaces affected. Dogs with the deep pyoderma often do not have other body sites affected, whereas other infectious conditions, such as demodicosis, involve other body areas. Deep pyoderma can be just pyoderma and will clear with the right antibiotic therapy, like in great Dane and mastiff dogs. Others dogs have deep pyoderma, like bulldogs, pit bulls, Labradors, and golden retrievers, which have the pyoderma secondary to allergic dermatitis or follicular cysts or both. In these

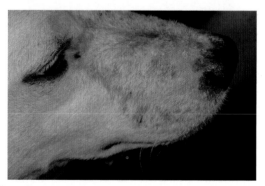

Fig. 21. Dermatophytosis.

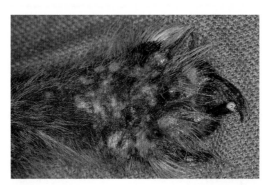

Fig. 22. Dermatophytosis.

dogs, treatment of the pyoderma is only part of the complete management because the other diseases complicate the management of the paws. If the pododermatitis seems to be idiopathic, referral to a dermatologist is recommended, as soon as possible. It is this author's experience that most cases of idiopathic pododermatitis are not idiopathic but the diagnosis is eluding the veterinarian.

2. Key features (See the article by Kinga elsewhere in this issue for further exploration of this topic.)
   a. Nodules
   b. Fistulas
   c. Multiple paws and multiple interdigital spaces
   d. Draining lesions, serosanguineous to purulent discharge (see **Figs. 5**, **15**, **17**, and **18**)
   e. Other body areas usually not affected
3. Treatment
   a. Systemic antibiotic chosen from the culture and sensitivity
   b. Systemic antibiotic for 4 to 8 weeks
   c. Avoid the use of corticosteroids during the antibiotic therapy
   d. Manage the other complicating underlying diseases.

Malassezia

1. This cause of pododermatitis is very common in the dog (see **Figs. 4** and **13**; **Figs. 23** and **24**). The *Malassezia* yeast is a common inhabitant of the canine skin, especially in the paws, ears, axillae, groin, and perineum. This yeast is capable of causing a reaction in the skin resulting in clinical signs of marked erythema, crusting, lichenification, hyperpigmentation, foul odor, and marked pruritus. This is most commonly seen in atopic dogs. *Malassezia* are normal organisms that are capable of becoming pathogens. Therefore, *Malassezia* dermatitis, or *Malassezia* pododermatitis, is never a primary disease; it is secondary to other skin diseases, usually atopy (see **Figs. 4**, **13**, **23**, and **24**). It is currently thought that defects in the normal epidermal barrier are the cause of atopic dermatitis and the associated secondary infections of *Malassezia* and pathogenic staphylococcal bacteria.[16] Atopic dogs develop both immediate type 1, IgE-mediated and cell-mediated hypersensitivity responses to *Malassezia,* which contribute to the severity of atopic dermatitis. Because the clinical lesions are the result of these hypersensitivity reactions, the number of organisms required can be very small. Thus, on cytologic sample from affected paws, large numbers of or only a few *Malassezia* yeasts may be found.

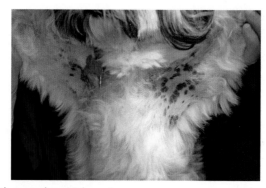

Fig. 23. Atopy with secondary *Malassezia.*

2. Key features
   a. Pruritus—usually marked
   b. Large patches and areas of erythema (see **Fig. 23**)
      i. Ventral cervical
      ii. Skin folds of the legs
      iii. Face
      iv. Paws (see **Figs. 4** and **24**)
   c. Greasy to waxy adherent scale crust
   d. Alopecia (see **Figs. 13** and **23**)
   e. Lichenification (see **Figs. 13** and **23**)
   f. Sometimes hyperpigmentation
   g. Musty odor
   h. Cytology is diagnostic
   i. Staphylococcal colonization is frequently present
3. Treatment
   a. Treat and control the underlying atopic disease
   b. In other diseases with *Malassezia* such as sarcoptic mange or demodicosis, treatment of the underlying disease is sufficient
   c. Oral ketoconazole 5 mg/kg/d
   d. Oral fluconazole 5 mg/kg/d
   e. Topical antifungals

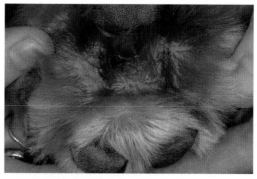

Fig. 24. Atopy with secondary *Malassezia.*

   i. Miconazole—in shampoos, sprays, and rinses
  ii. Climbazole—in shampoos and sprays
 iii. Ketoconazole—in shampoos and lotions

IMMUNOLOGIC DISEASE OF THE CANINE PAW
Pemphigus Foliaceus (Superficial Pemphigus)

1. This disease is characterized by serous crusting primarily of the paw pads, dorsal muzzle, planum nasale, pinnae, and periorbital areas (see **Fig. 7**; **Figs. 25–28**).[17] In records from referring veterinarians, there seems to be a focus on mucous membranes as possible sites for autoimmune disease. Mucous membranes are extremely uncommon sites for the most common autoimmune disease of dogs— superficial pemphigus. Paw pad lesions vary in severity but are almost always present. There are some dogs and cats in which pemphigus foliaceus is restricted to the paw pads.[18] Cytologic examination of either pustule contents or the exudate beneath the crusts will reveal numerous intact neutrophils and acantholytic cells without bacteria (see **Fig. 26**). Pemphigus is a pustular disease; however, the pustules are often microscopic and quickly become thick adherent crusts (see **Figs. 25** and **27**). These crusts are the most common clinical lesions of pemphigus foliaceus. Pemphigus foliaceus is usually a disease of middle-aged dogs; the mean age is 4 years. Superficial bacterial folliculitis is a major differential diagnosis for pemphigus foliaceus. Pustules seen in pemphigus are larger and more irregular than pustules of bacterial Folliculitis, which tend to be more circular (see **Fig. 27**). Histopathologic examination is required to confirm a diagnosis. Some caution is warranted when histopathologic examination alone is used to confirm a diagnosis of pemphigus foliaceus. Clinical lesions, cytologic examination, and history should be used with the histopathologic report to confirm a diagnosis. Usually, the clinician knows or has pemphigus in the list of differentials before taking the biopsy samples; this information must be given to the pathologist who will be doing the microscopic examination of the biopsy specimens for the pathologist to confirm a diagnosis of pemphigus. Simply finding acantholytic cells on the histopathologic examination is not a definitive diagnosis for pemphigus without the clinical and cytologic findings supportive of the disease. Ultimately, it is the clinician who is seeing the dog who has to make the diagnosis. If you are not familiar with this disease, refer the dog to a dermatologist. Conducting Internet research is not the correct way to deal with this disease.

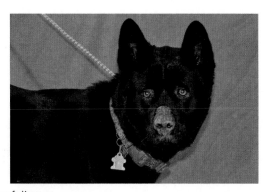

Fig. 25. Pemphigus foliaceus.

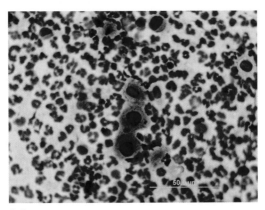

Fig. 26. Pemphigus foliaceus.

2. Key features
   a. Nonpruritic—pruritus can be present but it is not a striking feature of this disease
   b. Papules and pustules look similar to those of pyoderma
      i. Pyoderma does not typically affect the pinna, bridge of the nose, periocular area, or footpads
      ii. Cytologic examination of the pustules shows no bacteria present but does show intact neutrophils and acantholytic cells
   c. Paw pads have peripheral erythema and thick hypertrophic to cracked pads (see **Figs. 7** and **28**)
   d. Histopathologic findings alone are not diagnostic; they represent only a confirmatory test
      i. Biopsy samples must include the surface crusts
      ii. The pathologist should be told why you think this is pemphigus
         1. Physical examination findings
         2. Cytologic examination findings
      iii. Acantholytic cells in the biopsy samples must be combined with the clinical findings to make the diagnosis
   e. This disease is complicated in both making a diagnosis and in treatment, so if possible, these cases should be referred to a dermatologist for diagnosis and management

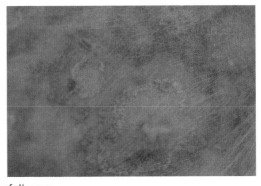

Fig. 27. Pemphigus foliaceus.

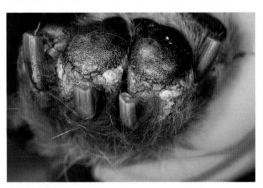

Fig. 28. Pemphigus foliaceus.

3. Treatment
   a. Usually with prednisone and azathioprine combination
   b. Begin both together, right in the beginning
   c. Do not start with low doses of prednisone and then gradually increase the dose.
   d. Begin with high doses of prednisone
   e. Monitor complete blood count and chemistry panel weekly until drug doses are low, then according to your clinical judgment
      i. Prednisone—starting dosage is 4 mg/kg/d and decrease as the disease is controlled via weekly reexaminations
      ii. Prednisone does not need to be given twice daily, unless you are dealing with large numbers of pills. You might divide the prednisone in the first few weeks, but once it is lowered, switching to once daily as soon as possible is better for the animal
      iii. Use gastrointestinal protectants such as sucralfate
      iv. Intestinal aids such as fructooligosaccharides (FOS, Nutri-flora), a prebiotic combined with probiotics, will help to prevent diarrhea
      v. The disease tends to cycle in waves so must give the disease time to cycle before making adjustments to drug doses
      vi. Make adjustments once per week based on clinical response
      vii. If lesions develop as you taper –
         1. Two possibilities—pemphigus or pyoderma
         2. Use cytologic examination to determine which is present (acantholytic cells = pemphigus, bacteria = pyoderma)
         3. Use antibiotic for the pyoderma; do not increase the prednisone
   f. Azathioprine—50 mg/m^2 once daily
      i. This drug dosage is kept the same until the prednisone has been tapered down to its lowest dose or has been discontinued
      ii. Once the dog has been stable for 1 or 2 months on the lowest dose of prednisone, then it is time to decrease the azathioprine to alternate days or less
   g. The long-term treatment goal is to discontinue all drugs
      i. Most dogs will need to stay on drugs for life
      ii. Many can go off the prednisone
      iii. Some can eventually be taken off all drugs[19]
4. This is a complicated disease to treat and referral to a dermatologist is recommended
   a. Especially if you do not get immediate control of the disease

b. Referral if the dog does not tolerate the drugs
c. Some dogs do not tolerate azathioprine
d. Should not treat pemphigus with prednisone alone
e. Most cases readily respond and the prednisone can be decreased in the first week
f. Keeping the prednisone at a high dose for longer than 4 weeks is not normal, and these cases need immediate referral.

Atopy

1. Dogs with atopy often have involvement of the paws; in some cases, only the paws are involved (see **Figs. 4**, **13**, **23**, and **24**; **Figs. 29–31**). Clinical lesions may not be present; the only clinical sign is the history of pruritus of the paws, face, axillae, ears, or flanks and groin or the perineum. In some cases, the clients are not aware of any clinical lesions; however, on close examination of the ventral aspect of the paws, subtle lesions may be seen (see **Fig. 24**). These may consist of erythema or can include variable amounts of alopecia and changes in the skin such as lichen-ification and excoriations (see **Figs. 13**, **29**, and **30**). Others have very obvious alopecia and skin changes both dorsally and ventrally. Atopic dogs most often have other body sites involved; these include the muzzle, perioral and periocular areas, pinna, axillae, flanks and groin, antebrachial folds, and perineum (see **Figs. 29** and **30**).
2. Key features of atopy
   a. Pruritus of the feet, face, ears, axillae, groin, and perineum
   b. Age of onset—6 months to 6 years
   c. Do not forget to obtain skin scrapings—demodicosis in the adult dog commonly tricks the veterinarian
   d. Collect cytologic samples for secondary infections caused by atopic disease
      i. Pyoderma
      ii. *Malassezia*
   e. Other paw diseases will look like atopy; be sure to rule them out
   f. Ear disease (see **Fig. 31**)—the most common reason for ear disease is atopy or food reactions
   g. A diagnosis of atopy is made by clinical signs, history, age of onset, and breed predisposition
   h. Corticosteroid response is nice to know about, but it is not used to make a diagnosis of atopic dermatitis or to determine the difference between atopy and food allergy

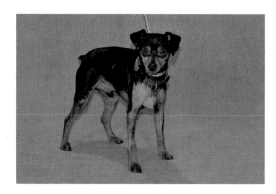

Fig. 29. Atopy.

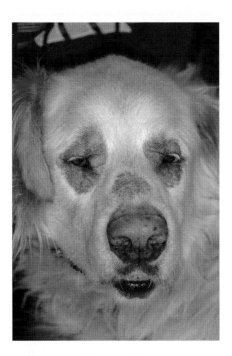

Fig. 30. Atopy.

     i. Some atopics do not respond to corticosteroids
     ii. Many dogs with food allergies respond to corticosteroids
  i. Allergy testing is not needed to make a diagnosis of atopy
     i. Allergy testing, preferably intradermal skin testing, is used to assist in choosing allergens for immunotherapy
     ii. Adverse food reactions are only found by an exclusionary diet; serum tests or skin tests for food allergens are not reliable
3. Treatment of atopy
  a. Food elimination diet trial to eliminate food as the only cause of the clinical signs
  b. Intradermal allergy testing—use in formulation of immunotherapy
  c. Allergen-specific immunotherapy

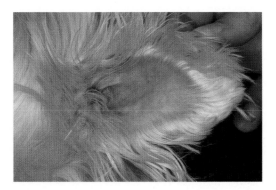

Fig. 31. Atopy.

d. Treat the secondary infections (bacterial, *Malassezia*)
   i. Oral antibiotics and antifungals (See the article by Cain elsewhere in this issue for further exploration of this topic.)
   ii. Topical preventatives—rinses, sprays, shampoos, and wipes (See the article by Jeffers elsewhere in this issue for further exploration of this topic.)
e. Manage the epidermal barrier abnormalities
   i. Replacement of the lack of normal ceramides, free fatty acids, and cholesterol sulfate
   ii. Topical spot-on products
   iii. Topical cream rinses and sprays
   iv. Topical shampoos
f. Oral antihistamines
g. Oral corticosteroids
h. Oral cyclosporine (See the article by Palmeiro elsewhere in this issue for further exploration of this topic.)
i. Atopy-like pemphigus is a complicated condition, and referral to a dermatologist is recommended.

Vasculitis

1. In this section on vasculitis, only the types of vasculitis involving the paw pads is discussed (see **Fig. 14**; **Figs. 32–35**). There are many types of vasculitis and the reader is advised to see the article by Innera elsewhere in this issue for a more in-depth discussion of vasculitis. Some cases of vasculitis involve the paw pads (see **Figs. 14** and **34**). The cause is multifactorial, viral infection, and drug or vaccine reactions are among the known causes, but most often the cause is not known. Clinical signs are swelling, erythema, and violaceous to erythematous plaques that may develop ulceration and necrosis. Lesions usually are on the tips of the tail, paw pads, and pinna, including the margins and multiple loci on the concave pinnae (see **Figs. 14**, **32**, **34**, and **35**). In some cases, there is a focal site of alopecia on the trunk (see **Fig. 33**) with surface crusting, ulceration, and subcutaneous swelling. These alopecic sites are locations of a previous vaccination. Vaccines implicated most frequently have been the rabies vaccine; however, the combination distemper/hepatitis/leptospirosis/parainfluenza/parvovirus vaccine also can cause these reactions. The nail beds can also be affected with shedding of multiple nails as the clinical sign. Pain is variable, and there are systemic signs of fever; malaise and anorexia are also reported. Skin biopsy is required to establish a diagnosis.

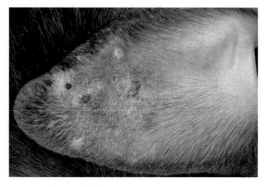

Fig. 32. Vasculitis.

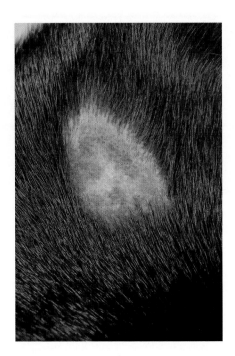

Fig. 33. Vasculitis.

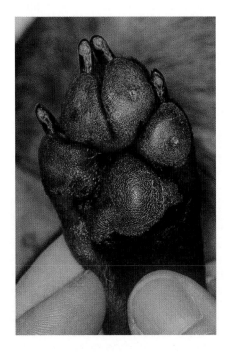

Fig. 34. Vasculitis.

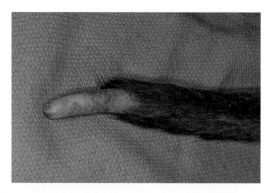

Fig. 35. Vasculitis.

For a more complete discussion of vasculitis, see the article by Innera elsewhere in this issue.

2. Key features
   a. Pinal lesions are the most obvious
   b. The paw pad lesions often very subtle—usually central portions of the paw pads (see **Fig. 34**)
   c. Tail tip—alopecia and ulceration can go unnoticed, especially in longer-haired dogs
   d. Look for a vaccine reaction site—alopecia with subcutaneous swelling, variable surface crusting, hyperpigmentation

3. Treatment of vasculitis
   a. Pentoxifylline 25 to 30 mg/kg twice to 3 times daily
   b. Corticosteroids—topical and systemic
   c. Tacrolimus (Protopic, Astellas Pharma, Inc, Deerfield, IL, USA)—topical
   d. Omega-3 fatty acids—30 mg/kg of the omega-3 fatty acids (DHA [docosahexaenoic acid] and EPA [eicosapentaenoic acid])
   e. If vaccine induced—subsequent vaccination could cause a more severe recrudescence of the condition
   f. Response to treatment is slow and can take months to resolve.

METABOLIC DISEASES OF THE CANINE PAW
Superficial Necrolytic Dermatitis (Hepatocutaneous Syndrome, Metabolic Epidermal Necrosis, Necrolytic Migratory Erythema)

1. This syndrome develops in dogs with chronic liver failure or with glucagon-secreting pancreatic tumors (see **Figs. 6** and **9**; **Fig. 36**).[20–22] Often there is very little to no metabolic changes on chemistry screen until very late in the stages of liver disease. The skin lesions are frequently the first sign that there is something seriously wrong internally. The skin signs are classic and frequently occur before liver changes are evident on chemistry screens. Metabolic alterations (amino acid deficiency) result in crusting and ulcerated lesions in the groin, perioral area, and paw pads (see **Figs. 6, 9**, and **36**). The paw pads are usually the most dramatic lesions. The paws are often sore, cracked, and fissured. The clinical lesions can be similar to those of pemphigus foliaceus. Skin biopsy and ultrasound of the liver have pathognomonic findings (references). The liver disease consists of a complete parenchymal collapse resulting in a severe amino acid deficiency. Prognosis is poor; however, some dogs will respond to intravenous amino acid therapy as needed, usually weekly to monthly. Amino acid therapy requires a central line catheter with slow intravenous infusion.

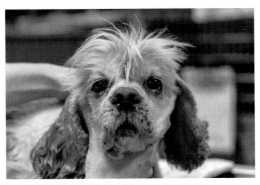

Fig. 36. Superficial necrolytic dermatitis.

2. Key features
   a. Old dog—usually older 10 years
   b. Striking footpad hyperkeratosis—so severe that the foot pads are very hard
   c. Pads often have cracks and fissures causing pain and signs of lameness (see **Figs. 6** and **9**)
   d. Some also have perioral and ventral abdominal crusted, hyperkeratotic lesions (see **Fig. 36**)
   e. Often is a secondary *Malassezia* infection in the paws
   f. Ultrasound of the liver in most cases has a "Swiss cheese" pattern
   g. Serum hypoaminoacidemia[23]
   h. Some have elevated glucose—rare sign
   i. Appetite is usually decreased
3. Treatment
   a. Intravenous amino acid therapy
   b. If dog has a glucagonoma, octeride[24–26] is effective
   c. Antifungal for the *Malassezia*—fluconazole
   d. Dietary management
      i. Oral amino acid supplements
      ii. Diets high in free amino acids such as Royal Canin's (Anergen, Royal Canin USA, St. Charles, MO, USA)
      iii. Egg yolks
      iv. Zinc supplement
   e. Glucocorticoids are contraindicated and can be very deleterious and lethal to the dog
   f. These dogs should be referred to an internal medicine specialist.

NEOPLASTIC DISEASES OF THE CANINE PAW
Nail Bed Squamous Cell Carcinoma

1. Nail bed squamous cell carcinoma is usually solitary but may affect multiple digits (**Figs. 37–39**). The author has seen standard poodles with nail bed squamous cell carcinomas in one digit on each of the front paws at the same time (synchronal). It is reported in the literature that multiple digits can be affected synchronously or meta-chronously.[27] Presenting signs include lameness, digital swelling, and deformity or loss of the nail (see **Figs. 37** and **38**). Radiographs may show evidence of phalangeal lysis. Early lesions are small and will be confined to the nail pulp and distal 3rd phalanx. Age of affected animals is 7 yrs. or older; however some are as young as

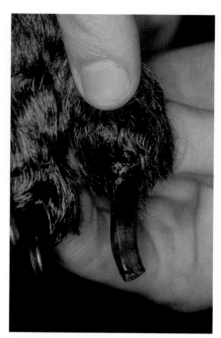

Fig. 37. Nail bed squamous cell carcinoma.

4 yrs. of age. Large breeds are predisposed (Labradors, standard poodles, rottweilers, giant schnauzers, Gordon setters, and Kerry blue terriers). In cases with multiple digital squamous cell carcinomas, a differential of metastatic carcinoma must be considered.

2. Key features
   a. Lameness
   b. Digital swelling of P3
   c. May have deformity of the nail
   d. May have loss of nail
   e. Bone lysis on radiographs
   f. Ulcerative tissue protruding under the nail plate (see **Fig. 39**)

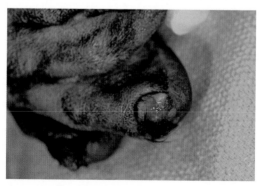

Fig. 38. Nail bed squamous cell carcinoma.

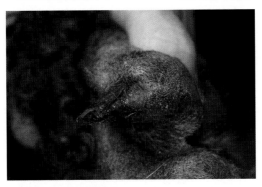

Fig. 39. Nail bed squamous cell carcinoma.

3. Treatment
   a. Amputation of P3
   b. Usually just P3
   c. Amputation is curative

Epitheliotropic Lymphoma

1. These patients are remarkably healthy except for the skin (see **Figs. 8** and **11**; **Figs. 40–43**). Usually, the condition is easily confused with conditions such as pyoderma, allergy, hypothyroidism, or autoimmune disease (see **Figs. 8** and **11**). The lesions consist of scale, erythema, and some slightly raised erythematous plaques (see **Fig. 40**). A diffuse depigmentation of the foot pads, lips, eye lids, and nasal planum caused by the infiltration of lymphocytes into the skin is a classic sign (see **Figs. 8, 11,**

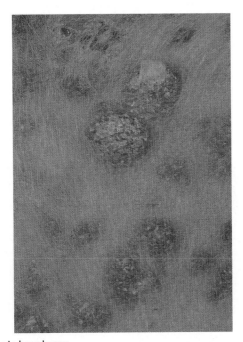

Fig. 40. Epitheliotropic lymphoma.

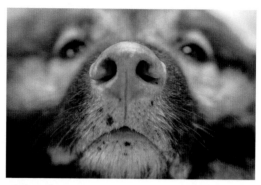

Fig. 41. Epitheliotropic lymphoma.

and **41–43**). Onset of this disease is subtle and slow, often beginning with just erythema, then gradually progressing to scale, then macular plaques. Early recognition is possible only to the trained eye. The inexperienced clinician will miss the early hallmark signs for this disease and treat it as a different disease before realizing it is not what they were originally led to believe it was. One of the synonyms for this disease in humans is mycosis fungoides, which reflects the previous misdiagnoses of this disease in humans. This disease can be a great imitator of other skin diseases.

2. Key features
   a. Age—older animals; 8 years and older
   b. Close look at the lesions reveals they are raised, "tumor"-like and are not typical pyoderma lesions (see **Fig. 40**)
   c. Often, there are small erythematous plaques present
   d. Many have a lot of scaling in the skin and in the hair coat
   e. Depigmentation is frequent (see **Figs. 41–43**)
      i. Nasal planum
      ii. Lips (see **Fig. 41**)
      iii. Eyelids
      iv. Foot pads (see **Figs. 42** and **43**)
   f. It may respond to prednisone, so for veterinarians who have the bad habit of using prednisone with antibiotics when treating skin infections, this will add one more level to the confusion if lymphoma is present and it is not a pyoderma

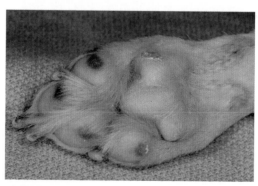

Fig. 42. Epitheliotropic lymphoma.

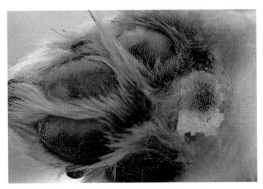

Fig. 43. Epitheliotropic lymphoma.

3. Treatment
   a. Prognosis is guarded to poor
   b. Some will respond to prednisone for awhile
   c. Other drugs that have suppressive effects on T cells (cyclosporine, leflunomide) might alleviate the lesions temporarily
   d. CCNU (Lomustine, Bristol-Meyers-Squibb Co, Princeton, NJ, USA) is an alkylating agent that may be considered
   e. No treatment is curative, only palliative, until the disease reaches the nonresponsive stage
   f. Should refer these to an oncologist

INHERITED/GENETIC DISEASES OF THE CANINE PAW
Familial Paw Pad Hyperkeratosis

1. This is a rare defect of keratinization, restricted to the paw pads of all 4 paws (see **Fig. 10**; **Fig. 44**). It may be a subgroup of ichthyosis (see the article by Mauldin elsewhere in this issue for a more in-depth discussion), which is a group of diseases that are caused by abnormalities in the development of various keratins in the epidermis. The paw pads of these dogs form thick, severe keratin proliferation. The pads produce thick keratin protrusions of horns, fronds, and thick hard pads (see **Figs. 10** and **44**). The pads form cracks and fissures, causing pain and signs of lameness. In some dogs, the claws also grow in abnormal curved patterns. The pads show these changes at a very young age (4–6 months),[28,29] and this defect

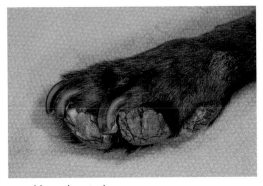

Fig. 44. Familial paw pad hyperkeratosis.

continues throughout life. If these lesions develop later in life, other diseases are more likely, such as pemphigus and superficial necrolytic dermatitis.

2. Key features
   a. Develop at 4 to 6 months of age
   b. No other body parts affected
   c. No systemic signs
   d. Affected breeds[30]
      i. Labrador retriever
      ii. Golden retriever
      iii. Dogue de Bordeaux
      iv. Irish terrier[28]
      v. Kerry blue terrier
   e. Biopsy confirms the diagnosis
3. Treatment
   a. Daily foot soaks in 50% propylene glycol[30] – help, but client compliance is poor.
   b. In the author's experience
      i. Daily oral acitretin (Soriatane, Stiefel, USA Research Triangle Park, NC, USA) 1 mg/kg/d helps but is not 100% effective.[31]
      ii. Dremel (Dremel USA, Racine, WI, USA) tool grinding off the keratin with the dog under sedation as needed (usually every 3–5 months)
   c. This is a lifelong disease and needs lifelong management.

FOREIGN BODY CONDITIONS THAT AFFECT THE CANINE PAW
Interdigital Follicular Cysts

1. A subtype of canine recurrent interdigital dermatitis recently described by the author (2008)[1] occurs when follicular cysts develop on the ventral (palmar or plantar) surface of the canine paw (**Figs. 45–48**). In some dogs, these cysts rupture and initiate a foreign body response, which eventuates from the ventral origin onto the dorsal interdigital space (see **Figs. 47** and **48**). The clinical lesions consist of recurrent nodules that are erythematous, and ulcerate and drain a purulent to serosanguineous exudate. The dog licks at the draining lesions, which rupture repeatedly, causing a recurrent interdigital disease. Many of the dogs that develop this condition have no other clinical disease and only the recurrent interdigital draining tracts. Usually, the tracts develop in the same interdigital spaces: front paws in the lateral interdigital space. The ventral lesions are usually not noticed because the dorsal disease is the most problematic. If one were to look at the ventral surface of the paws below the draining lesion, there is an area of alopecia between the digital and metacarpal

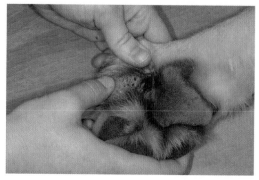

Fig. 45. Interdigital follicular cysts.

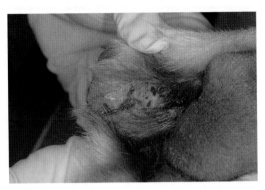

Fig. 46. Interdigital follicular cysts.

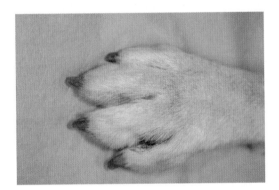

Fig. 47. Interdigital follicular cysts.

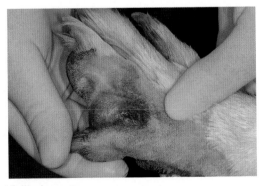

Fig. 48. Interdigital follicular cysts.

pads with varying amounts of hyperplastic to callous-like changes to the skin (see **Fig. 45**). There are usually comedones from which a semisolid, caseous to granular material can be expressed; the color may be white or various shades of light to dark gray (see **Fig. 46**). The interdigital space most often affected is the lateral space between digits IV and V, and the front feet are most commonly affected (see **Fig. 47**).

2. Key features
   a. Recurrent interdigital draining tracts; recur in the same interdigital space (see **Fig. 48**)
   b. Usually the front paws with the lateral interdigital spaces affected
   c. There is a failure to respond to antibiotic; new draining lesions develop while on antibiotics
   d. Usually, in the history it is evident that this problem started at a young age (1–3 years)
   e. Some dogs have other skin disease such as atopy, but most of these only have the interdigital draining lesions
3. Treatment
   a. Bacterial culture for antibiotic sensitivity
   b. Treatment with the right antibiotic for 4 to 8 weeks
   c. CO_2 laser ablation of the ventral cysts that remain after antibiotic treatment.

REFERENCES

1. Duclos DD, Jeffers JG, Shanley KJ. Prognosis for treatment of adult-onset demodicosis in dogs: 34 cases (1979-1990). J Am Vet Med Assoc 1994;204(4):616–9.
2. Gortel K. Update on canine demodicosis. Vet Clin North Am Small Anim Pract 2006;36(1):229–41, ix.
3. Saridomichelakis MN, Koutinas AF, Farmaki R, et al. Relative sensitivity of hair pluckings and exudate microscopy for the diagnosis of canine demodicosis. Vet Dermatol 2007;18(2):138–41.
4. Mueller RS. Treatment protocols for demodicosis: an evidence-based review. Vet Dermatol 2004;15(2):75–89.
5. Paradis M. New approaches to the treatment of canine demodicosis. Vet Clin North Am Small Anim Pract 1999;29(6):1425–36.
6. Barbet JL, Snook T, Gay JM, et al. ABCB1-1 Delta (MDR1-1 Delta) genotype is associated with adverse reactions in dogs treated with milbemycin oxime for generalized demodicosis. Vet Dermatol 2009;20(2):111–4.
7. Heine J, Krieger K, Dumont P, et al. Evaluation of the efficacy and safety of imidacloprid 10% plus moxidectin 2.5% spot-on in the treatment of generalized demodicosis in dogs: results of a European field study. Parasitol Res 2005; 97(Suppl 1):S89–96.
8. Mueller RS, Meyer D, Bensignor E, et al. Treatment of canine generalized demodicosis with a 'spot-on' formulation containing 10% moxidectin and 2.5% imidacloprid (Advocate, Bayer Healthcare). Vet Dermatol 2009;20(5–6):441–6.
9. Paterson TE, Halliwell RE, Fields PJ, et al. Treatment of canine-generalized demodicosis: a blind, randomized clinical trial comparing the efficacy of Advocate (Bayer Animal Health) with ivermectin. Vet Dermatol 2009;20(5–6):447–55.
10. Murayama N, Shibata K, Nagata M. Efficacy of weekly oral doramectin treatment in canine demodicosis. Vet Rec 2010;167(2):63–4.
11. Duclos D. Dermatophytosis. In: Jackson H, Marsella R, editors. BSAVA manual of canine and feline dermatology. 3rd edition. Gloucester (England): British Small Animal Veterinary Association; 2012. p. 188–97.

12. Fairley RA. The histological lesions of Trichophyton mentagrophytes var erinacei infection in dogs. Vet Dermatol 2001;12(2):119–22.

13. Nagino K, Shimohira H, Ogawa M, et al. Comparison of the therapeutic efficacy of oral doses of fluconazole and itraconazole in a guinea pig model of dermatophytosis. J Infect Chemother 2000;6(1):41–4.

14. Odds FC, Cheesman SL, Abbott AB. Antifungal effects of fluconazole (UK 49858), a new triazole antifungal, in vitro. J Antimicrob Chemother 1986;18(4):473–8.

15. Bieber T. Atopic dermatitis. Ann Dermatol 2010;22(2):125–37.

16. Olivry T. A review of autoimmune skin diseases in domestic animals: I, superficial pemphigus. Vet Dermatol 2006;17(5):291–305.

17. Ihrke PJ, Stannard AA, Ardans AA, et al. Pemphigus foliaceus of the footpads in three dogs. J Am Vet Med Assoc 1985;186(1):67–9.

18. Olivry T, Bergvall KE, Atlee BA. Prolonged remission after immunosuppressive therapy in six dogs with pemphigus foliaceus. Vet Dermatol 2004;15(4):245–52.

19. Bond R, McNeil PE, Evans H, et al. Metabolic epidermal necrosis in two dogs with different underlying diseases. Vet Rec 1995;136(18):466–71.

20. Brenseke BM, Belz KM, Saunders GK. Pathology in practice. Superficial necrolytic dermatitis and nodular hepatopathy (lesions consistent with hepatocutaneous syndrome). J Am Vet Med Assoc 2011;238(4):445–7.

21. Gross TL, Song MD, Havel PJ, et al. Superficial necrolytic dermatitis (necrolytic migratory erythema) in dogs. Vet Pathol 1993;30(1):75–81.

22. Outerbridge CA, Marks SL, Rogers QR. Plasma amino acid concentrations in 36 dogs with histologically confirmed superficial necrolytic dermatitis. Vet Dermatol 2002;13(4):177–86.

23. Mizuno T, Hiraoka H, Yoshioka C, et al. Superficial necrolytic dermatitis associated with extrapancreatic glucagonoma in a dog. Vet Dermatol 2009;20(1):72–9.

24. Oberkirchner U, Linder KE, Zadrozny L, et al. Successful treatment of canine necrolytic migratory erythema (superficial necrolytic dermatitis) due to metastatic glucagonoma with octreotide. Vet Dermatol 2010;21(5):510–6.

25. Papadogiannakis E, Frangia K, Matralis D. Superficial necrolytic dermatitis in a dog associated with hyperplasia of pancreatic neuroendocrine cells. J Small Anim Pract 2009;50(6):318.

26. Madewell BR, Pool RR, Theilen GH, et al. Multiple subungual squamous cell carcinomas in five dogs. J Am Vet Med Assoc 1982;180(7):731–4.

27. Binder H, Arnold S, Schelling C, et al. Palmoplantar hyperkeratosis in Irish terriers: evidence of autosomal recessive inheritance. J Small Anim Pract 2000; 41(2):52–5.

28. Schleifer SG, Versteeg SA, van OB, et al. Familial footpad hyperkeratosis and inheritance of keratin 2, keratin 9, and desmoglein 1 in two pedigrees of Irish terriers. Am J Vet Res 2003;64(6):715–20.

29. Scott DW, Miller WH, Griffin CE. Congenital and hereditary defects. In: Scott DW, Miller WH, Griffin CE, editors. Muller & Kirk's small animal dermatology. 6th edition. Philadelphia: WB Saunders; 2001. p. 913–1003.

30. Virtanen M, Gedde-Dahl T Jr, Mork NJ, et al. Phenotypic/genotypic correlations in patients with epidermolytic hyperkeratosis and the effects of retinoid therapy on keratin expression. Acta Derm Venereol 2001;81(3):163–70.

31. Duclos DD, Hargis AM, Hanley PW. Pathogenesis of canine interdigital palmar and plantar comedones and follicular cysts, and their response to laser surgery. Vet Dermatol 2008;19(3):134–41.

Canine Ichthyosis and Related Disorders of Cornification

Elizabeth A. Mauldin, DVM

KEYWORDS

- Canine • Cornification • Ichthyosis • Seborrhea • Scaling

KEY POINTS

- The stratum corneum, which is the outermost layer of the epidermis, serves as a primary barrier between the body and the environment. This layer functions to keep the body hydrated (ie, to retain water) and excludes pathogens and toxins.
- Disorders of cornification (DOC) arise when there is an inability to form a normal stratum corneum. Most DOC are secondary to alternations induced by allergic skin diseases, ectoparasitism, and endocrine/metabolic diseases. Primary DOC arise from spontaneous or inherited mutations in genes that regulate structural proteins, lipid metabolism, and transport.
- Few primary cornification disorders have been fully characterized in the dog. Mild forms of ichthyosis (fish scale disease) are common in the golden retriever and American bulldog.
- The stepwise diagnostic approach is fundamental to establishing a correct diagnosis, because there is no cure for ichthyosis. Treatment involves a lifetime regimen of topical therapy as well as medical care to address and prevent secondary bacterial and yeast infections.

INTRODUCTION

The term cornification (keratinization) is the process by which the epidermal cells undergo terminal differentiation from basal keratinocytes to the highly specialized corneocyte. The large surface area of the skin puts it in constant contact with environmental pollutants, irritants, and allergens; the outermost layer of the epidermis (the stratum corneum) serves as the first line of defense between these environmental hazards and the body.[1] Easily overlooked in histologic preparations, the normal corneal layer consists of more than 20 overlapping layers of bland, lightly staining, polyhedral, anucleate cells, most of which are lost during biopsy sampling, cutting, and processing.

Stratum Corneum Function

The stratum corneum is the key epidermal layer that restricts water movement into and out of the skin. In normal humans, approximately 0.5 L of water vapor is expelled

Department of Pathobiology, School of Veterinary Medicine, University of Pennsylvania, 3900 Delancey Street, Philadelphia, PA 19104-6051, USA
E-mail address: emauldin@vet.upenn.edu

Vet Clin Small Anim 43 (2013) 89–97
http://dx.doi.org/10.1016/j.cvsm.2012.09.005   vetsmall.theclinics.com
0195-5616/13/$ – see front matter © 2013 Elsevier Inc. All rights reserved.

through the stratum corneum per day. Even minor injuries to the corneal layer from tape stripping or applications of solvents result in increased transepidermal water loss.[2,3] Like humans, dogs with atopic skin disease have recently been shown to have an increased water loss through the corneal layer.[4]

Much of the barrier function is attributed to the physical property of continuous desquamation, which allows for the expulsion of pathogens. Furthermore, the stratum corneum is able to absorb ultraviolet light to protect the underlying tissue from free radical oxidation. This layer also contains natural antimicrobial peptides such as defensins and cathelicidins such that abnormalities in the corneal layer may predispose the patient (human or animal) to bacterial and yeast infections.[1]

DIAGNOSTIC APPROACH

Disorders of cornification (DOC) are divided into those with primary and secondary causes. In primary cornification disorders, the excessive scale is caused by a direct defect in 1 or more steps involved in the formation of the stratum corneum. Known defects are related to mutations in genes that encode the structural proteins that form the corneocyte (eg, transglutaminases), or enzymes involved in lipid formation or lipid transport.[1] Secondary disorders are those in which excessive scaling develops as a result of another condition (eg, flea bite hypersensitivity, sarcoptic mange, hypothyroidism, epitheliotropic lymphoma). More than 80% of scaling disorders arise from secondary causes.[3] Some investigators include abnormalities in sebaceous gland function (eg, sebaceous adenitis, sebaceous gland dysplasia) as primary cornification disorders as well. However, these disorders are not discussed in this article.

Primary DOC are generally diagnosed by ruling out all secondary causes. The signalment, age of onset, and presence or absence of pruritus aid in the formulation of a differential diagnosis and the diagnostic approach. In a standard veterinary practice, a minimum dermatologic database (eg, skin scrapings, acetate tape preparations, impression smears, trichograms, dermatophyte culture) along with routine blood work can effectively rule out most secondary disorders. However, skin biopsies are often needed to establish a definitive diagnosis. Primary cornification disorders are generally nonpruritic (when uncomplicated by secondary infections) and arise in young animals, but late-onset cases do occasionally occur. Ichthyosiform disorders have strong breed predilections; however, spontaneous mutations can arise in any breed or mixed-breed animals.

PATHOPHYSIOLOGY

The formation of the stratum corneum is an orchestrated and complex series of steps that occur concomitantly with a modified form of apoptosis. An alteration in any step can lead to disruption of barrier function and derangements in permeability. The scaling phenotype is an adaptive response to repair the injured stratum corneum barrier. When the barrier fails, lipid synthesis is upregulated and the epidermis becomes hyperplastic to deliver more lipid to the stratum corneum. Inflammation may also ensue.[1]

Several key steps must occur for normal cornification to proceed: (1) bundling of the keratin to establish the corneocyte core, (2) replacement of the cell membrane with a thick cornified envelope, (3) formation of lipid lamellar bilayers, and (4) desquamation. As the nucleus and intracellular organelles undergo proteolysis, profilaggrin (found in keratohyalin granules) in the granular cell layer is dephosphorylated into filaggrin. Filaggrin serves to bundle the loose keratin filaments in the cytosol to form the core of the corneocyte. Transglutaminases mediate calcium-dependent cross-linking of small peptides to replace the plasma membrane of the keratinocyte with a tough protein layer (corneocyte envelope). Lamellar bodies, small vesicular organelles containing lipid, are formed in the stratum spinosum. At the junction of the stratum granulosum and stratum corneum, the lipid is secreted into the intercellular space and undergoes processing into lamellar bilayers. Enzymes within the lamellar bodies modify polar lipids into nonpolar (hydrophobic) lipids. The resultant lipid in the stratum corneum is an equimolar mixture of cholesterol, long-chain fatty acids, and ceramides. The intercorneocyte adhesions (corneodesmosomes) are then cleaved by proteases to allow for desquamation and release of the keratin squames into the environment.[1]

The final product is a tough hydrophobic, but biochemically active, layer in a mortar-and-bricks arrangement, with the bricks being the corneocytes, which are sandwiched between layers of lipid (the mortar).[1]

ICHTHYOSIS: GENERAL

In veterinary medicine, the term ichthyosis has been limited to rare congenital or hereditary disorders thought to be caused by primary defects in the formation of the stratum corneum.[5,6] In human medicine, the term acquired ichthyosis is also used to denote similar clinical changes related to underlying diseases, but this confusing terminology has not been adopted by veterinary dermatologists. The diagnosis of ichthyosiform disorders is made via a detailed dermatologic examination (minimum dermatology database), in conjunction with signalment, history, and skin biopsy analysis. Genetic testing, when available, along with electron microscopy testing may be needed to further characterize the defect, but is not needed to establish a general diagnosis. Ichthyosis is currently subdivided into epidermolytic and nonepidermolytic forms based on light microscopy.[6]

EPIDERMOLYTIC ICHTHYOSIS

The word epidermolytic is based on the light microscopic findings of vacuoles and lysis of keratinocytes within the spinous and granular cell layers, which occur along with hypergranulosis and hyperkeratosis. Unlike nonepidermolytic ichthyosis (NI; discussed later), this finding uniquely corresponds with a defect in keratin formation (ie, formation of the corneocyte core). Epidermolytic ichthyosis (EI) in the Norfolk terrier is autosomal recessive and caused by a mutation in epidermal keratin (*KRT10*).[7] EI has been sporadically described in other dogs (Rhodesian ridgeback, Labrador cross).[6] The affected dogs have multifocal regions of pigmented scale with alopecia and roughening of the skin. EI (aka epidermolytic hyperkeratosis) can be diagnosed on light microscopy by an experienced dermatopathologist.

NONEPIDERMOLYTIC ICHTHYOSIS

To date, the nonepidermolytic forms of ichthyosis that have been characterized in dogs have been documented or presumed to be autosomal recessive traits. In humans, there are X-linked and dominant forms of NI; however, this has yet to be documented in the dog. The veterinary characterization of NI is still in its infancy. In humans, autosomal recessive congenital ichthyosis (ARCI) is the official classification for a heterogeneous group of disorders with overlapping phenotypes (eg, lamellar ichthyosis, congenital ichthyosiform erythroderma).[1] A variety of mutations affecting lipids and structural proteins cause similar clinical phenotypes as well as light microscopic changes. The current nomenclature used by pathologists in veterinary medicine labels these ARCI disorders by the breed predilection; this practice may change in the future.[6]

GOLDEN RETRIEVER ICHTHYOSIS

Although statistics are not known on the prevalence of this disorder, it seems to be common (relative to other forms of ichthyosis) and is unique in its clinical presentation. It is generally considered a mild form of scaling, but some owners may argue otherwise. Affected dogs develop large, soft, white-to-gray adherent scale that is prominent on the trunk and may be associated with ventral hyperpigmentation (**Fig. 1**). On histology, affected dogs have lesions typical of NI: diffuse lamellar orthokeratotic hyperkeratosis in the absence of epidermal hyperplasia and dermal inflammation.[8,9] Golden retrievers are typically diagnosed at less than 1 year of age; however, adult-onset cases are common.[8] Some dogs develop secondary bacterial folliculitis, which may lead to pruritus and clinical confusion with allergic skin disease. The disease may wax and wane with periodic bouts of exacerbation and remission.

A long-awaited publication recently documented a mutation in the *PNPLA1* gene as the cause of golden retriever ichthyosis.[10] The gene is thought to play a role in lipid organization and metabolism within the outer epidermis. A genetic test is currently offered by a European company (Antagen) and may be useful to assess for a carrier state in breeding dogs. In nonbreeding pets suspected of having the disease, a skin biopsy procedure with examination by an experienced dermatopathologist is sufficient for diagnosis.

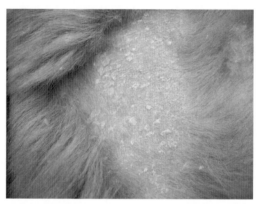

Fig. 1. Generalized large white scale in a golden retriever with nonepidermolytic ichthyosis.

AMERICAN BULLDOG ICHTHYOSIS

The author, in conjunction with Dr Margret Casal in the Medical Genetics section at the University of Pennsylvania School of Veterinary Medicine, has characterized a similar but more severe ichthyosiform disorder of American bulldogs.[11] Unlike the golden retriever, the bulldogs consistently develop clinical signs before weaning. Young puppies have a scruffy/disheveled hair coat compared with the smooth coat of normal littermates. The glabrous skin is erythematous with tightly adherent light brown scale, which gives the abdominal skin a wrinkled appearance. In the adult dog, the abdomen, axilla, and inguinal regions have a reddish brown discoloration (**Fig. 2**). Large white to light tan scales are distributed throughout the hair coat. *Malassezia* yeast overgrowth may be severe. The development of otitis externa, intertrigo, and pododermatitis corresponds with yeast proliferation and the onset of pruritus. The clinical presentation may be misinterpreted as nonseasonal atopic skin disease. Occasional adult dogs

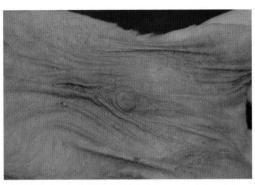

Fig. 2. Brown-red discoloration of the abdominal skin in 2-week-old American bulldog with ichthyosis.

may have footpad hyperkeratosis. Unlike golden retrievers, the skin lesions in bulldogs do not wax or wane and are generally more severe (manuscript in preparation). The disorder has been linked to *NIPAL-4 and leads* to decreased expression of the protein-icthyin. Similar to the *PNPLA-2* mutation in golden retrievers with NI ichthyosis, this gene has a role in lipid metabolism in the epidermis caused by a mutation.[1,10–12] The University of Pennsylvania School of Veterinary medicine, Section of Medical Genetics offers a genetic test to assess for carrier dogs.

JACK RUSSELL TERRIER ICHTHYOSIS

NI in Jack Russell terriers (JRT) is caused by a loss-of-function mutation in transglutaminase 1 (*TGM1*).[13] TGM1 mediates calcium-dependent cross-linking of peptides (eg, involucrin, loricrin) to form the cornified envelope; the strong exterior of the corneocyte. The phenotype in the JRT is characterized by large, thick, adherent, parchment paper–like scales. This phenotype is generally more severe than ichthyosis in American bulldogs and golden retrievers. The dogs develop severe *Malassezia* infections with corresponding inflammation and pruritus.

ICHTHYOSES NOT CHARACTERIZED

Several other breeds have been diagnosed on light microscopy and clinical examination (soft-coated Wheaten terriers and West Highland white terriers) with NI, but further molecular characterizations have not been documented.[6] Many cases are likely confirmed on skin biopsy and never receive further work-up. The author has confirmed cases in English springer spaniels, Labrador retrievers, and West Highland white terriers.

A congenital and familial form of keratoconjunctivitis sicca with scaling has been documented in Cavalier King Charles spaniel dogs. The dogs have a syndrome that includes the following features: keratoconjunctivitis noted from the beginning of eyelid opening, a roughened/curly hair coat, scaling with abdominal hyperpigmentation, footpad hyperkeratosis, and nail dystrophy. A recessive model of inheritance has been proposed; thus far, a candidate gene has not been identified.[14]

DIFFERENTIAL DIAGNOSIS FOR ICHTHYOSIFORM DISORDERS

The severe scaling of ichthyosiform disorders can be confused with several other diseases including sebaceous adenitis, atopy, parasitic disorders (cheyletiellosis, demodicosis, leishmaniasis), as well as hypothyroidism, epitheliotropic cutaneous lymphoma, or metabolic disease (eg, zinc-responsive dermatosis). A skin biopsy is helpful to establish the clinical diagnosis and ensure that other disorders (particularly sebaceous adenitis or sebaceous dysplasia) are not present.

TREATMENT OF PRIMARY DOC

In both human and veterinary medicine, research into the pathogenesis and molecular characterization of primary DOC has outpaced any significant therapeutic achievements. The goal of therapy must be to restore the stratum corneum barrier function to decrease the adaptive responses (hyperplasia, hyperkeratosis, inflammation). The best way to ensure effective therapy is to make sure the diagnosis is accurate, because there is no cure for ichthyosiform disorders. However, many of the diseases that can mimic them may be treated successfully. Corticosteroids may temporarily decrease the scale formation associated with ichthyosiform disorders, but steroids further impede the skin barrier function.

To date, topical therapy remains the treatment of choice for all forms of ichthyosis. The topical therapy may include keratolytic agents to remove excessive scale, moisturizers/emollients to restore the skin barrier (prevent water loss), and topical antimicrobials (eg, chlorhexidine and miconazole) for secondary bacterial or yeast infections. However, care should be exercised to avoid further damage to the skin barrier with harsh chemicals. The therapy must be tailored to the individual patient and requires good owner compliance. At first, baths may be required every other day to twice weekly. Shampoos containing 2% sulfur and salicylic acid help soften the scale and break apart the keratin squames. The shampoo should always be followed by a good moisturizer. Humectants (eg, Humilac, Virbac) may be helpful between baths. Avoid the use of harsh topical products that may further harm the skin barrier (eg, tar-based shampoos) and cause erythema or pruritus. Topical oil-based spot-ons such as Duoxo seborrhea spot-on (Sogeval), which contains 1% phytosphingosine (a major component of ceramides) and Allerderm spot-on (Virbac), which contains a combination of ceramides and fatty acids, are helpful between baths and may prolong the bath interval. Oral ω-3 and ω-6 fatty acids may also be beneficial, but the efficacy is difficult to quantify. The topical regimen is tailored to the degree of scale and then tapered based on the clinical response. Periodic rechecks are warranted to assess scale production, evidence of irritation or skin sensitivity, and secondary infection. American bulldogs and JRT may require oral antifungal therapy (eg, ketoconazole at 5–8 mg/kg once daily for 21 days) for secondary *Malassezia* infections. As research expands understanding of these disorders, there is hope for corrective therapy that may be targeted directly at the specific barrier defect.

UNCONFIRMED PRIMARY DOC
Vitamin A–Responsive Dermatosis

This disorder is most commonly seen in adult cocker spaniels, although cases are reported in Labrador retrievers, miniature schnauzers, and Gordon setters. Clinical lesions consist of hyperkeratotic plaques with follicular plugging and follicular casts on the ventral and lateral chest and abdomen. Affected dogs may have greasy hair coats with ceruminous otitis. In the author's opinion, this disorder has unique histologic features; however, the patients often have other conditions (eg, superficial spreading pyoderma, atopy, food allergy), which confuses the pathogenesis of the cornification defect (ie, cause or effect). The diagnosis is achieved by a skin biopsy analysis and response to vitamin A supplementation. The histologic features are marked orthokeratotic hyperkeratosis of the follicular ostea that is more severe than at the epidermal surface.[15] The standard vitamin A dose for a cocker spaniel is 10,000 IU/ d or 500 to 800 IU/kg/d.[5] A clinical response is typically seen in 3 to 8 weeks and dogs may require lifelong therapy.

GENERALIZED SEBACEOUS GLAND HYPERPLASIA OF TERRIERS

Idiopathic generalized sebaceous gland hyperplasia has been reported in both border terriers and wirehaired terriers.[16,17] It is unclear whether this disorder is a cornification defect or a manifestation of another disease process (eg, atopic dermatitis, demodicosis). This disorder is different from the nodules of sebaceous gland hyperplasia that arise in aging dogs. The terriers present with a greasy hair coat that is most severe on the dorsum. Some dogs, particularly the wirehaired terriers, have been documented with *Demodex injai* infestation.[16] These long-bodied *Demodex* mites are often found in sebaceous gland ducts in addition to hair follicles. The relationship of the sebaceous gland hyperplasia to the *Demodex* mites is unknown. Treatment of mite infestation improves the skin but does not reverse the sebaceous gland hyperplasia. It is plausible that the sebaceous gland hyperplasia is the primary lesion and predisposes the dogs to *Demodex* infestation.

PRIMARY SEBORRHEA: A CONTROVERSY

Use of the term seborrhea has been established in the veterinary dermatology literature for at least 5 decades. Seborrhea literally means flow of sebum, and it has been loosely correlated with abnormal sebaceous gland function. The term seborrhea is used clinically to describe excessive scaling, although, historically, seborrhea has been subdivided into those cases with dry scale (seborrhea sicca) or oily/greasy scale (seborrhea oleosa). The term seborrheic dermatitis has been used to describe scaling accompanied by inflammation. In the older literature, the diagnosis of seborrhea was based on gross morphology of skin lesions and, in general, histopathology and skin surface cytologic assessments were not included in the dermatologic work-up. From an etiopathologic viewpoint, the use of terms such as seborrhea and seborrheic dermatitis are nonspecific and should be used for clinical descriptive purposes only, and not to suggest a particular diagnosis.

Use of the term primary seborrhea has classically been reserved for cases in which all known causes of scaling have been ruled out (eg, ectoparasitism, metabolic diseases and endocrinopathies, allergic disease).[5,18] In the 1980s, this designation was potentially useful for treatment purposes, but it antedated the known significance of the role of *Malassezia* and staphylococcal infections as important promoters of secondary seborrhea and seborrheic dermatitis. Primary seborrhea has been reported to arise in adult springer and cocker spaniels.[5,19–21] Although consistently cited in textbooks, few peer-reviewed publications list scientific criteria for the diagnosis of primary seborrhea. Cases vary from early onset to adult onset and from those with mild scale to more severe seborrhea oleosa, which is considered to evolve over time. As dermatologic diagnostic criteria have expanded with time, and clinical/histopathologic accuracy has improved, many cases that would have been labeled primary seborrhea in the past are now readily diagnosed as pyoderma, malassezia dermatitis, sebaceous adenitis, allergic dermatitis, and so forth. This diagnosis is not to deny the presence of mild scale, which commonly occurs spontaneously (and often excessively) in canine and feline patients, or the influence of environment (eg, humidity, heat, diet) on scale formation; only that the scale formation is not pathognomonic for primary seborrhea.

In the cocker spaniel, it is likely that most cases of primary seborrhea would now be termed vitamin A–responsive dermatosis.

In brief, it is the author's opinion that primary seborrhea is an adaptive response rather than a constitutive change in the mechanisms of cornification, and that affected dogs most likely suffer from other dermatologic conditions. If primary seborrhea (eg, spaniel seborrhea) is a true entity, clear criteria should be established as a first step toward performing reasonable investigations to explore its etiopathogenesis. Until that time, the term primary seborrhea should be eliminated from the veterinary dermatology vernacular.

REFERENCES

1. Elias PM, Williams ML, Crumrine D, et al. Ichthyoses: current problems in dermatology. Ichthyoses; clinical, biochemical and diagnostic assessment, vol 39. Basel: Karger; 2010. p. 1–29.
2. Marks R. The stratum corneum barrier: the final frontier. J Nutr 2004;134: 2017S–21S.
3. Shimada K, Yoshihara T, Yamamoto M, et al. Transepidermal water loss (TEWL) reflects skin barrier function of dog. J Vet Med Sci 2008;70:841–3.
4. Shimada K, Yoon J, Yoshihara T, et al. Increased transepidermal water loss and decreased ceramide content in lesional and non-lesional skin of dogs with atopic dermatitis. Vet Dermatol 2009;20:541–6.
5. Scott DW, Miller WH, Griffin CE. Muller and Kirk's small animal dermatology. 6th edition. Philadelphia: WB Saunders; 2001. p. 913–20.
6. Credille KM. Primary cornification defects. In: Guaguère E, Prélaud P, editors. A practical guide to canine dermatology. Paris: Kalianxis; 2008. p. 425–38.
7. Credille KM, Barnhart KF, Minor JS, et al. Mild recessive epidermolytic hyperkeratosis with a novel keratin 10 donor splice-site mutation in a family of Norfolk terrier dogs. Br J Dermatol 2005;153(1):51–8.
8. Mauldin EA, Credille KM, Dunstan RW, et al. The clinical and morphologic features of non-epidermolytic ichthyosis in the golden retriever. Vet Pathol 2008; 45:174–80.
9. Cadiergues MC, Patel A, Shearer DH, et al. Cornification defect in the golden retriever: clinical, histopathological, ultrastructural and genetic characterisation. Vet Dermatol 2008;19(3):120–9.
10. Grall S, Guaguère E, Planchais S, et al. PNPLA1 mutations cause autosomal recessive congenital ichthyosis in golden retriever dogs and humans. Nat Genet 2012;44(2):140–7.
11. Casal ML, Mauldin EA. Canine models of ichthyosis. Philadelphia: American Society of Human genetics; 2008. p. 21894.
12. Dahlqvist J, Klar J, Hausser I, et al. Congenital ichthyosis: mutations in ichthyin are associated with specific structural abnormalities in the granular layer of the epidermis. J Med Genet 2007;44:615–20.
13. Credille K, Minor J, Barnhart K, et al. Transglutaminase 1-deficient recessive lamellar ichthyosis associated with a LINE-1 insertion in Jack Russell terrier dogs. Br J Dermatol 2009;161:265–72.
14. Hartley C, Donaldson D, Smith KC, et al. Congenital keratoconjunctivitis sicca and ichthyosiform dermatosis in 25 Cavalier King Charles spaniel dogs–part I: clinical signs, histopathology, and inheritance. Vet Ophthalmol 2012;15:327–32.
15. Ihrke PJ, Goldschmidt MH. Vitamin A-responsive dermatosis in the dog. J Am Vet Med Assoc 1983;182:687–90.

16. Ordeix L, Bardagí M, Scarampella F, et al. *Demodex injai* infestation and dorsal greasy skin and hair in eight wirehaired fox terrier dogs. Vet Dermatol 2009;20: 267–72.
17. Dedola C, Ressel L, Hill PB, et al. Idiopathic generalized sebaceous gland hyperplasia of the border terrier: a morphometric study. Vet Dermatol 2010;21: 494–502.
18. Ihrke PJ. Canine seborrheic disease complex. Vet Clin North Am Small Anim Pract 1979;9:93–106.
19. Austin VH. Congenital seborrhea of the springer spaniel. Mod Vet Pract 1973;54: 53–5.
20. Scott DW, Miller WH. Primary seborrhoea in English springer spaniels: a retrospective study of 14 cases. J Small Anim Pract 1996;37:173–8.
21. Scott DW. Granulomatous sebaceous adenitis in dogs. J Am Anim Hosp Assoc 1986;22:631–4.

Ischemic Dermatopathies

Daniel O. Morris, DVM, MPH

KEYWORDS

- Canine • Ischemic dermatopathy • Vasculopathy • Dermatomyositis
- Rabies vaccine

KEY POINTS

- Ischemic dermatopathies are typically characterized by atrophic lesions with erythema, scale/crust, erosions/ulcerations, and pigmentary changes. Lesions may affect the face, toes, nail beds, tail tip, pinnal margins, boney prominences, or any combination of these areas.
- Familial dermatomyositis (FDM), the archetype of generalized ischemic dermatopathy, most commonly occurs in juvenile collies and Shetland sheepdogs.
- Ischemic reactions to rabies vaccine may be either localized to the site of injection or may mimic the generalized distribution pattern typical of familial dermatomyositis. Therefore, patients of breed heritage atypical for FDM should be examined closely for a focal alopecic lesion at the site of prior vaccination.
- Other causes of focal or multifocal alopecia, such as demodicosis, bacterial folliculitis, and dermatophytosis, must be ruled out as either primary or secondary disease agents.
- A vasculopathy limited to the margins of the pinnae, which results in cyanosis and necrosis, is perhaps the most common form of ischemic dermatopathy seen in clinical practice. Although this condition is often idiopathic, it may also result from a variety of antigenic triggers.
- The most reliable symptomatic therapy for ischemic dermatopathy of any type is the combination of pentoxifylline and vitamin E.

INTRODUCTION

The ischemic dermatopathies are a group of vasculopathic skin diseases that share similar end-stream clinical and histologic features, despite arising from different primary causes. Regardless of the inciting cause, the injury occurs because of interruption of adequate delivery of oxygenated blood through damaged vessels, which results in protracted atrophy of recipient tissues (an analogy is fruit withering on the vine during a drought). Direct histologic evidence of vessel wall inflammation is often absent, and, for this reason, the ischemic dermatopathies are often described as examples of cell-poor vasculitis.

Department of Clinical Studies - PHL, School of Veterinary Medicine, University of Pennsylvania, 3900 Delancey Street, Philadelphia, PA 19104, USA
E-mail address: domorris@vet.upenn.edu

Vet Clin Small Anim 43 (2013) 99–111
http://dx.doi.org/10.1016/j.cvsm.2012.09.008
0195-5616/13/$ – see front matter © 2013 Elsevier Inc. All rights reserved.

vetsmall.theclinics.com

Unlike cases of true vasculitis (see the article by Innera elsewhere in this issue), hemorrhage within and necrosis of affected tissues are not common features of these diseases. The primary histologic changes noted are fading of hair follicles, smudging of dermal collagen, and clefting at the basement membrane zone (which is usually caused by vacuolar change of the basal keratinocytes). Individual keratinocytes throughout the epidermis may also be damaged and die, resulting in a compensatory hyperkeratotic response of the epidermis. Accumulation of mild inflammatory cell infiltrates at the dermal-epidermal junction, coupled with basal keratinocyte damage, may be reported as cell-poor interface dermatitis by the pathologist.[1–3]

This constellation of pathologic changes results grossly in alopecia, thinning of the skin, and hyperkeratosis/scale. In addition, the thinned skin may be easily damaged by mild trauma, resulting in erosions and ulcers that are slow to heal. In chronic cases, the anoxic insult results in eventual scarring and pigmentary changes; either postinflammatory hyperpigmentation or depigmentation (leukoderma) are possible. Several ischemic dermatopathies of known or unknown cause are considered here.

CANINE FAMILIAL DERMATOMYOSITIS: DISEASE OVERVIEW

Canine familial dermatomyositis (FDM) is an ischemic dermatopathy and myopathy that occurs most commonly in rough collies and Shetland sheepdogs.[1,4] It has also been documented in a group of Beauceron shepherds,[5] and has been described in several individual cases involving other dog breeds. Canine FDM is thought to represent a homolog to juvenile dermatomyositis (JDM) in children, because of overlap of clinicopathologic features.[1] It is the archetypal disease of the ischemic dermatopathy group, because it is the best documented. However, it may be clinically and histologically indistinguishable from other diseases in this category, such as rabies vaccine–associated ischemic dermatopathy (discussed later).

Historical Considerations

Canine FDM was first described in collie dogs in the mid-1980s, although it was likely present in this population during preceding decades. In retrospect, initial reports of a mechanical blistering disease of collies and shelties in the 1970s, which was suggested to resemble epidermolysis bullosa simplex (EB) of people,[6] could have been either FDM[7] or a separate and distinct entity now known as vesicular cutaneous lupus erythematosus (VCLE) of the collie and sheltie.

Clinical Features

Chronic canine FDM is characterized by scarring alopecia of the face, distal extremities, tail tip, and other boney prominences that are subject to mechanical trauma. The earliest lesions include erythema, alopecia, scales, and crusts. With progression, erosions and ulcerations are common, and secondary pyoderma may be superimposed on erosive lesions (**Fig. 1**).[8] Secondary pyoderma may cause pruritus and be mistaken for allergic dermatitis. Demodicosis has also been described in cases of canine FDM, and is thought to occur in association with immunosuppression of the skin.[8] Primary vesicles and bullae are rarely appreciated in clinical practice, because of their fragility. In breeding studies of affected collies, the earliest lesions of FDM appeared between 7 and 11 weeks of age on the inner surfaces of pinnae. Oral and facial vesicles were noted early in the course of the disease, as were footpad erosions in severely affected dogs.[1] Spontaneous resolution of skin lesions was also documented.[9]

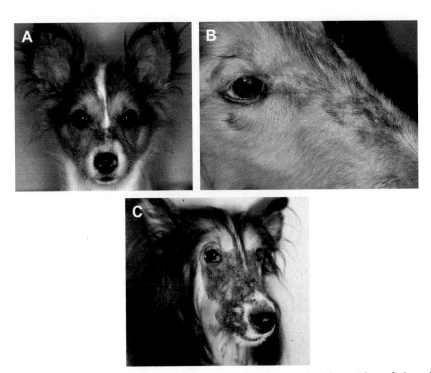

Fig. 1. (*A*) A juvenile collie with early lesions of FDM, characterized by patches of alopecia with erythema and postinflammatory hyperpigmentation, affecting the periocular region. (*B*) Young adult collie with chronic/active lesions of FDM, characterized by patches of scarring alopecia with cutaneous atrophy, erythema, and hyperpigmentation. Note the punctate ulcers on the bridge of the muzzle, which is an acute injury. (*C*) Geriatric Shetland sheepdog with chronic lesions of FDM, characterized by regionally extensive scarring alopecia, erythema, and hyperpigmentation. Note the dished-out appearance of the face, caused by marked facial muscle atrophy.

Although dermatitis may occur without clinical signs of muscle weakness, histologic and electromyographic evidence of myositis may still be apparent.[8–10] In breeding studies of collies, muscle changes were observed between 13 and 19 weeks of age.[1] Electromyographic abnormalities may include fibrillation potentials (most commonly), positive sharp waves, and bizarre high-frequency discharges.[8,9] When clinical signs of myositis are present, the most commonly affected group is the muscles of mastication, and the most consistent clinical signs related to this are difficulty prehending food, chewing, and lapping water. In mild cases, owners may describe only a dirty water bowl with floating food particles. Megaesophagus is a less common feature, but a concerning one because of the threat of regurgitation and aspiration pneumonia. When peripheral muscles are affected, generalized weakness of the limbs is typically noted, characterized by difficulty jumping and climbing stairs. Symptomatic muscle disease seems to be less common in Shetland sheepdogs than in collies.[11,12]

Adult-onset dermatomyositis (DM) in dogs is rare, but perhaps more common in shelties than in collies. Adult-onset lesions are said to occur after a precipitating event, such as estrus, parturition, lactation, trauma, or intense ultraviolet (UV) light exposure.[11] Spontaneous resolution of juvenile-onset FDM has been described anecdotally, but is rare in the author's experience.

Differential Diagnosis

Once FDM had been documented in collies and shelties in the 1980s, confusion persisted in the literature regarding the existence of more than 1 phenotype of familial skin disease in these breeds; 1 with features of human JDM, and 1 with a distinct pattern of adult-onset ulcerations that lacked clinical signs of myositis. The term ulcerative dermatosis of the collie and sheltie eventually replaced the earlier term epidermolysis bullosa, because it became apparent that this ulcerative disease was not a reasonable homolog to human EB. However, throughout the 1990s it was still thought that it might represent a milder form of adult-onset dermatomyositis in these breeds.[11,13] More recently, this ulcerative dermatosis has been shown to be histologically and immunopathologically distinct from FDM, and to represent a reasonable homolog of subacute cutaneous lupus erythematosus of humans, from which the term VCLE is derived.[14] Canine VCLE is characterized by sharply demarcated erosions and ulcerations of the groin and axilla, mucocutaneous junctions, and footpads. Unlike canine FDM, onset of this disease occurs in adulthood, and symptomatic muscle disease is not a feature.[15]

Because canine FDM is characterized by alopecia, and especially because early or mild lesions may be erythematous and scaly, there are several important differentials for such lesions regardless of the age of the dog. These differentials include bacterial folliculitis, demodicosis, and dermatophytosis as primary follicular pathogens, and other inflammatory dermatoses (such as allergic dermatitis) with secondary pyoderma or *Malassezia* yeast overgrowth. As mentioned previously, there is also some evidence that localized cutaneous immunosuppression associated with dermatomyositis can result in secondary bacterial pyoderma and demodicosis, so these conditions must be ruled out regardless of the final primary diagnosis. In dogs of an atypical breed heritage for FDM, rabies vaccine–associated ischemic dermatopathy is the major differential.

Pathophysiology

The pathophysiology of dermatomyositis in dogs remains unclear. Based on the analogous human diseases, both autoimmune and infectious causes have been postulated. In children, JDM is thought to represent a genetically mediated autoimmune disease that is triggered by environmental factors, such as infectious agents, drugs, and vaccines.[16] Environmental factors may trigger the disease through molecular mimicry, which occurs when a foreign antigen cross-reacts with a self-protein. Environmental triggers for dogs are also obvious, as outlined earlier; skin lesions may wax and wane with flares associated with estrous or UV light exposure.[8] Malignancy is a common trigger in adult-onset DM of people, causing 24% of cases,[17] but such a cause has not been reported in dogs.

The familial nature of the disease in dogs strongly supports a genetically mediated predisposition. In rough collies, an autosomal dominant mode of inheritance with incomplete penetrance has been suggested through breeding trials,[8,9] but similar studies have not been reported in shelties. However, a genomic screening technique using microsatellite markers has suggested that a risk gene may map to a region on canine chromosome 35 of shelties.[12]

Regardless of its genetic predisposition, the immunologic basis of the disease remains unclear. In people, both humoral and cell-mediated immune factors are thought to contribute to disease pathogenesis, and autoantibodies have been detected in about 40% of children with JDM.[18] Dysregulation of several cytokines and interferons, which affect inflammatory responses, have been described in human patients compared with healthy controls.[19] In a study of shelties that used gene transcript profiling and molecular techniques for autoantibody analysis, a large number of gene transcripts were shown to be differentially expressed between normal and affected dogs.[20] A significant number of these genes are known to play critical roles in immunoregulation. However, disease-specific autoantibodies were not detected by molecular methods, and tissue immunohistochemistry failed to identify the dramatic degree of T-cell activation that has been described for the human disease.[20] In addition, earlier studies of collies with DM failed to show complement deficiency as has been documented for human patients,[21] and Kunkle and colleagues[8] reported negative or equivocal anti-nuclear antibody (ANA) results for all dogs tested. In practice, veterinary dermatologists rarely order immunologic tests to evaluate clinical cases. Therefore, the immune-mediated basis for the canine disease remains elusive.

There is some evidence that JDM of children may be associated with certain infectious disease agents. Some of the epidemiologic aspects of FDM also fit well with a viral trigger in dogs.[22] Perhaps the most compelling report to support a viral cause was the description of crystalline virus-like structures identified in muscle tissues of collies, which were compatible in size and appearance with picornaviruses.[23] Since this initial study, additional reports that might implicate an infectious cause have not been published.

Diagnostic Considerations

The diagnosis of canine FDM, as with any ischemic dermatopathy, relies on recognition of typical clinical changes with confirmation by histopathology. Breed signalment and the early age of onset are usually helpful. It is also important to search for evidence of other primary or secondary conditions, such as demodicosis, dermatophytosis, and superimposed bacterial pyoderma and/or *Malassezia* yeast overgrowth. A minimum of 4 biopsy samples should be collected, because it is possible that not every sample will contain histologic changes that are definitive for the diagnosis. It is often helpful to select lesions that are thought to be early (acute), fully developed, and late (chronic). Biopsy specimens should be a minimum of 6 mm in size, if a biopsy punch is used. When haired skin is sampled by biopsy punch, a thin black line should be drawn on the skin with a permanent ink marker, in the direction of hair growth. The punch is then centered over the black line, which allows the pathologist to properly orient the biopsy specimen for sectioning, so that the hair follicles are cut longitudinally. This technique is helpful for any disease process that results in alopecia, because it maximizes visualization of the length of hair follicles.[24]

The cutaneous histopathology of FDM is typically characterized as a cell-poor interface dermatitis with attendant follicular atrophy.[1,2] The most clear and consistent injury is follicular atrophy, which may be accompanied by variable degrees of perifollicular inflammation.[2] Less consistent changes may include vesiculation at the level of the basement membrane, individual necrosis of keratinocytes (which form shrunken, irregular, and brightly eosinophilic structures known as colloid bodies), or both.[2,10] These changes are interpreted as representing an anoxic injury, and are seen in other types of ischemic dermatopathy. Depending on the stage of disease during which skin biopsies are collected, true small-vessel vasculitis (an acute injury) or variable degrees of dermal fibrosis (a chronic change) may be present.[1,2] In clinical practice, patients are often presented and biopsied during the more chronic phase of the disease, in which follicular atrophy and scarring with minimal inflammation are the prominent features.

The gross appearance of affected muscles has been described as pale tan and slightly soft tissue (as opposed to the reddish brown of normal muscle).[21] Muscle biopsy is rarely performed in clinical practice, but the histopathology includes variable lymphocytic, suppurative, and plasmacytic inflammation of myofibers, and variable fragmentation, loss of cross-striation, and fibrosis of muscle fibers.[1] Muscle fiber necrosis has also been reported.[7] Muscle enzyme determinations are insensitive indicators of active myositis in canine FDM.[25] Perhaps the most sensitive indicator of myositis is electromyography, which can reveal abnormal tracings even in the absence of clinical signs.

Management

Pharmacologic intervention may be indicated for moderate to severe cases. The safety profile of the primary therapies used (discussed later) allow the clinician to recommend treatment of even mild cases when the pet owner is overtly concerned. Because of the mechanical trauma component of the disease, affected dogs should be encouraged to lie on soft/cushioned surfaces, and protective footwear can be used when the pads are eroded/ulcerated. Secondary infections and demodicosis must be properly diagnosed and treated to avoid confusing clinical signs of these with flares of the primary disease process.

RABIES VACCINE–INDUCED VASCULITIS WITH ALOPECIA: DISEASE OVERVIEW

This disease is characterized by a localized inflammatory or ischemic reaction to subcutaneously administered rabies vaccine. It was originally reported to occur most commonly in miniature poodles,[26] but, in the author's experience, more often affects other small breed dogs (Bichons, shih tzus, miniature pinschers, Maltese, Chihuahuas, Yorkshire terriers, and Jack Russell terriers). The strong breed predilection coupled with anecdotal reports of cases occurring among littermates supports a genetic mode of susceptibility.

Clinical Features

Lesions associated with localized rabies vaccine reactions are typically atrophic, depressed, alopecic patches arising at the site of (or just dependent to the site of) vaccine injection. The clinical lesion is erythemic at onset, with peripheral scale and progressive alopecia. Many owners do not notice the lesion for several months following vaccination, until alopecia draws their attention. Chronic lesions may become darkly hyperpigmented, and are usually atrophic to some degree (**Fig. 2**).

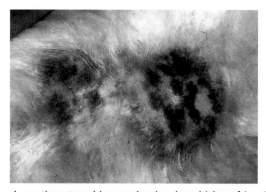

Fig. 2. Two localized reactions to rabies vaccination in a bichon frise. The vaccines were administered 3 years apart. The lesion on the left is the older, nonactive lesion with residual scarring alopecia and hyperpigmentation. The lesion on the right is a chronic/active lesion, in which the alopecia continues to expand in circumference. The latter lesion was mitigated by pharmacologic intervention with pentoxifylline.

Differential Diagnosis

The differential diagnosis should include other causes of focal alopecia, such as staphylococcal folliculitis, demodicosis, dermatophytosis, and alopecia areata.

Pathophysiology

The causal pathomechanism remains unknown, but formation of antigen-antibody complexes that become lodged in vessel walls (a type III hypersensitivity response) has been postulated.[26]

Diagnostic Considerations

Some cases are characterized by deep dermal and subcuticular arteriolitis histologically, whereas others show only subtle vasculopathic change. Other changes may include septal panniculitis, fat necrosis, and focal lymphocytic nodules.[26] Adnexal atrophy is present histologically in most cases, which explains the clinical observation of alopecia and poor hair regrowth. In many cases, a pale-blue foreign material can be appreciated histologically, which is thought to represent persistence of vaccine adjuvant within the subcutis.

Management

In some cases, continued expansion of lesions requires pharmacologic intervention (discussed later).[27] The author bases this therapeutic decision on client reports and histologic evidence of persistent inflammation. Cases have also been reported in which new reactions have occurred at the sites of repeat vaccinations, and the author has noted 1 case that developed severe and generalized (life-threatening) skin lesions on subsequent vaccine exposure, when only a localized reaction had occurred previously. Documentation of the serologic titer to rabies vaccine is not considered a legal substitute for vaccination in most municipalities. Therefore, when an animal's health is thought to be in jeopardy from repeat vaccination, local public health officials should be consulted.

VACCINE-ASSOCIATED ISCHEMIC DERMATOPATHY: DISEASE OVERVIEW

This form of postvaccinal dermatopathy is a multifocal disease that is clinically similar to familial dermatomyositis. However, the original focus of alopecia (ie, at an injection site) must also be appreciated to suggest a cause-and-effect relationship with vaccination and to differentiate it from idiopathic ischemic dermatopathy (**Fig. 3**).[3] Although most cases seem to be associated with rabies vaccine, polyvalent vaccines have also been implicated in the literature and anecdotally.[28]

Clinical Features

Like FDM, the disease affects predominantly the periorificial skin and areas that overlie boney prominences or are most subject to mechanical trauma. In the author's experience, the lesions are typically more severe than the standard FDM case, and exhibit more significant atrophy and crusting (**Fig. 4**). In addition, many cases exhibit a moderate to marked degree of muscle atrophy underlying the affected skin. Histologic evidence of myositis has been documented.[3]

Differential Diagnosis

The differential diagnosis must include FDM and idiopathic ischemic dermatopathy if the primary vaccine reaction site cannot be documented. In this case, other causes for vasculopathy/vasculitis (see the article by Innera elsewhere in this issue) should also

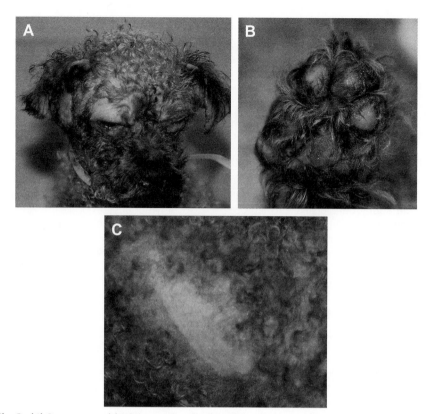

Fig. 3. (*A*) Seven-year-old miniature poodle mix with vaccine-associated ischemic dermatopathy 5 months following rabies vaccination. Note the alopecia, edema, and atrophy of the periocular skin and pinnal margins, and the ulceration/crusting of pinnal margins. (*B*) Ulcerative footpads of the patient in (*A*). (*C*) Rabies vaccination site of the patient in (*A*), characterized by alopecia and mild erythema.

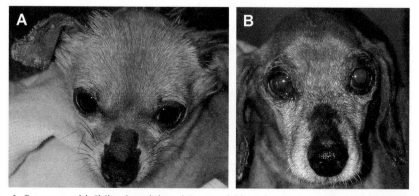

Fig. 4. Four-year-old Chihuahua (*A*) and 9-year-old beagle mix (*B*) with vaccine-associated ischemic dermatopathy following rabies vaccination. Both cases exhibit chronic/active scarring alopecia with hyperpigmentation of the face and head, and marked atrophy with necrosis and crusting of the pinnal margins.

be excluded before making the diagnosis of idiopathic ischemic dermatopathy (discussed later).

Pathophysiology

Reduced density of dermal blood vessels and deposition of complement (C_{5b-9}/membrance attack complex) in muscle and vessel walls has been shown in tissue biopsies from dogs affected by postvaccinal ischemic dermatopathy, suggesting complement-mediated microangiopathy.[3]

Diagnostic Considerations

The diagnosis is based on clinical presentation, the presence of a primary (injection site) lesion, and supportive histopathology.

Management

Pharmacologic intervention is always indicated.

OTHER ISCHEMIC DERMATOPATHIES: OVERVIEWS
Idiopathic Ischemic Dermatopathy

Cases of ischemic dermatopathy without a clear temporal association with vaccination and that occur in adult dogs of breeds atypical for FDM are occasionally identified in clinical practice (**Fig. 5**). Although a careful search for some source of antigenic stimulation should be pursued (eg, infectious diseases, adverse food reaction), a causal association is rarely identified. If the histopathology is consistent with the changes described for FDM or vaccine-associated ischemic dermatopathy, analogous treatment regimens should be pursued (discussed later).

Familial Cutaneous Vasculopathy of the German Shepherd

This genodermatosis has been recognized primarily in a group of Canadian shepherds,[29] but sporadic cases have also been reported from the United States and Europe. Therefore, veterinary clinicians should be aware of the clinical presentation,

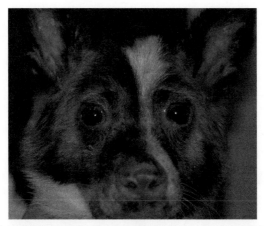

Fig. 5. Six-year-old cattle dog cross with idiopathic ischemic dermatopathy characterized by alopecia and edema of the eyelids, alopecia and scaling of the skin of the temporal regions and concave surfaces of the pinnae, and depigmentation with erosions of the nasal planum. No vaccine site reaction could be appreciated, and extensive testing for other inciting causes of the vasculopathy/vasculitis (see article by Innera elsewhere in this issue) was negative.

which manifests in puppies as fever and lethargy accompanied by footpad swelling, depigmentation of pads and nasal planum, and crusting/ulceration of the pinnal margins and tail tip. Lesion onset is often temporally related to routine vaccination of puppies (with multivalent vaccines). Concurrent demodicosis has also been described in some cases. Pedigree analysis of the Canadian dogs suggests an autosomal mode of genetic susceptibility.

Proliferative Thrombovascular Necrosis of the Pinnae (Pinnal Margin Vasculopathy)

This disorder is poorly documented in the veterinary literature, despite being common in clinical dermatology practice. Lesions typically begin on the apical margins of the pinnae and progress proximally. Crusting, erythema, and cyanosis are present in the acute phase, and the pinnal margins become notched or serrated with chronicity (**Fig. 6**). Although potentially seen in any breed, dachshunds and Rhodesian ridgebacks seem to be over-represented in the author's group practice. Although most cases are diagnosed as idiopathic by exclusion, the author has noted an association with adverse food reaction/food allergy or recent vaccination (several cases each). Other causes of vasculitis/vasculopathy (see the article by Innera elsewhere in this issue) should also be excluded. Successful treatment with pentoxifylline or tetracycline/niacinamide has been reported anecdotally (discussed later).

Pharmacologic Therapies for Ischemic Vasculopathies

For JDM of children, most rheumatologists in North America report prescribing oral corticosteroids as the mainstay of therapy. Observational studies of this disease have suggested that early intervention with high-dose corticosteroids is associated with an improved prognosis. The most commonly used adjunctive agent prescribed for children is methotrexate, which is used for its steroid-sparing properties.[30] Other adjunctive immunosuppressive therapies reported for human DM include intravenous immunoglobulin (for severe flares/ulceration), hydroxychloroquine (for refractory cases or those without muscle involvement), cyclosporine A, mycophenolate mofetil, systemic tacrolimus, cyclophosphamide, and tumor-necrosis factor α antagonists.[30] Although many of these therapies could potentially be considered for canine FDM and other ischemic dermatopathies, veterinary dermatologists generally try to avoid the use of corticosteroids because they may potentiate the skin and muscle atrophy that are features of these diseases. In addition, anecdotal reports of nonsteroidal

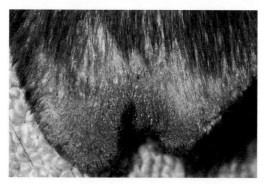

Fig. 6. Idiopathic thrombovascular necrosis of the pinnal margin, characterized by a large focus of necrosis flanked by cyanosis. On the more proximal pinna, active inflammation (erythema and scale) persists, with progressive alopecia. Note the serrated-edge appearance of the pinnal margin beyond the large defect.

immunosuppressive therapies for ischemic dermatopathies of dogs suggest that response is typically marginal. The author has found that a tapering/pulsed course of predniso(lo)ne or methylprednisolone can be useful for severe flares and ulcerative lesions associated with these dermatopathies, but is often counterproductive with extended use. The mainstay for pharmacologic management of ischemic dermatopathies is pentoxifylline in combination with vitamin E.[3]

Pentoxifylline belongs to the methylxanthine class of drugs, and is a derivative of theobromine, although it lacks the cardiac and bronchodilatory effects of other drugs in its class.[31] A myriad of pharmacodynamic effects have been described for pentoxifylline in humans, including antiinflammatory and hemorrheologic properties. The latter is described as the ability to reduce blood viscosity through small vascular spaces, whereas the immunomodulatory properties are diverse and include inhibition of many proinflammatory cytokines and leukocyte-mediated effects.[31] Pentoxifylline has been described as a successful therapy for ischemic dermatopathies including canine rabies vaccine–associated dermatopathy, pinnal margin vasculopathy, and FDM.[3,27,32] Pharmacokinetic studies have suggested that therapeutic concentrations (based on human response data) are achieved in dogs with a dosage ranging from 15 mg/kg every 8 hours by mouth[33] to 30 mg/kg every 12 hours by mouth.[34] In a prospective, 12-week, open-label clinical trial in 10 dogs with FDM, a dose of 25 mg/kg every 12 hours promoted a complete clinical response in 4 dogs and a partial (but acceptable) response in the other 6.[32] There were no adverse effects noted in any of these studies based on clinical chemistries, hematology, urinalyses, or physical examination findings.[32–34]

Vitamin E (in its most active form as α-tocopherol) is a potent antioxidant that quenches oxygen free radicals and other molecules that contribute to oxidative stress during various physiologic and pathologic processes (in the skin and many other tissues).[35] Vitamin E is an important constituent of sebum, which is secreted continuously for delivery to the epidermis.[35] It has known benefits in the management of allergic diseases, exercise-associated stress, and skin damage by UV light.[35] Vitamin E has also been shown to provide a protective effect against ischemic injury in a canine coronary artery infarct model,[36] which is perhaps the best evidence to support its use for the treatment of ischemic dermatopathies. The levels of vitamin E detected within the skin are directly correlated to dietary intake,[35] however vitamin E applied topically is rapidly depleted in a dose-dependent manner by UV-B radiation.[37] The ideal oral dosage of α-tocopherol for maximum cutaneous protection has not been elucidated, but it has a wide margin of safety for oral supplementation.[38] Doses used in veterinary dermatology practice range from 200 to 800 IU every 12 hours, depending on the pet's size.[39] Its use in conjunction with pentoxifylline has been reported in the successful treatment of vaccine-associated ischemic dermatopathy.[3] The author routinely uses vitamin E in therapeutic regimens for all types of ischemic injury, at an oral dosage of 200 IU (small breeds), 400 IU (medium breeds), or 600 IU (large breeds), every 12 hours.

Tetracycline and niacinamide exhibit synergistic and leukocyte-specific antiinflammatory properties.[40] This combination may be useful for some milder cases of ischemic dermatopathy, especially pinnal margin vasculopathy. See the article by Innera elsewhere in this issue for details on mechanisms of action and dose regimens.

REFERENCES

1. Hargis AM, Haupt KH, Hegreberg GA, et al. Familial canine dermatomyositis. Initial characterization of the cutaneous and muscular lesions. Am J Pathol 1984;116:234–44.

2. Gross TL, Kunkle GA. The cutaneous histology of dermatomyositis in collie dogs. Vet Pathol 1987;24:11–5.
3. Vitale CB, Gross TL, Magro CM. Vaccine-induced ischemic dermatopathy in the dog. Vet Dermatol 1999;10:131–42.
4. Hargis AM, Haupt KH, Prieur DJ, et al. A skin disorder in three Shetland sheepdogs: comparison with familial canine dermatomyositis of collies. Compend Cont Ed Pract Vet 1985;7:306–15.
5. Guaguere E, Magnol JP, Cauzinille L, et al. Familial canine dermatomyositis in eight Beauceron shepherds. In: Kwochka KW, Willemse T, Von Tscharner C, editors. Advances in veterinary dermatology. New York: Pergamon Press; 1996. p. 527–8.
6. Scott DW, Schultz RD. Epidermolysis bullosa simplex in the collie dog. J Am Vet Med Assoc 1977;171:721–3.
7. Hargis AM, Haupt KH, Prieur DJ, et al. Animal model of human disease: dermatomyositis; familial canine dermatomyositis. Am J Pathol 1985;120:323–5.
8. Kunkle GA, Chrisman CL, Gross TL, et al. Dermatomyositis in collie dogs. Compend Contin Ed Pract Vet 1985;7:185–92.
9. Haupt KH, Prieur DJ, Moore MP, et al. Familial canine dermatomyositis: clinical, electrodiagnostic, and genetic studies. Am J Vet Res 1985;46:1861–9.
10. Ferguson EA, Cerundolo R, Lloyd DH, et al. Dermatomyositis in five Shetland sheepdogs in the United Kingdom. Vet Rec 2000;146:214–7.
11. Hargis AM, Mundell AC. Familial canine dermatomyositis. Compend Contin Ed Pract Vet 1992;4:855–64.
12. Clark LA, Credille KM, Murphy KE, et al. Linkage of dermatomyositis in the Shetland sheepdog to chromosome 35. Vet Dermatol 2005;16:392–4.
13. Ihrke PJ, Gross TL. Ulcerative dermatosis of Shetland sheepdogs and collies. In: Bonagura JD, editor. Kirk's current veterinary therapy XII. Philadelphia: WB Saunders; 1995. p. 639–40.
14. Jackson HA, Olivry T. Ulcerative dermatosis of the Shetland sheepdog and rough collie may represent a novel vesicular variant of cutaneous lupus erythematosus. Vet Dermatol 2001;12:18–27.
15. Jackson HA, Olivry T, Berget F, et al. Immunopathology of vesicular cutaneous lupus erythematosus in the rough collie and Shetland sheepdog: a canine homologue of subacute cutaneous lupus erythematosus in humans. Vet Dermatol 2004;15:230–9.
16. Batthish M, Feldman BM. Juvenile dermatomyositis. Curr Rheumatol Rep 2011;13:216–24.
17. Zahr ZA, Baer AN. Malignancy in myositis. Curr Rheumatol Rep 2011;13:208–15.
18. Khanna S, Reed AM. Immunopathogenesis of juvenile dermatomyositis. Muscle Nerve 2010;41:581–92.
19. Kao L, Chung L, Fiorentino DF. Pathogenesis of dermatomyositis: role of cytokines and interferon. Curr Rheumatol Rep 2011;13:225–32.
20. Wahl JM, Clark LA, Scalli O, et al. Analysis of gene transcript profiling and immunobiology in Shetland sheepdogs with dermatomyositis. Vet Dermatol 2008;19:52–8.
21. Hargis AM, Prieur DJ, Haupt KH, et al. Prospective study of familial canine dermatomyositis. Correlation of the severity of dermatomyositis and circulating immune complex levels. Am J Pathol 1986;123:465–79.
22. Kunkle GA, Schmeitzel LP. Canine dermatomyositis. A disease with an infectious origin. An immune-mediated disease with a link to canine lupus erythematosus. Compend Cont Ed Pract Vet 1992;4:866–71.

23. Hargis AM, Prieur DJ, Haupt KH, et al. Postmortem findings in four litters of dogs with familial canine dermatomyositis. Am J Pathol 1986;123:480–96.

24. Mauldin EA, Castle S, Davenport GM, et al. A simple biopsy technique to improve dermatopathologic interpretation. Vet Med April 2002;286–8.

25. Haupt KH, Prieur DJ, Hargis AM, et al. Familial canine dermatomyositis: clinicopathologic, immunologic, and serologic studies. Am J Vet Res 1985;46:1870–5.

26. Wilcock BP, Yager JA. Focal cutaneous vasculitis and alopecia at sites of rabies vaccination in dogs. J Am Vet Med Assoc 1986;188:1174–7.

27. Nichols PR, Morris DO, Beale KM. A retrospective study of canine and feline cutaneous vasculitis. Vet Dermatol 2001;12:255–64.

28. Kim HJ, Kang MH, Kim JW, et al. Long-term management of vaccine-induced refractory ischemic dermatopathy in a miniature pinscher puppy. J Vet Med Sci 2011;73:1237–40.

29. Weir JA, Yager JA, Caswell JL, et al. Familial cutaneous vasculopathy of German shepherds: clinical, genetic, and preliminary pathological and immunological studies. Can Vet J 1994;35:763–9.

30. Stringer E, Bohnsack J, Bowyer SL, et al. Treatment approaches to juvenile dermatomyositis (JDM) across North America: the Childhood Arthritis and Rheumatology Research Alliance (CARRA) JDM treatment survey. J Rheumatol 2010;37:1953–61.

31. Marks SL, Merchant S, Foil C. Pentoxifylline: wonder drug? J Am Anim Hosp Assoc 2001;37:218–9.

32. Rees C, Boothe DM. Therapeutic response to pentoxifylline and its active metabolites in dogs with familial canine dermatomyositis. Vet Ther 2003;4:234–41.

33. Marsalla R, Nicklin CF, Munson JW, et al. Pharmacokinetics of pentoxifylline in dogs after oral and intravenous administration. Am J Vet Res 2000;61:631–7.

34. Rees C, Boothe DM, Boeckh A, et al. Dosing regimen and hematologic effect of pentoxifylline and its active metabolites in normal dogs. Vet Ther 2003;4:188–96.

35. Jewell DE, Yu S, Joshi DK. Effects of serum vitamin E levels on skin vitamin E levels in dogs and cats. Vet Ther 2002;3:235–43.

36. Tripathi Y, Hegde BM. Effect of alpha-tocopherol pretreatment on infarct size following 90 minutes of ischemia and 4 hours of reperfusion in dogs. Indian J Physiol Pharmacol 1997;41:241–7.

37. Krol ES, Kramer-Stickland KA, Liebler DC. Photoprotective actions of topically applied vitamin E. Drug Metab Rev 2000;32:413–20.

38. Gross KL, Wedekind KJ, Cowell CS, et al. Nutrients: vitamin E. In: Hand MS, Thatcher CD, Remillard RL, et al, editors. Small animal clinical nutrition. 4th edition. Marceline (MO): Walsworth Publishing; 2000. p. 86–7.

39. Rosencrantz WR. Discoid lupus erythematosus. In: Griffin CE, Kwochka KW, MacDonald JM, editors. Current veterinary dermatology. St. Louis (MO): Mosby-Year Book; 1993. p. 149–53.

40. Fivenson DP. Nicotinamide and tetracycline therapy of bullous pemphigoid. Arch Dermatol 1994;130:753–8.

Cutaneous Vasculitis in Small Animals

Marie Innerå, Dr med Vet

KEYWORDS

- Cutaneous vasculitis • Necrotizing vasculitis • Neutrophilic vasculitis
- Immune mediated • Cutaneous adverse drug reactions • Canine • Dog • Cat

KEY POINTS

- Cutaneous vasculitis is a reaction pattern and not a disease in itself.
- A thorough workup to identify underlying triggers should always be made.
- The diagnosis must be confirmed histologically, and one should obtain deep tissue samples to make sure vascular damage is not missed.
- If a drug is suspected or confirmed as the cause of vasculitis, withdrawal and future avoidance is the most important treatment.
- Very high doses of steroids may not be the best treatment for patients presenting with large areas of ulcerated skin, because this increases the risk of secondary wound infections and delays wound healing.

Vasculitis is a reaction pattern, characterized by an aberrant immune response directed toward blood vessels.[1] The pathophysiology is not fully understood, and is most likely complex, involving a variety of mechanisms acting in concert to induce necrotizing inflammatory changes in the blood vessel wall.[2]

Clinical presentation of patients affected by this multifactorial reaction pattern depends mainly on the extent of vascular destruction, and both cutaneous and systemic forms have been reported.[1] Impaired vascular function may lead to edema formation, hemorrhage, and purpura. Full-thickness skin necrosis and crateriform ulcers may follow. Patients affected with systemic or cutaneous vasculitis are most often sick, presenting with constitutional signs. A varying degree of pain is common and may range from mild to severe. Extensive ulcerations of large areas of skin predispose these patients to secondary bacterial wound infections and sepsis, much like a patient presenting with extensive burns, so proper wound management is essential.

Numerous triggering factors have been identified as a cause of vasculitides in dogs and cats; therefore, a thorough drug history and early workup for underlying ongoing disease processes are important steps when presented with these patients.[1,3] Diagnosis should be based on history and clinical findings along with compatible histopathology reports.

Disclosure: The authors have nothing to disclose.
Finnsnes Dyreklinikk, Postboks 228, Finnsnes 9305, Norway
E-mail address: marie_inneraa@hotmail.com

Treatment must be tailored to the individual patient, and should be based on underlying triggering factors as well as the extent and severity of cutaneous lesions.

Vasculitic diseases currently recognized in dogs and cats, including cutaneous necrotizing vasculitis or neutrophilic immunologic vasculitis, are covered herein. Specific familial vasculitides will also be reviewed briefly. For information about ischemic dermatopathies please refer to the article by Morris elsewhere in this issue.

IMMUNOPATHOGENESIS

The primary immunopathogenic events that initiate the process of vascular inflammation and blood vessel damage are poorly understood in both people and animals; however, immunologic mechanisms appear to play an active role.[2]

Applying the traditional Gell-Coombs classification of hypersensitivity reactions, it is thought that immediate hypersensitivity reactions as well as type II and type III reactions may all be involved in the immunopathogenesis of vasculitic diseases.[4] This immunologic heterogeneity also illustrates the importance of not viewing vasculitic diseases as a diagnosis in itself, but a reaction pattern that warrants further investigations to achieve a proper diagnosis and prognosis for the individual patient.

Type I Hypersensitivity Reactions

Immediate hypersensitivity reactions, characterized by the formation of immunoglobulin E antibodies have been stated to be involved especially in the early stages of cutaneous vasculitides in animals[5]; however, type I reactions are unlikely to be the major player in most cases of canine and feline vasculitides.[1]

Type II Hypersensitivity Reactions

In a classical type II hypersensitivity reactions, antigen–antibody interactions result in the local production of anaphylotoxin (C5a), the recruitment of polymorphonuclear leukocytes, and subsequent tissue injury owing to the release of hydrolytic neutrophil enzymes after their autolysis. In human medicine, a subset of vasculitides are characterized by the formation of autoantibodies; so called antineutrophil cytoplasmic antibodies (ANCA) and the diseases associated with the production of these antibodies are referred to as ANCA vasculitides. In ANCA vasculitides (Wegener's granulomatosis [WG], Churg–Strauss syndrome, and polyarteritis nodosa), ANCA bind directly to neutrophil granules and the release of toxic mediators leads to a direct damage of vessel walls.[1,2]

Human antibody-associated vasculitides, where antibodies bind directly to the vessel walls, are thus classical examples of type II reactions.[2]

Type III Hypersensitivity

Immune complex reactions occur when antibodies present in the blood result in the formation and deposition of antigen–antibody complexes. The very presence of these complexes lodged in blood vessels, in addition to the polymorphonuclear leukocytes attracted by complement activation, results in tissue injury and compromised function. Vasculitis associated with connective tissue diseases such as systemic lupus erythematosus are examples of a type III hypersensitivity reaction.[1,6] This is currently the most widely accepted pathomechanism of cutaneous vasculitis in animals.

HISTOLOGIC FEATURES

Histologic examination is needed to confirm a diagnosis of cutaneous vasculitis, and samples from affected patients show pathologic changes in the vascular structures of the dermis or sometimes deep panniculus, as well as secondary changes that can be related to tissue hypoxia.[5] True vasculitis is separated histologically from *vasculopathy*, the latter being a term used to describe thromboembolic accidents and occlusion of vessels by fibrin thrombi, usually as a result of sepsis and vascular toxins.[7]

In cases of "true" vasculitis, a differentiation between leukocytoclastic and non-leukocytoclastic vasculitis is made. Leukocytoclasia is a histologic term referring to pyknosis and karyorrhexis of nuclei. This can be visualized histologically as fragmented nuclear debris around blood vessels, often referred to as "nuclear dust." Leukocytoclasia may range from subtle to severe and can sometimes be the only evidence of a vascular insult[5]; however, a diagnosis of leukocytoclastic vasculitis requires several other criteria to be satisfied: Intramural inflammation (visualized as inflammatory cells transmigrating the vessel histologically), endothelial cell swelling, leukocytoclasia, hemorrhage, and fibrinoid necrosis of the vessel wall.[7] The dominant inflammatory infiltrate may be neutrophilic (majority of cases), eosinophilic, or lymphocytic. Leukocytoclasia is normally a feature of vasculitis affecting small or medium sized vessels.[5]

Damage to dermal vessels usually leads to the development of hemorrhage and edema within the tissues. Hypoxic changes with pale collagen ("smudging of the collagen") along with faded hair follicles and adnexal structures may be seen as well. Epidermal lesions such as exudation, crusting, and ulceration may also develop owing to tissue ischemia.[7]

CLASSIFICATION

Classification of vasculitides in animals has traditionally been based on histologic inflammatory patterns. Currently, no classification system taking into account the clinical presentation of the individual patient is recognized in veterinary medicine. Based on such histologic classification, vasculitides in animals are categorized as either leukocytoclastic or non-leukocytoclastic, and then subdivided as neutrophilic, eosinophilic, or lymphocytic.[5] Correlations have also been made between histologic classifications and the different triggering factors leading to the vasculitic event; however, one should keep in mind that histologic lesions may evolve and change over time.[7] This has been thoroughly documented in human patients, where serial evaluations of human leukocytoclastic cutaneous vasculitis has shown that the granulocytic infiltrate gives way to a predominantly mononuclear population within 48 hours.[7]

It is the personal opinion of the author that the current classification alone is unsatisfactory from a clinical standpoint, because it does not help to predict the outcome of the disease for the individual patient.

CLINICAL FINDINGS
Dermatologic Presentation

Disruption of adequate blood flow and tissue oxygenation may lead to a wide range of clinical signs. Dermatologic lesions may be the only clinical sign, but it is not uncommon for constitutional signs to antedate cutaneous changes.[8]

Palpable purpura, plaques and hemorrhagic bullae, and wheals and serpentine papules, alone or in combination with pitting edema, are common presenting signs.[1] Purpura, a symptom indicating an ongoing hemorrhagic event in the skin, may also become darker with time.[8] It is imperative that purpura is differentiated from erythema. This can easily be done by applying a glass slide to the lesion with slight pressure. If the lesion does not blanch, purpura can be confirmed. This diagnostic test is commonly referred to as diascopy (**Fig. 1**).[5]

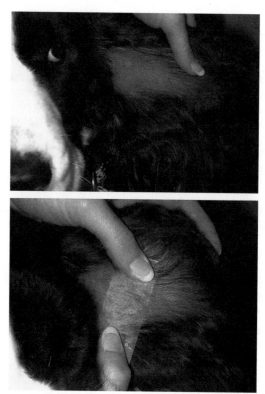

Fig. 1. Diascopy is performed by pressing a transparent glass slide onto the skin. Using this simple diagnostic test will help to differentiate between erythema and purpura (hemorrhage).

With severe vascular injury and subsequent hypoxia or ischemia of the tissue, resulting lesions in the form of full-thickness necrosis and "punched out" crateriform ulcers or even eschars may develop. Devitalized tissue may be firm, discolored, and cool to the touch.

If the vasculitic event targets vessels of subcutaneous adipose tissue, a process referred to as *septal vasculitis*, palpable, firm subcutaneous nodules, and swellings may be present.[5] Acrocyanosis, a bluish discoloration of the extremities, has also been reported in some affected dogs.[8]

Atypical presentation with target lesions and a clinical picture mimicking erythema multiforme was observed in 1 patient with confirmed vasculitis histologically (personal observation). Some patients, especially if food allergy is an inciting trigger of the vasculitis, may also present with a generalized, sometimes chronic urticaria.[3]

Lesions may develop at any site of the body, including the oral cavity and mucous membranes. Independent of body site, it is not uncommon that lesions are distributed in a linear fashion, reflecting the vascular anatomy of the patient. This may be a striking feature, especially when the tail or extremities are affected, that should alert the clinician to a possible ongoing vasculitic event.[8] The clinician needs to keep in mind that the cutaneous lesions resulting from an ischemic event in the skin may evolve over time. Patients presenting early may develop ulcers only several days later, and pitting edema along with constitutional clinical signs, which may be the only finding in the early stage of the disease. See **Figs. 2–6** for examples of dermatologic presentations.

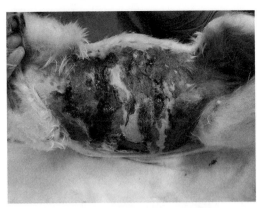

Fig. 2. Severe necrotizing vasculitis in a 7-year-old Jack Russell Terrier mix. Note the extensive deep ulceration, devitalized tissue in the cranial parts of the abdomen, and a punched out eschar on the right lateral aspect of the umbilicus region.

Palpation of the skin is imperative to detect pitting edema, unusual firmness of the skin, or temperature changes that may occur as a result of a deficient blood supply. Patients with a long hair coat should be clipped to allow better visualization of the affected skin and thus better monitoring of disease progression and response to treatment. Marking the edges of the lesions with a waterproof marker is a simple but effective tool for monitoring progression of disease when lesions are extensive.

Systemic Clinical Signs

Patients may present with a range of clinical symptoms and constitutional signs, such as anorexia, depression, malaise, and pyrexia.[8] In a retrospective evaluation of 36 patients with histologically confirmed cutaneous necrotizing vasculitis, 34 of 36 patients presented with signs of systemic illness (Marie Innerå, unpublished data, 2011). In the same group, a majority of patients suffering from vasculitis also displayed

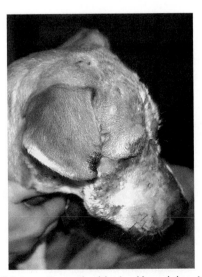

Fig. 3. Generalized vasculitis in an 8-month-old mixed breed dog. No triggers could be identified in this patient, but the dog was managed on 5 mg/kg cyclosporine.

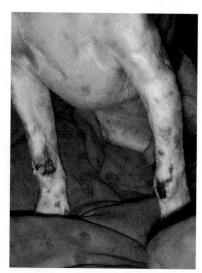

Fig. 4. Same dog as in **Fig. 3**. Full-thickness ulceration of the front legs below the anastomosis of the proximal palmar venous arch and the accessory cephalic arch (where the vessels are narrower). The lesions follow the vasculature in a linear and symmetric fashion. This is commonly seen in patients suffering from cutaneous vasculitis.

signs of generalized or diffuse pain. This is particularly common during the initial phase of the disease; however, degree of pain may be highly individual. Pain may be related to the skin as a single organ system and in certain cases may be so severe that it becomes difficult to evaluate whether or not other organs are involved, for example, involvement of the ventral abdomen may cause the animal to walk with a stiff gait or avoid lying down. It may also be challenging to palpate the abdomen or perform a routine abdominal ultrasound, even under sedation, when the skin of the abdomen is severely affected

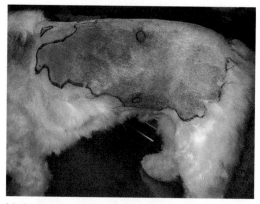

Fig. 5. This 5-year-old Shi Tzu originally presented as an emergency owing to ocular vasculitis and hyphema a day after visiting the groomer. On recheck with the ophthalmologist 3 weeks later, the dog developed these confluent purpuric lesions that rapidly expanded while being examined by the ophthalmologist. A thorough drug history revealed that the owner would give the dog acepromazine before car rides. Acepromazin was thus the likely trigger in this dog, because it had been administered both before the visit to the groomer and before seeing the ophthalmologist for a recheck.

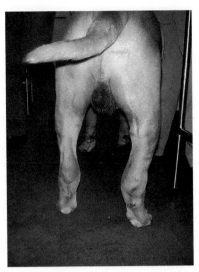

Fig. 6. Pitting edema is a common finding in vasculitis patients. This 9-year-old Mastiff presented with pitting edema of both hind legs and intensely painful purpuric lesions of the groin and scrotum. The dog was diagnosed with lymphoma.

and painful. Dogs with a thick hair coat may only show signs of severe pain when touched or handled and the lesions may not become evident to the owners or clinician until the skin itself is more thoroughly examined. Oral lesions, when present, may cause the animal to salivate, become anorexic, or to be reluctant to open its mouth.

Polyarthropathy, myopathy, and neuropathy has also been described in patients with cutaneous necrotizing vasculitis. It is common to see moderate elevations liver enzymes (50% of patients in an unpublished study, Marie Innerå, 2011). Glomerular disease, pleuritis, pericarditis, and gastrointestinal inflammation may also be present. These findings correspond with what is seen in human cases of leukocytoclastic cutaneous vasculitis.[8]

In contrast with ischemic dermatopathies (also known as cell-poor vasculopathy or cell-poor vasculitis), patients presenting with true cutaneous vasculitis are usually sick dogs that require a thorough workup and careful monitoring. Early recognition of clinical symptoms and a tentative working diagnosis of cutaneous vasculitis allows for a better prognosis for the patient, so that appropriate actions can be taken in the early stage of the disease process.

DIAGNOSIS

A thorough history should always be obtained when vasculitis is suspected and should include information about exposure to drugs and/or xenobiotic substances administered to the pet either systemically, topically or added to the animals diet within the last 2 to 4 months (Dr Edmund Rosser, personal communication, 2009). A drug history should also include routine vaccinations and dietary supplements. Information should also be obtained with regard to current and previous diets (including treats and people food) that the animal has been exposed to, so that an appropriate elimination diet can be selected if necessary.

A comprehensive physical examination must be performed, including a thorough dermatologic examination. A minimum database should include a complete blood count with differential, a serum chemistry profile, and urinalysis. Tick titers should be evaluated, especially when the patient is living in or traveling to areas where tick-borne illnesses are endemic.

Cutaneous hemorrhagic events may be the only symptom of certain coagulation disorders or ongoing immune-mediated hematologic processes. Such diseases are important differentials for cutaneous vasculitis, and a coagulation profile as well as more specific immunologic testing may be necessary (antinuclear antibody testing, Coombs tests, and rheumatoid arthritis factor).

One of the most important and critical steps in the workup of patients suffering from vasculitis is differentiating between infectious and non-infectious disease processes. If sepsis is suspected, blood cultures are indicated. However, it can often take some time to get the results of these tests and the same is true for histopathology reports. When faced with acutely ill patients, additional diagnostic tools can therefore be of value in an emergency setting. The author finds fine-needle aspiration biopsies from edematous areas to be a helpful in such situations. Aspiration of edematous skin lesions and subsequent staining with a Romanowsky type stain such as Diff Quick or Hemacolor can provide an impression of the nature of the cutaneous infiltrate. More important, bacterial organisms may be visualized on such smears.

D-Dimer, if available, may also be of value in this early stage of decision making, because this test predicts thrombus formation in dogs with cutaneous vasculitis.[9-11] This test, however, will not differentiate between infectious and non-infectious processes so a positive D-dimer only reflects thrombus formation and does not replace histopathology as a means of diagnosing vasculitis.

Histology is essential to confirm the diagnosis, regardless of fine-needle aspiration biopsy results, and it is advised to obtain biopsies that are representative of different stages of the disease process. One should make an effort to include the deeper layers of the skin as well as the epidermis in the biopsy, because vascular disease processes may be more easily observed here. Taking skin biopsies at an early stage allows for a more rapid diagnosis. A sterile punch biopsy should be obtained simultaneously and submitted for macerated tissue culture and susceptibility testing (bacterial and fungal) to rule out infectious processes (**Box 1**).

DIFFERENTIAL DIAGNOSES

Several diseases may mimic cutaneous vasculitis both clinically and histologically. Vascular damage, vasculopathy, and thrombosis of blood vessels are features of several infectious diseases. This highlights the importance of ruling out infectious causes of vasculitis before making a diagnosis of true vasculitis.

The principal clinical differentials that needs to be considered before making a diagnosis of true vasculitis includes sepsis (which can lead to thrombosis and/or vasculopathy), disseminated intravascular coagulation, cryoglobulinemia, cryofibrinogenemia (cold agglutinin disease), and frostbite.[5] Sepsis can lead to thrombosis and vasculopathy secondary to infections of the skin, such as deep pyoderma when it complicates demodicosis, or as a result of internal infections such as bacterial endocarditis.[5] Other, less common differentials include erysopleothrix rhusiopathie infections and Rocky Mountain spotted fever. These diagnoses are, however, not common in dogs.[5,12]

TRIGGERS AND UNDERLYING DISEASES

The list of underlying causes that can result in an aberrant immune response directed toward the vascular endothelium is exhausting and summarized in **Box 2**.[1,3,5]

Box 1
Diagnostic testing for cutaneous and systemic vasculitis in dogs

Minimum Database

- Complete blood count with differential
- Serum chemistry assay
- Urinalysis
- Tick titers
- Cytology (fine-needle aspiration biopsy)
- Histopathology
- Culture (fungal and bacterial)

Additional diagnostic tests

- Coagulation profile
- Blood cultures
- Coombs test
- Antinuclear antibody test (ANA)
- Rheumatoid arthritis factor
- Diagnostic imaging
- Elimination diet

Drugs

Drugs may act as antigens triggering a number of cutaneous adverse drug reactions. The antigen may be the drug itself, one of its metabolites, or a drug–protein or metabolite–protein complex.[6] In all cases of cutaneous adverse drug reactions, a drug could

---

Box 2
Underlying causes of vasculitis in dogs

1. Drugs
2. Insect bites
3. Infectious causes
   a. Viral
   b. Bacterial
   c. Mycobacterial
   d. Fungal
   e. Protozoal
   f. Rickettsial
4. Neoplastic processes
5. Adverse reactions to food
6. Autoimmune diseases
7. Genetic/familial forms
8. Idiopathic forms

also be defined as any "drug-like substance" and not necessarily only licensed medication intended for the treatment of animals. This is important, because the trend for supplementing and treating companion animals with holistic or alternative medications is gaining popularity. Such supplements might sometimes be included in the animal's diet. In addition, with the recent technological developments, owners are relying more on information from various other sources than their regular veterinarian when it comes to treatment of various maladies in their pets. The list of remedies an animal may have been exposed to before an adverse event could therefore be extensive.

When presented with a patient suffering from an adverse drug reaction, a thorough drug history is of crucial importance, because the most important therapy is drug withdrawal, including all drugs or drug-like substances administered to the patient within the last 4 to 6 months.[6]

Determining whether or not a drug is in fact the trigger may be problematic, especially in patients receiving multiple medications, and there are few solid reports of specific drugs implicated as triggers of vasculitis. This may stem from the fact that proving a relationship between a drug and a specific adverse drug reaction can be challenging. Patients commonly receive multiple drugs simultaneously and when a reaction to a drug produces a severe life-threatening reaction, rechallenge runs the risk of being fatal and is therefore not advisable. Specific diagnostic tests aimed at documenting immunologically based reactions to specific medications are not commercially available for dogs and cats at the moment. This "lack of solid proof" may well be one of the reasons for the sparse amount of literature being published on the subject of cutaneous vasculitis and one can probably make the assumption that these diseases are underreported. Much of the currently available information is thus based on an association between previous drug exposure and development of clinical signs along with exclusion of other possible triggers.

Itraconazole is a well-known, dose-dependent trigger of vasculitis in dogs. In a report from 1996, Legendre and coworkers reported that 7.5% of dogs receiving a 10 mg/kg dose of itraconazole developed vasculitis, whereas dogs receiving lower doses (5 mg/kg) did not develop lesions.[13]

Recently, nonsteroidal anti-inflammatory drugs have been associated with vasculitis in dogs. Meloxicam was suspected as a trigger of vasculitis in a 10-year-old mixed breed dog from Portugal treated with the drug awaiting surgical repair of a cranial cruciate ligament injury.[14]

An association between meloxicam exposure and cutaneous vasculitis was seen in 3 of 36 dogs in an unpublished retrospective review of canine cutaneous vasculitis (Marie Innerå, unpublished data, 2011); however, a true connection between the drug and the clinical disease was difficult to assess in 2 out of 3 cases because 1 patient had a history of recent exposure to both meloxicam and deracoxib, and another dog received allergen-specific immunotherapy for atopic dermatitis as well as cephalexin at the time of the vasculitic event. A true connection between nonsteroidal anti-inflammatory drugs and cutaneous vasculitis may thus be difficult to assess, owing to the common practice of co-administering of additional medications. However, in the same retrospective study, a 5-year-old Shih Tzu developed cutaneous eosinophilic vasculitis 3 days post administration of beef-flavored chewable firocoxib tablets. Eosinophilic vasculitis has previously been associated with food antigens as a trigger of vasculitis.[3] Whether or not the drug or the flavoring ingredient was the true trigger in this patient remains unknown.

Drugs that have been associated with cutaneous vasculitis in dogs are listed in **Box 3**.

Box 3
Drugs Associated with Cutaneous Vasculitis in Dogs and Cats

- Antibiotics (Cephalexin)
- Ivermectin
- Vaccines
- Metronidazole
- Phenobarbital
- Furosemide
- Itraconazole
- Phenylbutazone
- Enalapril
- Imodium
- Metoclopramide
- Fenbendazole
- NSAIDs (Meloxicam)
- Acempromazin

Refs.[14,57]

Feline vasculitides have also been associated with drugs. A case of systemic vasculitis with cutaneous involvement was reported in a cat after having received fenbendazole[15] and another cat was reported to have developed cutaneous vasculitis as a result of oral cimetidine administration.[16]

Insect Bites

In addition to having an important role as vectors of certain diseases, biting, stinging, or hematophagous insects and ticks may elicit numerous immune responses when stinging or feeding on their hosts.[8] Venomous insects express toxins that may damage tissues directly. When bees and wasps sting, they deposit the tip of their abdomen into the skin and the entire poison apparatus is left in the wound. Salivary antigens from different insects and ticks may also be deposited into the skin during feeding. Thus, there are numerous ways in which insects can introduce foreign antigens into the skin, and in this way trigger immune responses in their hosts.[8]

Infectious Causes

Infectious causes of cutaneous or systemic vasculitis may develop owing to direct invasion of the vessel wall by a pathogen, as a result of immune complex deposition on the vascular endothelium, or via activation of B or T cells.[17]

In human medicine, a distinction is often made between primary and secondary vasculitides, with primary vasculitis representing immunologic or autoimmune diseases with no identifiable infectious agent, and secondary vasculitis representing those vasculitic diseases that should be considered a symptom or clinical feature of an infectious disease by itself.[17] Before the development of advanced molecular diagnostic methods, idiopathic human vasculitides were considered common. However, with recent developments in diagnostic methods, an increasing body of evidence is mounting for the potential role of microbial agents and infections in the pathogenesis of diseases previously considered to be strictly immune mediated.[18] To exemplify this, tissue destruction caused by different microbial agents during an infectious process may lead to formation of autoantibodies directed against various cells, including vascular endothelium. The role of viruses, heat shock proteins, superantigens, and various underlying comorbidities as possible initiators of different immune-mediated diseases is still not fully understood. However, new insight into this area may substantially increase our understanding of these diseases in the future.[17,19]

Viral infections
In dogs, the list of infectious diseases associated with cutaneous vasculitis is extensive. However, a true relationship between viral diseases and cutaneous vasculitis has not been made in canines. In cats, on the other hand, cases of cutaneous vasculitis have been documented in patients suffering from feline infectious peritonitis.

Progression from feline coronavirus infection to the development of feline infectious peritonitis is determined not only by mutations of the virus, but by the animal's immune response and characterized by Immune complex deposition in various organs.[20] Although rare, cats suffering from feline infectious peritonitis have presented with dermatologic clinical signs consisting of slightly raised demarcated and erythematous intradermal nodules or non-pruritic papules along with other organ system involvement.[21–23] In 1 cat, lesions were transient and probably recognized because the affected cat belonged to a hairless breed.[23]

A leukocytoclastic immunologic vasculitis was reported in one of these cases, whereas a pyogranulomatous infiltrate was described in 2 others. Changes restricted to the mid and deep dermis with severe edema and multifocal pyogranulomas, often centered around vessels, along with dermal necrosis and hemorrhage was observed. In addition to dermal vascular pathology, adnexal structures were affected in all 3 cases.[21–23] In 2 out of 3 cases, feline coronavirus antigen was confirmed in both kidney and skin tissues using a mouse monoclonal antibody.[21,22]

Bacterial infections
Bacterial pyoderma was reported to be associated with canine vasculitis in 1978 and a hypersensitivity reaction to bacterial antigens was proposed as the most likely triggering event.[24] In people, nasal carriage of *Staphylococcus aureus* (including methicillin-resistant *S aureus*) has a known affinity for vascular endothelium, and *Staphylococcus aureus* carriage is capable of modulating the expression of WG, a type of human neutrophilic vasculitis. Patients suffering from WG are also more likely to carry *S aureus* (nasal colonization) than normal healthy individuals. Although the majority of patients suffering from WG are nasal carriers of *S aureus*, the corresponding prevalence for the general population is approximately 25%.[25]

The exact pathomechanisms leading to an increased carriage of *S aureus* in human patients suffering from this type of vasculitis and the role of *S aureus* as a cause of exacerbations and flares of WG is unknown. However, several hypotheses have been proposed, including molecular mimicry, binding of cationic staphylococcal enzymes to glomerular endothelial cells, and a direct activation or priming of neutrophils. Patients carrying strains of *Staphylococcus* that produce superantigens, such as toxic shock syndrome superantigen-1 carry a particular strong risk for relapse of their vasculitic disease.[18,25]

Whether or not staphylococcal organisms are of importance in immune-mediated diseases in dogs and cats is not known; however, *Staphylococcus pseudintermedius*, the dominant staphylococcal organism of dogs and cats, has the capacity of producing exotoxins with superantigenic properties.[26]

Gram-negative toxin-producing bacteria has been linked with a specific form of systemic vasculitis mainly occurring in racing Greyhounds fed a diet consisting of undercooked beef. In idiopathic cutaneous and renal glomerular vasculopathy in racing Greyhounds (also known as green track disease and Alabama rot), an association has been made between verotoxin-producing strains of *Escherichia coli* O157:H7 and idiopathic cutaneous and renal glomerular vasculopathy in racing Greyhounds.[1] A purely infectious nature of this syndrome could, however, not be confirmed because oral and intravenous inoculation of adult greyhounds with high doses of idiopathic cutaneous and renal glomerular vasculopathy in racing Greyhounds-producing strains of *E coli* alone failed to produce the disease.[27] Unidentified genetic factors may also be involved, but this acute and potentially lethal syndrome has also been recognized in other breeds such as Great Danes.[28] The true etiology of this disease thus remains unproved.

Affected dogs present with cutaneous lesions consisting of multifocal erythematous cutaneous swellings that may drain a serosanguinous fluid, and affected animals are usually lethargic and febrile. Lesions evolve into sharply demarcated ulcers, and pitting edema of the distal limbs may be present in some dogs. The ventral abdomen and extremities are most commonly affected, sparing the head and dorsum. Gastrointestinal symptoms and signs of acute renal failure may also be present. Some cases present with strictly cutaneous involvement.[1,8]

Fibrinoid necrosis of small dermal arterioles along with full thickness necrosis of the epidermis is the typical dermatohistopathologic finding and renal biopsy specimens usually reveal glomerular lesions with thrombotic microangiopathy and necrosis. Glomerular changes resemble the childhood form of hemorrhagic uremic syndrome in humans; however, children do not develop cutaneous clinical signs.[29]

Bartonella infections may lead to a condition called bacillary angiomatosis in dogs and people. This is a disease in which the vessels are directly invaded by the bacteria, producing lesions that may resemble vasculitis (*pseudovasculitis*). Bacillary angiomatosis was recently described in an immunosuppressed dog, and may in fact be an underdiagnosed disease because it requires special staining to detect the organisms in tissue sections[30]

Tick-transmitted pathogens Associations between different tick-borne diseases and cutaneous vasculitides has long been proposed, but solid evidence of a true correlation between the 2 may be difficult to prove scientifically. There are several reasons for this. First, there may be a failure to recognize the importance of ticks as disease agents themselves.[31] Also, a substantial number of animals may be seropositive for specific tick-borne pathogens in endemic areas, making a true correlation between vasculitic diseases and tick-transmitted pathogens difficult to prove.[32]

Classical symptoms of the different tick-borne illnesses are usually easily recognized in endemic areas. However, animals with an incomplete protective immune response commonly develop persistent subclinical infection, which can recrudesce with stress or concurrent disease.[33] In these cases, low numbers of organisms and cryptic infections make diagnosis difficult using standard methods. Continued antigenemia can lead to the induction of polysystemic, immune-mediated disease such as cyclic anemia, thrombocytopenia, polyarthropathy, uveitis, and vasculitis. Infected animals commonly have high serum globulin levels with monoclonal or polyclonal gammopathies and immune complex formation.[34]

The true prevalence of tick-transmitted pathogens as triggers of canine cutaneous vasculitis is unknown. However, in a recent review of 36 cases of cutaneous necrotizing vasculitis, tick titers were performed as part of the workup for their vasculitic disease in 10 of the 36 dogs. Three of these 10 dogs showed significant elevation in tick titers. One had elevated *Ehrlichia* titers, 1 had a significantly elevated *Anaplasma phagocytophilum* titer, and 1 young dog presented with a *Borrelia burgdorferi* titer of 1:2560 (reference range >80 considered negative). In the latter dog, a convalescent tick titer was performed 4 weeks after initiating treatment with anti-inflammatory doses of prednisolone and standard doses of doxycycline, and a significant titer reduction was observed along with clinical resolution of cutaneous clinical signs.

Another retrospective study involving 21 cases of cutaneous vasculitis failed to identify cases associated with elevated tick titers, but this study also included a substantial number of patients suffering from ischemic dermatopathies.[3]

Although tick-transmitted pathogens have different target cells, most of them are deposited directly into the skin of their host during a blood meal. *B burgdorferi* in particular replicate in the skin before systemic dissemination.[35]

Beagles experimentally infected with *B burgdorferi* organisms were shown to harbor *B burgdorferi* in their skin as measured by polymerase chain reaction and skin cultures as late as 14 months (end of study) after initial inoculation. An even longer period of tissue replication could potentially be expected, which would mean that these patients experience chronic ongoing antigen stimulation lasting several months to several years.[33]

An established relationship between canine granulocytic anaplasmosis and cutaneous vasculitis has yet to be documented, but anecdotal reports of cases presenting with cutaneous vasculitis and significantly elevated *A phagocytophilum* antibody titer are occasionally encountered by clinicians in different countries.

A study evaluating a possible association between *A phagocytophilum* infection as measured by positive serologic antibody titers and skin lesions in dogs was recently conducted. Of 12 seropositive dogs presenting with skin lesions, DNA for *A phagocytophilum* could be detected in the cutaneous tissue of 3 dogs using molecular diagnostic techniques (polymerase chain reaction). The histologic findings of these dogs were characterized by moderate to severe edema with variable hemorrhage. A superficial and periadnexal mixed cell infiltrate and multifocal nodules, composed of neutrophils and macrophages were seen as well. Established vasculitic criteria, however, could not be confirmed on examined skin biopsies from these dogs.[36]

Neoplastic Processes

Vasculitis presenting as a paraneoplastic syndrome secondary to various underlying malignancies, both solid tumors and hematopoietic cancers does occur but is inconsistently documented most likely owing to the inability of collecting larger case series for systematic reviews. In general, paraneoplastic syndromes may antedate the neoplasm, may occur simultaneously, or may become apparent during the late stages of the malignant disease.[37] Diagnostic imaging at the time of initial presentation is advised in older patients presenting with cutaneous necrotizing vasculitis, because treatment with immunosuppressive agents may delay a diagnosis of hematopoietic cancers particularly.

No definite connection has been made between particular neoplastic processes and the development of vasculitides in canine or feline patients so far.

Adverse Reactions to Food

Cutaneous vasculitis may be the only presenting clinical sign of an adverse reaction to food in dogs.[3] It has so far not been described in the cat.

The mechanism by which food antigens trigger this cutaneous reaction pattern is not known. The majority of these food allergic dogs have presented with an urticarial form of vasculitis with dermatologic findings presenting as intense erythroderma and generalized erythematous serpentine wheals that fail to blanch on diascopy (**Fig. 1**).[3] A chronic angioedema that often fails to respond to glucocorticoid treatment may be the dominant clinical symptom in some patients, and gastrointestinal signs with soft stools, large bowel diarrhea, flatulence, and frequent bowel movements (>3 per day) may or may not accompany the dermatologic signs. More typical signs of cutaneous necrotizing vasculitis with erythroderma skin necrosis and deep crateriform cutaneous ulcers have also been observed (author's unpublished observations, 2007).

In cases where urticarial vasculitis was the primary presenting clinical sign, histology often revealed an eosinophilic infiltrate; however vasculitis triggered by food may as well be neutrophilic (author's unpublished observations, 2009–2011).

When presented with cases of cutaneous vasculitis, 1 or more elimination and provocation diets should be performed if other triggers cannot be identified. A home-cooked, novel protein diet is recommended; however, hydrolyzed protein diets may also be attempted.

Autoimmune Diseases

Multisystemic involvement associated with cutaneous lesions compatible with vasculitis should alert the clinician to a possible systemic autoimmune disease process as systemic and cutaneous vasculitis may be a feature of such diseases. In dogs, vasculitis has been associated with systemic lupus erythematosus, discoid lupus erythematosus, and rheumatoid arthritis.[7]

Genetic/Familial Forms

Familial pyogranuloma and vasculitis of Scottish Terriers

In 1991, Pedersen and Scott reported a disease in related Scottish Terriers from Denmark in which young animals presented with severe non-painful ulcerations affecting both the nasal planum and the nasal cartilage itself. Affected dogs ranged in age from 3 weeks to 6 months and also showed constitutional signs such as lethargy, depression, and intermittent fever. Both genders were affected and all dogs were from the same breeder. Histologic findings consisted of pyogranulomatous inflammation along with a leukocytoclastic vasculitis. Attempted treatment with prednisolone in 1 case proved to be ineffective and all dogs were eventually humanely killed.[38]

Additional cases have since been reported in other countries—1 case from Argentina and 1 from the United States. The ethiopathogenesis of this disease is currently unknown. Based on preliminary pedigree analyses, the disease is suspected to represent an autosomal-dominant genodermatosis.[39]

Acute febrile neutrophilic vasculitis of the skin of young Shar-Pei dogs

In 2002, Malik and coworkers described 3 cases of necrotizing neutrophilic vasculitis in young Shar Pei dogs. All the affected dogs presented with constitutional signs of before the onset of, or along with the development of, cutaneous lesions. Extensive edema, especially of the face and extremities, that subsequently developed into multifocal, full-thickness skin necrosis and deep cutaneous ulcerations was seen dermatologically. Two dogs responded to treatment with steroids and various antibiotics, whereas 1 dog showed a better response to enrofloxacin than a combination of immunosuppressive treatment, clavulanate-potentiated amoxicillin, and cephalexin along with injectable dexamethasone. A pedigree analysis was not possible to perform in these cases and a genetic etiology could not be confirmed. Two of these 3 dogs had been vaccinated with a live virus vaccine 3 weeks before the onset of illness, and 2 dog dogs had also been exposed to antibacterial treatment with a combination of amoxicillin and clavulanic acid. Whether this disease represents a genodermatosis in the Chinese Shar Pei is currently unknown. Additional cases have not been reported so far.[40]

Proliferative arteritis of the nasal philtrum

A highly distinctive arteritis affecting only the nasal philtrum was originally described in 4 St Bernards and a Giant Schnauzer.[41] Subsequently, the disease has also been described in a Newfoundland and a Basset Hound. A genetic predisposition seems to exist in the St Bernard.[5,42]

The typical appearance is of a solitary, well-circumscribed, round, or sometimes V-shaped ulcer that is neither painful nor pruritic. Episodes of arterial bleeding may occur in affected dogs, a situation that often warrants emergency interventions.[5,42]

The visual appearance of this distinct disease of the St. Bernard is striking, but diagnosis should still be confirmed histologically to differentiate it from other disease processes that may affect the nasal cartilage.

Histologically, changes are highly characteristic and not comparable with the other vasculitides covered within this article. The disease targets the deep dermal arteries, and subendothelial spindle cell proliferation is seen within these vessels. A marked extracellular matrix deposition containing mucin and collagen may also be seen subjacent to the ulcer. This leads to intimal thickening and stenosis of dermal arteries and arterioles. Immunohistochemical studies have shown that spindle cells proliferating within this thickened area of vascular intima are positive for smooth muscle actin and vimentin and negative for factor VIII-related antigen, suggesting either myofibroblast or smooth muscle-like differentiation of the proliferating cells. Superficial changes have included neutrophilic dermal inflammation and lymphoplasmacytic dermatitis.[7]

Long-term treatment with immunosuppressive therapies have been used, including prednisolone, topical fluocinolone in dimethyl sulphoxide, a combination of tetracycline and niacinamide, and fish oil.[42] In the author's experience, topical tacrolimus ointment applied 2 or 3 times a day for extended period has been effective as well. Surgical treatment options for this disease has also been proposed[42]

Idiopathic

Idiopathic vasculitis is clearly a diagnosis of exclusion. If no triggering agent can be detected, a diagnosis of idiopathic vasculitis can be made. In a retrospective study of vasculitis in dogs and cats, the diagnosis was idiopathic in 10 of 21 cases. The corresponding numbers from a recent unpublished study concluded with idiopathy in 9 of 36 cases.

TREATMENT

Treatment must be tailored to the individual patient and should be based on history, clinical findings, identification of the inciting cause, and whether or not the disease is progressing or regressing. In patients suffering severe and extensive cutaneous ulcerations, adequate wound care is essential to prevent secondary bacterial infections and sepsis.

Treatment should not lead to a worsening of the patient's prognosis and care should be taken to make sure underlying diseases and comorbidities that may affect the outcome are not missed.[1] Treatment may in some cases be guided by the histologic inflammatory pattern.[3,7]

Avoidance of Triggers

If drugs or "drug-like substances" are suspected, the most important treatment is removal and future avoidance of such agents. Keep in mind that the inciting agent can also be the vehicle of a drug and not only the drug itself (eg, capsules containing gelatin may be the triggering factor of hypersensitivity vasculitis in a beef-allergic dog). In patients suffering from vasculitis triggered by an adverse reaction to drugs, removal of the drug along with close patient monitoring may in fact be the only treatment necessary. This may also be true for patients presenting with severe and extensive ulcerations of the skin. As an example, a patient presenting with severe ulcerations affecting 20% of the total body surface with a particular drug as the only triggering factor may not benefit from glucocorticoid treatment unless the disease is progressing, because this may only serve to delay wound healing and increase the risk of wound infection and sepsis. Such patients may benefit more from drug withdrawal and proper wound care along with future avoidance of the offending drug.

Care should, therefore, be taken when planning treatment of these patients and therapy should be based on the individual patient's needs. Close monitoring of the patient during the early phase of the disease is essential to decide on a proper treatment regiment suitable for each individual case.

Glucocorticoids

If no underlying trigger of vasculitis can be identified, and the disease is progressing during the initial 24 to 48 hours of monitoring glucocorticoid therapy should be considered. Older literature has recommended immunosuppressive doses ranging between 2 and 4 mg/kg of prednisolone.[8] However, the author prefers starting at a lower dose of 0.5 to 1 mg/kg of prednisolone. Starting at lower doses makes sense because prednisolone doses can easily be increased if necessary, higher doses are associated with severe side effects and poor wound healing, and significant immunosuppression may predispose animals with severe and extensive cutaneous ulcerations to secondary (wound) infections and sepsis. Furthermore, in the early phase of the disease, several diagnostic tests may still be pending, including tests for infectious conditions (blood cultures, tick titers, and tissue cultures). Administering high doses of steroids during this phase of disease could therefore have detrimental effects and negatively affect treatment outcome if it is later discovered that the animal was suffering from an infectious condition.

When a dose sufficient of halting progression of clinical signs has been established, the patient is kept on this dose until clinical remission is achieved. Slow tapering with a 25% dose reduction every 14 days is then attempted.[1]

Oral prednisone or prednisolone are both alternatives for dogs; however, prednisone has a relative bioavailability of 65% compared with prednisolone because it needs to be actively converted in the liver.[43] Oral prednisolone is the drug of choice in cats.[44] Cases refractory to prednisolone may benefit from triamcinolone or dexamethasone.

Patient follow-up Patients on long-term glucocorticoid treatment should have a complete blood count, serum chemistry profile, urinalysis, and a urine culture performed at least every 6 months[45,46]

Calcineurin inhibitors

Cyclosporine A is a systemic immunosuppressant licensed for systemic administration to both dogs and cats. In recent years, it has been used off label for the treatment of an increasing spectrum of immune-mediated and inflammatory diseases. Cyclosporine exerts its effect by blocking transcription of genes required for T-cell activation.[47,48] See article by Palmeiro elsewhere in this issue for details on mechanisms of action and dose regimens. There are, however, no solid studies evaluating efficacy of this medication for the treatment of cutaneous vasculitis in dogs and cats. Based on anecdotal reports, cyclosporine may be effective in the treatment of some cases of cutaneous vasculitis.[1,7] The author would consider this drug in patients that require long-term medical management of idiopathic vasculitis, especially in patients that cannot tolerate glucocorticoid therapy.

Cytotoxic agents

Use of cytotoxic agents for the treatment of cutaneous vasculitis may be necessary when other therapeutic measures have failed or are otherwise contraindicated[1,7]

Azathioprine, a prodrug of 6-mercaptopurine, is an immunosuppressant and corticosteroid-sparing agent used for the treatment of several immune mediated diseases in dogs. Thiopurine antimetabolites compete with endogenous purines for incorporation into RNA and DNA, resulting in nonsense sequences. DNA and RNA syntheses are thus inhibited, and mitosis and cellular metabolism disrupted.[49]

Azathioprine is a potent cytotoxic agent that may be considered as a steroid-sparing agent in cases refractory to empiric anti-inflammatory therapy to reduce side effects associated with persistent high-dose corticosteroid therapy. Some dogs may experience life-threatening myelosupression, consisting of profound neutropenias, lymphopenias, and thrombocytopenias, as a result of standard azathioprine dosing.[50] Weekly or biweekly complete blood counts should be performed in all patients treated with azathioprine. Other uncommon adverse effects include hepatotoxicity, pancreatitis and gastrointestinal distress.[47] Myelosupression occurs more frequently in the cat preventing the widespread use of this drug in feline patients.[49]

The clinician needs to keep in mind that there may be a considerable lag time before full effect of this drug is reached; 1 to 6 weeks have been reported.[1,51] Once the patient is clinically stable, tapering to the lowest necessary dose should be attempted to minimize side effects.[1] The author prefers to start with a dose of 1 to 2 mg/kg, and uses the lower range of the dose in schnauzers or related breeds.[52] The dose is then tapered down slowly (every 14–21 days) to a dose of 1 or 0.5 mg/kg before tapering down further to every 48 hours and if possible every 72 hours.

Patient follow-up A complete blood count, serum chemistry profile, and urinalysis is performed before starting therapy. A complete blood count is then performed weekly in the initial phase of treatment.[1]

Chlorambucil may be used in cases incapable of tolerating azathioprine. The starting dose is 0.1 to 0.2 mg/kg orally once daily or every other day. Side effects and patient follow-up are as for azathioprine.[1]

Xanthin derivatives

Pentoxiphylline is a methylxanthine derivative with both hemorheologic (changes the conformation of erythrocytes, improves microcirculatory blood flow, and tissue oxygenation) and immunomodulatory effects that traditionally has been recommended as a suitable treatment option for cutaneous vasculitides.[8] Its value in the treatment of true cutaneous vasculitis is difficult to assess, because it is more commonly used in combination with other treatments. Some clinicians, including the author, find it to be a valuable drug when dealing with ischemic dermatopathies (see article by Morris elsewhere in this issue), but it is rarely effective as a single agent for the treatment of neutrophilic vasculitis.[53] The onset of action is slow, and several weeks to months may be required before clinical response is seen.[1,54] Pentoxiphylline is, however, a safe drug, is associated with few side effects in dogs, and should not be discarded as a steroid-sparing agent in patients that require long-term management of their disease. Gastrointestinal irritation, although rare, has been reported as a side effect.

Drugs targeting neutrophil function

Tetracycline/niacinamide The combination of tetracycline and niacinamide could be considered a treatment in milder cases of cutaneous vasculitis.[1,7] Tetracyclines (tetracycline, doxycycline, monocycline) exert a variety of anti-inflammatory and immunomodulating properties by themselves or in combination with niacinamide (synonyms are nicotinamide and nicotinic acid amide). The combination of tetracyclines and niacinamide has the ability to inhibit blast transformation of lymphocytes and chemotaxis of neutrophils and eosinophils; however, their exact mechanism of action in immune-mediated diseases is not completely understood.[55]

Dosing alternatives

Tetracycline/niacinamide For dogs weighing less than 10 kg, give 250 mg/dog of each drug orally every 8 hours with food. For dogs weighing more than 10 kg, give 500 mg/dog of each drug orally every 8 hours with food.[56] Alternatively, a dosage of 22 mg/kg every 8 to 12 hours, rounded to the nearest convenient tablet size (tablets are easily halved or quartered), may be calculated (Dr Daniel O. Morris, personal communication, 2012). Tetracycline has recently become unavailable in the United States, and doxycycline may be substituted for it at a dosage of 5 to 10 mg/kg every 12 hours. Niacinamide should still be administered every 8 hours when possible, until remission is established, but can often be tapered thereafter.

Patient follow-up This drug combination is usually well-tolerated by most dogs, but side effects have been reported, most commonly owing to niacinamide. Vomiting, lethargy, anorexia, diarrhea, and elevated liver values have been observed.[57] Tetracyclines are also capable of lowering seizure thresholds in epileptics and may induce hepatopathy.[1]

Sulfasalazine and dapsone Sulfonamide drugs can be highly effective in treatment of neutrophilic cutaneous vasculitis failing to respond to other alternative therapies. Sulfasalazine is usually preferred over dapsone, because the latter has been associated with more severe hepatotoxicities[3,7]

Side effects associated with sulfa drugs are well-documented in dogs and includes anemia, leukopenia, keratoconjunctivitis sicca, and hepatotoxicity. Blood dyscrasias, cutaneous eruptions, nephrotoxicity, and neuropathies can also occur. Keratoconjunctivitis sicca has been shown to be reversible with reduction of either dosage or frequency of administration.[7]

For sulfasalazine, a dose of 25 mg/kg 3 times per day has been recommended. It is advised not to exceed a total dose of 3 g per day. Dapsone is dosed at 1 mg/kg by mouth once daily.

Patient follow-up A complete blood count, serum chemistry profile, and Schirmer tear test should be performed every 2 weeks for the initial 2 months of treatment. If no adverse events are observed during this period, follow-up can be reduced to once every 30 days for 2 months and then every 3 months as long as the dog remains on the treatment.[1]

SUMMARY

Cutaneous vasculitis is an inflammatory process targeting blood vessels. A number of underlying factors may be associated with vasculitides in dogs and cats, including drugs, infectious diseases, adverse reactions to food, malignancies, and immune-mediated diseases. Vasculitis should thus be regarded as a reaction pattern that warrants an extensive workup of the patient to identify such triggers. Affected patients present with a variety of symptoms, such as purpura, pitting edema, and ulcerations of the skin. Constitutional signs such as fever, depression, and anorexia are common and seem to be present in the majority of patients. Once a diagnosis is confirmed by compatible histologic findings, treatment, and follow-up must be tailored to the individual patient. High doses of immunosuppressive medications are only recommended once infectious diseases capable of producing a similar constellation of clinical signs have been ruled out.

REFERENCES

1. Bloom PB. Cutaneous vasculitis: what it is and how you treat it. In the 25th Proceedings of the North American Veterinary Dermatology Forum. Portland, April 14–17, 2010.
2. Cuchacovich R. Immunopathogenesis of vasculitis. Curr Rheumatol Rep 2002;4: 9–17.
3. Nichols PR, Morris DO, Beale KM. A retrospective study of canine and feline cutaneous vasculitis. Vet Dermatol 2001;12:255–64.
4. Rajan TV. The Gell–Coombs classification of hypersensitivity reactions: a re-interpretation. Trends Immunol 2003;24(7):376–9.
5. Gross TL, Ihrke PJ, Walder EJ, et al. Skin diseases of the dog and cat: clinical and histopathologic diagnosis. 2nd edition. Oxford (UK): Blackwell Science Ltd; 2005. p. 238–47.
6. Voie KL, Campbell KL, Lavergne SN. Drug Hypersensitivity reactions targeting the skin in dogs and cats. J Vet Intern Med 2012;26(4):863–74.
7. Morris D. Cutaneous vasculitis. In: Proceedings of the 25th annual Congress of the ESVD-ECVD. Brussels, September 8–10, 2011.
8. Scott DW, Miller WH, Griffin CE. Muller & Kirk's small animal dermatology. 6th edition. Philadelphia: W.B. Saunders; 2001. p. 506–7, 742–56.
9. Rosser EJ Jr. Use of the D-dimer assay for diagnosing thrombosis in cases of canine cutaneous vasculitis. Vet Dermatol 2009;20(5–6):586–90.
10. Nelson OL, Andreasen C. The utility of plasma D-dimer to identify thromboembolic disease in dogs. J Vet Intern Med 2003;7:830–84.
11. Monreal L. D-dimer as a new test for the diagnosis of DIC and thromboembolic disease [editorial]. J Vet Intern Med 2003;17:757–79.
12. Gasser AM, Birkenheuer AJ, Breitschwerdt EB. Canine rocky mountain spotted fever: a retrospective study of 30 cases. J Am Anim Hosp Assoc 2001;(1): 41–8.
13. Legendre AM, Rohrbach BW, Toal RL, et al. Treatment of blastomycosis with itraconazole in 112 dogs. J Vet Intern Med 1996;10:365.
14. Niza MM, Felix N, Vilela CL, et al. Cutaneous and ocular adverse reactions in a dog following meloxicam administration. Vet Dermatol 2007;18:45–9.
15. Jasani S, Boag AK, Smith KC. Systemic vasculitis with severe cutaneous manifestation as a suspected idiosyncratic hypersensitivity reaction to fenbendazole in a cat. J Vet Intern Med 2008;22:666–70.
16. McEwan NA, McNeil PE, Kirkham D, et al. Drug eruption in a cat resembling pemphigus foliaceus. J Small Anim Pract 1987;28:713–20.
17. Mohan N, Kerr G. Infectious etiology of vasculitis: diagnosis and management. Curr Rheumatol Rep 2003;5:136–41.
18. Kallenberg CG, Tadema H. Vasculitis and infections: contribution to the issue of autoimmunity reviews devoted to "autoimmunity and infection". Autoimmune Rev 2008;8(1):29–32.
19. Oyoo O, Espinoza LR. Infection-related vasculitis. Curr Rheumatol Rep 2005;7(4): 281–7.
20. Hartmann K. Feline infectious peritonitis. Vet Clin North Am Small Anim Pract 2005;35:39–79.

21. Cannon MJ, Silkstone MA, Kipar AM. Cutaneous lesions associated with coronavirus-induced vasculitis in a cat with feline infectious peritonitis and concurrent feline immunodeficiency virus infection. J Feline Med Surg 2005; 7(4):233–6.
22. Declerq J, De Bosschere H, Schwarzkopf I, et al. Papular cutaneous lesions in a cat associated with feline infectious peritonitis. Vet Dermatol 2008;19(5):255–8.
23. Gross TL. Pyogranulomatous vasculitis and mural folliculitis associated with feline infectious peritonitis in a sphinx cat. Vet Pathol 1999;36:507.
24. Scott DW, MacDonald JM, Schultz RD. Staphylococcal hypersensitivity in the dog. J Am Anim Hosp Assoc 1978;14:766–79.
25. Popa ER, Stegeman CA, Abdulahad WH, et al. Staphylococcal toxic-shock-syndrome-toxin-1 as a risk factor for disease relapse in Wegener's granulomatosis. Rheumatology (Oxford) 2007;46:1029–133.
26. Yoon JW, Lee GJ, Lee SY, et al. Prevalence of genes for enterotoxins, toxic shock syndrome toxin 1 and exfoliative toxin among clinical isolates of Staphylococcus pseudintermedius from canine origin. Vet Dermatol 2010;21(5):484–9.
27. Renninger MR, White MR, Saeed AM, et al. Oral and intravenous inoculation of greyhound dogs with Escherichia coli O157:H7 did not result in cutaneous renal glomerular vasculopathy. Abstracts from the American Association of Veterinary Laboratory Diagnosticians 43rd Annual Meeting. October 21–23, 2000.
28. Rotermund A, Peters M, Hewicker-Trautwein M, et al. Cutaneous and renal glomerular vasculopathy in a great Dane resembling "Alabama rot" of greyhounds. Vet Rec 2002;151:510–52.
29. Hertzke DM, Cowan LA, Schoning P, et al. Glomerular ultrastructural lesions of idiopathic cutaneous and renal glomerular vasculopathy of greyhounds. Vet Pathol 1995;32:451–9.
30. Yager JA, Best SJ, Maggi RG, et al. Bacillary angiomatosis in an immunosuppressed dog. Vet Dermatol 2010;21(4):420–48.
31. Willadsen P, Jongejan F. Immunology of the tick-host interaction and the control of ticks and tick borne diseases. Parasitol Today 1999;15(7):258–62.
32. Bowman D, Little SE, Lorentzen L, et al. Prevalence and geographic distribution of Dirofilaria immitis, Borrelia burgdorferi, Ehrlichia canis and Anaplasma phagocytophilum in dog in the United States: results of a national clinic-bases serologic survey. Vet Parasitol 2009;160(1–2):138–48.
33. Straubinger RK, Summers BA, Chang YF, et al. Persistence of Borrelia burgdorferi in experimentally infected dogs after antibiotic treatment. J Clin Microbiol 1997;35:111–6.
34. Shaw SE, Day MJ, Birtles RJ, et al. Tick-borne infectious diseases of dogs. Trends Parasitol 2001;17:74–80.
35. Straubinger RK, Alix F, Straubinger AF, et al. Status of borrelia burgdorferi infection after antibiotic treatment and the effects of corticosteroids: an experimental study. J Infect Dis 2000;181(3):1069–181.
36. Berzina I, Müller N, Krudewig C, et al. PCR-based detection of A. phagocytophilum DNA in paraffin embedded skin biopsies from dogs seropositive against A. phagocytophilum –Abstract accepted for presentation at ECVCP & ISACP Conference. July 3–7, 2012.
37. Turek MM. Cutaneous paraneoplastic syndromes in dogs and cats: a review of the literature. Vet Dermatol 2003;14:279.
38. Pedersen K, Scott DW. Idiopathic pyogranulomatous inflammation and leukocytoclastic vasculitis of the nasal planum and nostrils and nasal mucosa in Scottish terriers in Denmark. Vet Dermatol 1991;2(2):85–9.

39. Tonelli EA, Benson CJ, Scott DW, et al. Hereditary pyogranuloma and vasculitis of the nasal plane in Scottish terriers: two new cases from Argentina and the United States. Jpn J Vet Dermatol 2009;15(2):69–73.

40. Malik R, Foster SF, Martin P, et al. Acute febrile neutrophilic vasculitis of the skin of young Shar-Pei dogs. Aust Vet J 2002;80:200–26.

41. Torres SM, Brien TO, Scott DW. Dermal arteritis of the nasal philtrum in a Giant Schnauzer and three Saint Bernard dogs. Vet Dermatol 2002;13(5):275–81.

42. Pratschke KM, Hill PB. Dermal arteritis of the nasal philtrum: surgery as an alternative to long-term medical therapy in two dogs. J Small Anim Pract 2009;50(2):99–103.

43. Colburn WA, Sibley CR, Buller RH. Comparative serum prednisone and prednisolone concentrations following prednisone or prednisolone administration to beagle dogs. J Pharm Sci 1976;65:997–1001.

44. Graham-Mize CA, Rosser EJ. Bioavailability and activity of prednisone and prednisolone in the feline patient. Plenary Session Abstracts. Vet Dermatol 2004; 25(Suppl 1):1–19.

45. Ihrke PJ, Norton AL, Ling GV, et al. Urinary tract infections associated with long-term corticosteroid administration in dogs with chronic skin disease. J Am Vet Med Assoc 1992;200:1497–500.

46. Torres SM, Diaz SF, Nogueira SA. Frequency of urinary tract infections among dogs with pruritic disorders receiving long term glucocorticoid treatment. J Am Vet Med Assoc 2005;227:239–43.

47. Whitley NT, Day MJ. Immunomodulatory drugs and their application to the management of canine immune-mediated disease. J Small Anim Pract 2011;52:70–85.

48. Gaugere E, Steffan J, Olivry T, et al. a new drug in the field of canine dermatology. Vet Dermatol 2005;15:61–74.

49. Beale KM. Azathioprine for treatment of immune-mediated diseases of dogs and cats. J Am Vet Med Assoc 1988;192:1316–8.

50. Rinkardt NE, Kruth SA. Azathioprine-induced bone marrow toxicity in four dogs. Can Vet J 1996;37:612–3.

51. Houston DM, Taylor JA. Acute pancreatitis and bone marrow suppression in a dog given azathioprine. Can Vet J 1991;32:496–7.

52. Rodriguez DB, Mackin A, Easley R. Relationship between red blood cell thiopurine methyltransferase activity and myelotoxicity in dogs receiving azathioprine. J Vet Intern Med 2004;18:339–45.

53. DeBoer DJ, Affolter VK, Hill PB. Workshop: "Variabilities in Vasculitis," In: Advances in veterinary dermatology. vol. 6. Proceedings of the Sixth World Congress of Veterinary Dermatology Hong Kong. 2008. p. 408–13.

54. Rothstein E, Scott DW, Riis RC. Tetracycline and niacinamide for the treatment of sterile pyogranuloma/granuloma syndrome in a dog. J Am Anim Hosp Assoc 1997;33(6):540–3.

55. Scott DW, Miller WJ, Griffin GE. Miscellaneous skin diseases. In: Scott Danny W, Miller William H Jr, Griffin Craig E, editors. Small animal dermatology. Philadelphia: WB Saunders; 2001. p. 1136–40.

56. White SD, Rosychuk RA, Reinke SI, et al. Tetracycline and Niacinamide for treatment of autoimmune skin diseases in 31 dogs. J Am Vet Med Assoc 1992;200: 1497–500.

57. Scott DW, Miller WJ, Griffin GE. Miscellaneous skin diseases. In: Scott Danny W, Miller William H Jr, Griffin Craig E, editors. Small animal dermatology. Philadelphia: WB Saunders; 2001. p. 754.

Cutaneous Manifestations of Internal Diseases

Catherine A. Outerbridge, DVM, MVSc

KEYWORDS

- Cutaneous markers of internal disease • Paraneoplastic skin disease
- Metabolic skin disease • Endocrine skin disease

KEY POINTS

- The skin's appearance and integrity is influenced by internal factors, such as hormonal levels and overall health of the animal. Consequently, changes in the skin can be a critical sentinel for internal disease.
- Recognizing those skin changes that are clinical markers for internal disease can expedite the diagnosis and timely management of certain systemic diseases.
- The skin changes seen with endocrine disease are good examples of the connection between the skin and internal disease.
- Paraneoplastic skin diseases, such as feline paraneoplastic alopecia, provide clinically distinct, cutaneous clues to the clinician about internal neoplasia.
- Several systemic infectious diseases can be associated with skin lesions, and biopsies of the skin can, in some cases, provide the diagnostic information to confirm the diagnosis.

INTRODUCTION

The skin's functions in providing innate protection and maintaining homeostasis along with the systemic factors that can influence its integrity make it a critical sentinel for internal disease. Some cutaneous changes are so intimately associated with a particular underlying organ dysfunction or disorder that they are immediate visual clues to evaluate for specific diseases. Evaluation for disturbances in hemostasis or vascular integrity is clearly indicated when petechiations or ecchymoses are identified on the skin or mucosal surfaces of patients. The color change seen in an animal with icteric mucous membranes is a clear indicator to evaluate for causes of jaundice in that patient. Changes in the appearance of the skin may be markers of pathology occurring in another organ system or they may represent a disease process that is multisystemic, such as seen with some infectious diseases or in systemic lupus erythematosus. Both the appearance and integrity of the skin are influenced by several systemic factors. These factors include the nutritional status, hormonal levels and interactions,

Department of Veterinary Medicine and Epidemiology, William Pritchard Veterinary Medical Teaching Hospital, University of California Davis, One Shields Avenue, Davis, CA 95616, USA
E-mail address: caouterbridge@ucdavis.edu

Vet Clin Small Anim 43 (2013) 135–152
http://dx.doi.org/10.1016/j.cvsm.2012.09.010
0195-5616/13/$ – see front matter © 2013 Elsevier Inc. All rights reserved.

perfusion and vascular integrity, and the overall health and systemic organ function of the individual animal. The skin is also readily accessible for diagnostic sampling and can in some cases provide the necessary information for making the diagnosis of internal disease.

CUTANEOUS CHANGES ASSOCIATED WITH HORMONAL DISTURBANCES

Endocrine diseases provide excellent examples of the connection between internal disease and the skin. Hypothyroidism, hyperadrenocorticism (HAC), and sex hormone imbalances from testicular neoplasia, ovarian tumors, or adrenal tumors (see later discussion) can alter the skin's appearance and function.

Hypothyroidism

Thyroid hormones are important to the skin and promote the initiation of the anagen phase of the hair follicle cycle.[1,2] Consequently, many hypothyroid dogs have some degree of alopecia. This alopecia is often first noted in areas of wear (neck under collar, dorsal tail, pressure points, lateral trunk). The extent and pattern of alopecia can vary among breeds of dogs and individual animals. For example, Rhodesian Ridgebacks can develop a pronounced striping pattern (**Fig. 1**).[2] The persisting hair coat is often dry and brittle and can be dull or faded.[3] Failure to regrow hair coat after clipping is sometimes a presenting complaint of hypothyroid dogs.[2,3] Hypothyroidism results in disturbances in cornification and melanosis, an increase in the number of hair follicles in telogen, and accumulation of glycosaminoglycans in the dermis.[2,3] Clinically, this results in alopecia, a dull, dry hair coat, variable hyperpigmentation, scaling, and myxedematous changes. Pinnal margin seborrhea may be seen in some dogs (**Fig. 2**).[2] In hypothyroidism, the normal barrier function of the epidermis is likely impaired, and in animal models impaired neutrophil and lymphocyte function has been reported. Consequently, recurrent pyoderma and otitis externa often occur.[3] In some cases, recurrent or refractory otitis externa or recurrent pyoderma may be the only presenting clinical signs in a dog with hypothyroidism.

Hyperadrenocorticism

Dermatologic changes seen in dogs with HAC occur because glucocorticoids cause cornification abnormalities, inhibition of fibroblast proliferation and collagen production, and pilosebaceous gland atrophy. Clinically, excessive cortisol (endogenous or exogenous) also results in disturbances in cornification, dermal thinning, and delayed

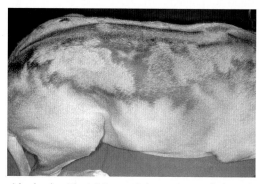

Fig. 1. A Rhodesian ridgeback with striking, striping pattern of alopecia secondary to hypothyroidism. (*Courtesy of* Dr. Stephen White.)

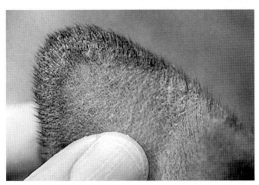

Fig. 2. A hypothyroid dog with pinnal margin seborrhea characterized by follicular casting and adherence of keratinized debris along the pinnal margin. (*Courtesy of* University of California Davis, Veterinary Dermatology Service.)

wound healing. Dogs with HAC or iatrogenic hypercortisolism can develop bilaterally symmetric alopecia, thin hypotonic skin susceptible to bruising, easily visible dermal vasculature, phlebectasias, comedones, calcinosis cutis, increased susceptibility to recurrent pyoderma and adult onset demodicosis.[3]

Calcinosis cutis

This is a broad term and includes all forms of dystrophic or metastatic calcification of the skin. More specifically, the term is often used for the dystrophic calcification seen in dogs secondary to hyperadrenocorticism or iatrogenic hyperglucocorticoidism. Erythematous papules coalesce into firm, gritty plaques that may ulcerate and develop hemorrhagic crusts. Lesions often develop in areas prone to chronic flexure movement, and the dorsal cervical, axillary, or inguinal areas are common lesional sites (**Fig. 3**). Dystrophic calcification can also involve mucosal membranes and the tongue. Metastatic calcification producing nodular calcium deposits in the skin, especially foot-pads, has been reported in dogs and cats with chronic renal failure.[2] The author has documented calcinosis cutis lesions in the inguinal region of a dog supplemented chronically with calcitriol postparathyroidectomy. Lesions of calcinosis cutis typically resolve in time if the underlying metabolic disturbance can be removed. In some cases, osseous metaplasia can occur. The resulting osteoma cutis lesions will not regress.

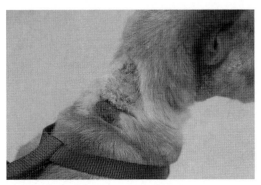

Fig. 3. Calcinosis cutis lesion is present in the dorsal cervical region of this dog. Erythematous plaque was indurated on palpation and had some hemorrhagic crusting associated with it. (*Courtesy of* University of California Davis, Veterinary Dermatology Service.)

Feline-acquired skin fragility

Acquired skin fragility in cats is associated with hyperadrenocorticism (often adrenal tumors), iatrogenic hyperglucocorticoidism, or excessive levels of progestational compounds from either adrenal tumors or the iatrogenic effect of administered progestational compounds. Affected cats have extremely thin, fragile skin that easily bruises and can be torn with simple manipulations, often during restraint or handling. There are also rare reports of feline skin fragility being associated with hepatic lipidosis and hepatic neoplasia.[2]

CUTANEOUS PARANEOPLASTIC MARKERS

Paraneoplastic skin diseases represent a group of skin disorders that, if recognized, alert the clinician to underlying internal neoplastic disease. These disorders include cutaneous changes and feminization seen with testicular tumors, feline paraneoplastic alopecia, feline thymoma-associated exfoliative dermatitis, nodular dermatofibrosis, paraneoplastic pemphigus, and superficial necrolytic dermatitis associated with glucagonoma.

Testicular Tumors (Hyperestrogenism)

Increased estrogen can arise from cystic ovaries, granulosa cell tumors, or testicular tumors (Sertoli cell tumors most commonly) or iatrogenically from estrogen supplementation for urinary incontinence or chronic exposure to human topical estrogen products. Estrogen inhibits anagen initiation of hair follicles, which results in alopecia. Hyperpigmentation often is present and can be diffuse or macular. In male dogs with testicular tumors (with presumed hyperestrogenism), a visually distinctive lesion of linear preputial hyperpigmentation with varying degrees of erythema often is seen (**Fig. 4**). Hyperestrogenism can also cause feminization in the male dog and in severe cases bone marrow suppression and aplastic anemia. Intact animals should be neutered. Already neutered animals should be evaluated for possible exogenous sources of estrogen (diethylstilbestrol) as may be used for urinary incontinence or exposure to human use of estrogen topical therapy.

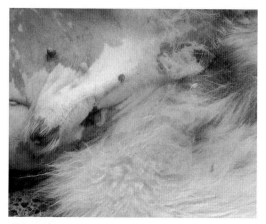

Fig. 4. Linear preputial erythema present along the midline of the prepuce in a dog with testicular neoplasia (sertoli cell tumor and seminoma). (*Courtesy of* University of California Davis, Veterinary Dermatology Service.)

Feline Paraneoplastic Alopecia

There is an association with pancreatic adenocarcinoma and a bilaterally symmetrical, ventrally pronounced distribution of alopecia in which the skin appears shiny but is not fragile (**Fig. 5**). Some of these cats may also have dry, scaly, or fissured footpads (**Fig. 6**). On necropsy, exocrine pancreatic adenocarcinoma with hepatic metastases is the most common tumor found, but bile duct carcinoma has been reported in 2 cases.[4] The disease affects older cats, and the chief clinical complaint is often the acute and dramatic alopecia that affects the ventral trunk, medial aspects of the limbs, and the ventral cervical region. Secondary *Malassezia* infections are common and may contribute to why some affected cats groom excessively. Histopathology of a skin biopsy shows epidermal hyperplasia with marked follicular and adnexal atrophy. Any cat with a tentative diagnosis of paraneoplastic alopecia should undergo an abdominal ultrasound scan to evaluate for the presence of a pancreatic or hepatic mass. Temporary resolution of the cutaneous disease was reported in one cat after the primary pancreatic tumor had been removed; the lesions recurred with development of metastatic disease.[5]

Feline Thymoma-associated Exfoliative Dermatitis

A rare, exfoliative dermatitis has been described in middle-age to older cats with thymomas.[4] The exact pathogenesis is not known but is thought to be immunologic with an erythema multiforme or graft-versus-host type of reaction having been proposed. Skin lesions tend to begin on the head and pinnae but can quickly generalize to involve the entire cat. Generalized erythema and marked scaling are present. Secondary infections with bacteria and *Malassezia* may develop. Respiratory signs secondary to the cranial mediastinal mass may be present at the time of presentation, but in most cases skin changes precede any other systemic signs. Histopathology of representative skin lesions shows a cell-poor, hydropic interface with apoptosis (single cell necrosis) of basal cell keratinocytes. If detected and diagnosed, removal of the thymic tumor will lead to resolution of the dermatologic clinical signs.[4,6,7]

Nodular Dermatofibrosis

A syndrome characterized by the development of a generalized nodular dermatofibrosis with associated renal cystadenocarcinomas or cystadenomas has been described

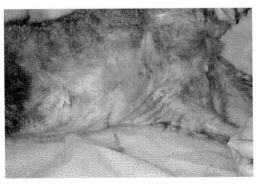

Fig. 5. A cat with marked ventral alopecia characteristic of feline paraneoplastic alopecia. The skin has a shiny appearance to it yet is not fragile. There are excoriations present that indicate self trauma. Cat had concurrent *Malassezia* dermatitis. (*Courtesy of* University of California Davis, Veterinary Dermatology Service.)

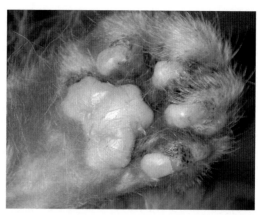

Fig. 6. A cat with feline paraneoplastic alopecia that has dry, scaling foot pads that have a shiny appearance to the epidermal surface. (*Courtesy of* University of California Davis, Veterinary Dermatology Services.)

most often in German Shepherd dogs and their crosses.[4] There does not seem to be a sex predilection, and the syndrome is diagnosed in middle-age dogs, typically between 6 and 8 years of age. In the German Shepherd dog, the development of this syndrome is suggested to have an autosomal dominant mode of inheritance.[8] In affected intact female dogs, uterine leiomyomas can develop. The pathogenesis linking nodular cutaneous lesions and renal and uterine tumors remains obscure. Nodules are found most often on distal extremities and can ulcerate or result in lameness. As the disease progresses, numerous nodules may develop involving the trunk and head as well. Nodules range in size from several millimeters to centimeters in diameter and are typically firm on palpation with variable amounts of pigmentation and hair present on the epithelial surface. Histopathologic evaluation of the cutaneous nodules finds dense collagenous hyperplasia. Ultrasonography is warranted in all cases of nodular dermatofibrosis. If the original ultrasound scan is normal, it should be repeated at serial intervals. Female dogs should be spayed to avoid development of uterine leiomyomas. Renal function should be monitored. Affected dogs usually have clinical signs of renal dysfunction within 2.5–5 years after skin lesions are first noticed.[9] Cutaneous lesions that are problematic for the dog can be surgically excised.

Paraneoplastic Pemphigus

Paraneoplastic pemphigus (PNP) is a rare and severe blistering disease that involves mucosal surfaces (oral, urogenital), mucocutaneous junctions, and haired skin seen in association with internal neoplasia. There are rare reports of this disease in the dog.[10] It has been reported in association with thymic lymphoma and splenic sarcoma.[2] The lesions are clinically similar to those of pemphigus vulgaris. Human patients have autoantibodies that target a variety of proteins responsible for connections between keratinocytes: specifically, plakin and desmoglein (Dsg) proteins.[2] It has been shown in the dog that antibodies target desmoplakin, envoplakin, periplakin, and Dsg 1 and Dsg 3.[10,11] Histologic lesions include suprabasilar clefting (as seen in pemphigus vulgaris) with intraepidermal keratinocyte apoptosis (as seen in erythema multiforme) and intraepidermal pustulation with acantholytic keratinocytes (as seen in pemphigus foliaceus).[10] This unusual mixture of lesions is the key to making the diagnosis and warrants a full evaluation of the patient for underlying neoplasia. Immunopathologically compatible cases in which neoplasia was not found have been recognized, and, in those cases, drug reactions were suspected.[10] PNP associated with neoplasia carries a grave prognosis. Definitive diagnosis of actual PNP is made with compatible histopathology in an animal with concurrent neoplasia and immunologic studies to identify the targeted antigens.

CUTANEOUS MANIFESTATIONS OF NUTRITIONAL OR METABOLIC PERTURBATIONS

The skin can develop lesions secondary to nutritional deficiencies; however, this is uncommon in a patient that has a good appetite and is eating a well-balanced commercial food. Some cutaneous manifestations of nutritional deficiencies are recognized in particular breeds, suggesting perhaps an alteration in absorption or metabolism, whereas others have been linked to inadequate or unbalanced diets. Superficial necrolytic dermatitis can be a paraneoplastic skin marker if associated with glucagonoma, but it is more commonly associated with some yet-to-be-determined alterations in metabolism that causes depletion of amino acids. Underlying disturbances in lipid metabolism can result in the development of cutaneous xanthomas.

Zinc Responsive Dermatosis

The skin contains approximately 20% of the total body zinc (Zn) stores, and the highest concentrations of Zn are found in the keratinized tissue of the nasal planum, tongue, and footpad.[12] There are several recognized syndromes associated with either Zn deficiency or disturbances in Zn assimilation that present with cutaneous signs.

Syndrome I has been identified in Siberian huskies, Alaskan malamutes, and occasionally other breeds. Affected dogs typically present with erythema followed by variable alopecia with fine silver scale that becomes adherent or develops into crusting involving the mucocutaneous junctions of the face (periocular, perioral), pressure points (elbows, hocks), and footpad margins (**Fig. 7**). Dogs with this disease manifest signs even on well-balanced diets. Diagnosis is based on signalment, typical cutaneous lesions, and histopathology of skin biopsies that shows marked follicular and

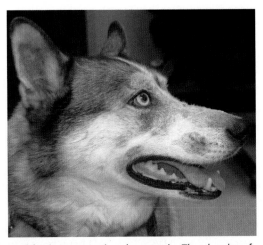

Fig. 7. A Husky dog with zinc responsive dermatosis. The dog has focal areas of partial alopecia with adherent fine, silvery scale present on the dorsal and lateral muzzle, commissure of the lip, upper eyelid, and beneath the eye. (*Courtesy of* University of California Davis, Veterinary Dermatology Service.)

epidermal parakeratotic hyperkeratosis. Therapy requires Zn supplementation with a recommended dosage of 2–3 mg/kg of elemental Zn in the form of zinc sulfate, zinc gluconate, or zinc methionine. There was not a detected difference between the different Zn salts in one study[13] Clinical signs are typically improved within 4–6 weeks.

Syndrome II occurs in rapidly growing puppies that are being fed a poor-quality dog food or are being oversupplemented with calcium. These dogs are thought to have a relative Zn deficiency caused by a combination of low Zn intake and calcium or cereal phytate binding of Zn. Affected dogs have generalized crusting plaques with extensive crusting and fissuring of the foot pads. Diagnosis is based on compatible history, clinical signs, and histopathology (similar to those of syndrome I). Response to Zn supplementation is dramatic but is not needed once the dog has reached maturity, unlike most syndrome I dogs. Many dogs will respond to a higher quality diet.

There has been a recent report of zinc-responsive dermatitis in related Pharaoh hound puppies.[14] Dogs developed cutaneous lesions, including exfoliative, erythematous lesions of the foot pads in the first months of life that histologically were suggestive of an underlying Zn deficiency. Affected puppies also had systemic signs of lethargy, poor growth, and mental dullness. Dogs did not respond to oral supplementation, and intravenous supplementation with zinc sulfate was required to ameliorate clinical signs.

Generic Dog Food Dermatosis

A dermatosis associated with the exclusive feeding of a poor-quality dog food was reported in the mid to late 1980s.[15,16] This disease is seen less commonly in North America since the institution of pet food certification programs. Many affected dogs were typically less than a year of age and undergoing a period of rapid growth. Affected dogs develop well-demarcated, thick, crusted plaques with fissures and erosions.[16] These lesions are typically located on the muzzle, on mucocutaneous junctions, over pressure points, and on distal extremities. Histopathology of representative skin lesions shows an acanthotic epidermis with parakeratosis, crusting, and spongiosis.[2] Diagnosis is based on compatible dietary history and histopathologic evaluation of skin biopsies. Anecdotal reports of a similar disease occurring in dogs fed vegan diets have also surfaced. Lesions resolve with feeding a better-quality diet.

Lethal Acrodermatitis

Lethal acrodermatitis (LAD) is an autosomal recessive disease seen in white bull terriers. The disease has some clinical similarities to the human disease acrodermatitis enteropathica.[2,17–19] The homozygously affected puppies show clinical signs in the first few weeks of life and have a median survival of 7 months, typically succumbing to bronchopneumonia and sepsis. Bull terriers that are heterozygously affected may have increased risk for pyoderma.[2]

Affected dogs are characterized by a progressive crusting dermatitis of the distal extremities and mucocutaneous junctions. Abnormal keratinization of paw pads can result in splaying of the feet. Claw dystrophy and paronychia may also be present. Secondary infections of the skin with bacteria and Malassezia yeast are common.[2,18] Dogs with LAD also often have an abnormally arched hard palate, retarded skeletal growth, abnormal mentation, diarrhea, and bronchopneumonia. In a report of 28 affected dogs, all had difficulty eating, stunted growth, splayed digits, and developed skin lesions by 12 weeks of age.[18] Dogs with LAD have been shown to have significantly lower IgA levels than a control group of dogs.[20] A diagnosis of LAD can be strongly suspected in any bull terrier showing a combination of the aforementioned signs from an early age. Skin biopsy results show a marked parakeratotic hyperkeratosis. Although many of the clinical signs and the histopathology of this condition suggest Zn deficiency, Zn supplementation is of little benefit. There is no effective therapy. A recent report of a proteomic analysis of liver tissue in 2 affected bull terriers documented that 13 proteins involved in a variety of cellular functions were abnormally expressed in affected pups compared with a normal bull terrier.[18] Diagnosis is based on compatible signalment, physical examination findings, and skin biopsy results.

Superficial Necrolytic Dermatitis

Superficial necrolytic dermatitis (SND) (synonym, metabolic epidermal necrosis) is an uncommon skin disease associated with systemic metabolic disease(s). Affected dogs most commonly have a characteristic concurrent hepatopathy, thus, the popular use of the term *hepatocutaneous syndrome* (HCS) to describe the skin condition. However, other disease processes, including glucagonoma of the pancreas, vacuolar hepatopathy, phenobarbital administration, and intestinal disease have been reported to cause similar histologic skin lesions. Therefore, it may be more appropriate to refer to the skin disease as *SND* and to reserve the term *HCS* for cases with the characteristic liver pathology. The disease is typically diagnosed in older dogs. The mean age of reported cases is 10 years, with a range of 4–16 years[21] Sixty-four percent of all reported cases are male dogs,[21] Shetland sheepdogs, West Highland white terriers, Cocker spaniels and Scottish terriers may have a predisposition to HCS because they seem to be overrepresented in the literature.[21]

Footpads develop marked crusting, fissuring, and ulcerations (**Fig. 8**). Erythema, crusting, exudation, ulceration, and alopecia can also involve the periocular or perioral regions, pressure points on the limbs, and scrotum. Secondary cutaneous infections with bacteria, yeast (*Malassezia*, *Candida*), or dermatophytes, particularly involving the feet, often are present in dogs with SND. Lameness secondary to footpad lesions, inappetance, and weight loss can also be associated with SND. Polydipsia and polyuria may be present when there is concurrent diabetes mellitus or if significant liver dysfunction is present. Diabetes mellitus has been reported to occur in 25%–40% of dogs with the hepatic form of SND.[21]

Diagnosis of SND is based on obtaining skin biopsies with the typical histopathologic changes of a marked parakeratotic epidermis with striking intercellular and intracellular edema in the upper epidermis and hyperplastic basal cells, creating the red,

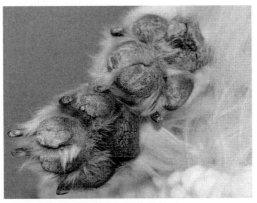

Fig. 8. Marked hyperkeratosis and fissuring that is affecting all foot pads and is characteristic of the foot pad lesions seen in dogs with superficial necrolytic dermatitis. (*Courtesy of* University of California Davis, Veterinary Dermatology Service.)

white and blue lesion that is diagnostic of this disease. Abdominal ultrasound scan can provide further support for the diagnosis if the characteristic honeycomb pattern consisting of variable-sized hypoechoic regions surrounded by hyperechoic borders is documented. If this ultrasonographic pattern to the liver is not visualized in a dog with a confirmed histologic diagnosis of SND on skin biopsy, evaluation for a possible pancreatic tumor or protein-losing enteropathy is warranted. Pancreatic tumors may not be readily visible with an abdominal ultrasound examination; therefore, measurement of plasma glucagon is also recommended. Elevation of liver enzymes and hypoalbuminemia are the most common clinicopathologic changes in one retrospective study.[22] Glucosuria and hyperglycemia may be documented if diabetes mellitus is present. Plasma amino acids, if measured, should document a characteristic severe hypoaminoacidemia. Because severe hypoaminoacidemia is documented to occur in all cases of SND in which plasma amino acids have been measured, regardless of associated disease, it is likely that this metabolic derangement is directly contributing to the cutaneous lesions seen in affected dogs. The liver plays a critical role in amino acid balance. With both chronic and acute hepatitis, compromised hepatic metabolism results in increased concentrations of many plasma amino acids, but this is not seen in dogs with SND, because most individual plasma amino acid concentrations are less than 60% of normal.[22] These differences suggest that the pathogenesis of hypoaminoacidemia in dogs with SND cannot be explained by compromised hepatic metabolism. It seems probable that an as yet unexplained increase in hepatic catabolism of amino acids might account for the severity of hypoaminoacidemia documented in the dogs with SND.

The most effective symptomatic or palliative therapy for dogs with the hepatic form of SND seems to be the administration of intravenous (IV) amino acids. Several crystalline amino acid solutions are commercially available that vary in their concentration and the inclusion of electrolytes. Although there are minor differences in the amounts of essential and nonessential amino acids between manufacturers, there are no data to suggest that one product is more efficacious than another. Solutions without additional electrolytes are preferred. Ten percent Aminosyn solution (Abbott Laboratories, Abbot Park, North Carolina), Travasol 8.5% without electrolytes (Baxter Healthcare Corp, Clintec Nutrition Company, Deerfield, IL), and ProcalAmine (B. Braun Medical Inc, Irvine, CA), 3% amino acids with 3% glycerine and electrolytes, have all been used for IV infusions in treating dogs who have SND. These hypertonic amino acid solutions should ideally be administered via a central vein to diminish the chance of thrombophlebitis. Inducing a hyperosmolar state is possible if administration is too aggressive. Dogs should be monitored for neurologic signs and the infusion discontinued if these occur. If compromised hepatic or renal function is present, the administration of intravenous amino acids may exacerbate hepatic encephalopathy or augment increases in blood urea nitrogen. Such dogs warrant close monitoring with serial measurements of ammonia, blood urea nitrogen, and osmolality during IV amino acid administration. Some dogs show dramatic improvement in attitude with resolution of skin lesions after receiving amino acid infusions. There are no defined protocols for the administration of amino acid infusions in these dogs, and repeat infusions are performed bimonthly, monthly, or when clinical signs return.

Oral nutrition should include a high-quality protein diet that can be supplemented additionally with an amino acid powder. Unless significant hepatic dysfunction with hyperammonemia has been documented, suggesting the presence of some other concurrent liver disease and necessitating a low-protein diet, most dogs with SND cannot be fed enough protein to overcome the hypoaminoacidemia occurring in this disease. Zinc, essential fatty acid supplementation, and egg yolks have been recommended in the literature to be beneficial.[23,24] These supplements might provide micronutrients that have some as-yet unknown role in this disease, but to maximize additional protein from an egg source, egg whites should be included. Secondary infections should be treated with appropriate antibiotic and antifungal therapy with careful consideration of those drugs that may be hepatotoxic or require hepatic metabolism. Topical therapy with antimicrobial shampoos can also be of benefit in some dogs in helping manage secondary infections. Therapy with glucocorticoids is not recommended. Although antiinflammatory therapy for the skin lesions may be helpful to improve comfort, the risk of precipitating or exacerbating diabetes mellitus in these dogs makes the use of glucocorticoids contraindicated. Diabetes mellitus, if present, requires appropriate management. Surgical removal of a glucagonoma has been reported to result in resolution of lesions in one dog. Serial treatments with octreotide in a dog with glucagonoma associated SND was palliative in one case report.[25]

The prognosis for dogs with SND is generally poor and most dogs have survival times of less than 6 months. However, 20% of dogs in one study were maintained for 12 months or more with oral protein hyperalimentation and periodic parenteral IV amino acid infusions.[22]

Cutaneous Xanthomas

Cutaneous xanthomas are rare and occur when there is underlying hereditary defects in lipid metabolism or acquired dyslipoproteinemia secondary to diabetes mellitus, or use of megestrol acetate. These skin lesions result from the accumulation of lipid-laden macrophages within the dermis. Feline cutaneous xanthomas may develop in cats with hereditary hyperchylomicronemia, megestrol acetate–induced diabetes mellitus, or naturally occurring diabetes mellitus. Cutaneous xanthomas have been reported in a dog with diabetes mellitus.[26] Often affected animals are consuming a diet rich in fats or triglycerides at the time lesions develop.

Clinically, cutaneous xanthomas present as multiple pale yellow to white plaques, papules, or nodules with erythematous borders. They often are located on the head, particularly the preauricular area or pinnae. Lesions can develop in paw pads and over boney prominences on limbs (**Fig. 9**). Lesions may bruise readily, and larger masses may, in rare cases, ulcerate and exude inspissated necrotic material.[2] Cats with inherited hyperchylomicronemia may also show peripheral neurologic signs because of nerve compression from subcutaneous xanthoma formation. Histologic evaluation of skin biopsies shows large foamy macrophages and giant cells. Serum biochemistry evaluations for diabetes mellitus, hypercholesterolemia, and hypertriglyceridemia should be obtained. Feeding of a low-fat diet and identification and correction of the underlying disturbance in lipid metabolism is recommended for patients that have had cutaneous xanthomas identified.

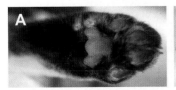 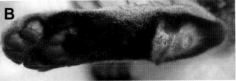

Fig. 9. (*A*) Cutaneous xanthomas present as multifocal nodular pinkish plaques on multiple feet in this cat that had an underlying disturbance in lipid metabolism. (*B*) Lesions over the metatarsal regions are inflamed and developing serocellular crusting caused by pressure and compromised integrity of the overlying skin. (*Courtesy of* University of California Davis, Veterinary Dermatology Service.)

CUTANEOUS MANIFESTATIONS OF SYSTEMIC INFECTIOUS DISEASES
Leishmaniasis

This protozoal disease has been reported in dogs in the United States that have been imported or spent time in the Mediterranean basin/southern Europe (*Leishmania infantum*) or South America (*Leishmania chagasi*) but also from autochthonous foci in many states and 2 provinces in Canada.[27] In North America, foxhounds seem to be predisposed. The first signs of this disease noticed by owners are often skin lesions. Alopecia, erythema, and scaling with ulceration are common lesions involving the pinnae, dorsal muzzle, and mucocutaneous junctions. Affected dogs may be systemically unwell with concurrent lymphadenopathy, hyperproteinemia, hyperglobulinemia, nonregenerative anemia, azotemia, and proteinuria. Diagnosis is made by demonstration of the organism in aspirates of lymph nodes, bone marrow or synovial fluid, or histology of skin biopsies or culture, or looking for evidence of the infection via a variety of immunologic or serologic tests or polymerase chain reaction (PCR).[28] Recommended therapy is antimonial compounds, such as meglumine antimoniate in Europe and sodium stibogluconate in the United States (available from the CDC for use in dogs) along with oral administration of allopurinol.[29] Treatment failures and relapses are common.

Systemic Mycosis

Many systemic or deep mycoses (blastomycosis, coccidioidomycosis, cryptococcosis, histoplasmosis, aspergillosis) can present with cutaneous lesions. These lesions include papules, nodules, draining tracts, and ulceration and typically result from hematogenous dissemination of the fungal organism to the skin. Although rare, direct inoculation of fungal organisms into a cutaneous wound could result in a solitary lesion. Skin lesions are seen most commonly in feline cryptococcal infections and in canine blastomycosis and are reported to occur in approximately 20%–40% of cases of these fungal infections. Typically, there are other systemic clinical signs. Nasal aspergillosis can cause depigmentation and ulceration often beneath the nares as a result of a drainage board effect from the chronic nasal discharge (**Fig. 10**). Diagnosis of any of the fungal infections is based on demonstration of the organism within

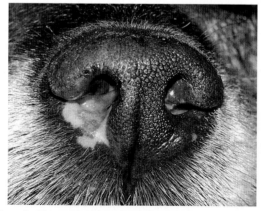

Fig. 10. Drainage board effect with depigmentation and erosions, and ulceration is present on the rostral muzzle and nares on the side of the nasal cavity that had pronounced nasal discharge resulting from nasal aspergillosis. (*Courtesy of* University of California Davis, Veterinary Dermatology Service.)

biopsied tissue or fungal culture. Suspicious cutaneous lesions can provide easy and rapid diagnostic information in the evaluation of animals with systemic mycoses. Appropriate antifungal therapy is chosen based on type of organism and overall health of the animal.

Viral Diseases

Canine distemper virus

Distemper virus has long been associated with hard pad disease. Hard pad disease represents an uncommon manifestation of canine distemper virus infection with a still unknown pathogenesis. Dogs develop excessive keratinous material on the foot pads and nasal planum. Diagnosis is suspected when the cutaneous lesions develop in a dog that shows other systemic signs of canine distemper virus. Canine distemper is an epitheliotropic virus that initially targets the gastrointestinal system, then respiratory tract, and then the central nervous system. Diagnosis can be confirmed by immunohistochemical demonstration of the virus within skin biopsies.[30]

Feline retroviruses

Opportunistic skin infections, oral ulcerations, and gingivitis have been associated with feline leukemia virus (FeLV) and feline immunodeficiency virus. Cutaneous horns can develop on the paw pads of cats with FeLV. In severe cases, lameness and discomfort can be marked. Diagnosis is confirmed with a positive FeLV status and skin biopsy. Immunohistochemistry can show the presence of the virus within a skin biopsy. Cutaneous lymphoma and giant cell dermatosis have also been reported in FeLV positive cats.[31]

Feline herpes virus

Feline herpes virus ulcerative dermatitis typically involves the dorsal muzzle, but lesions may extend to involve the nasal planum (**Fig. 11**). Cats do not have to have concurrent ocular or upper respiratory tract signs. Histologically, the lesion is a necrotizing, ulcerative dermatitis most often with a concurrent marked eosinophilic inflammation, but the inflammatory pattern may be strongly neutrophilic in some cases. The

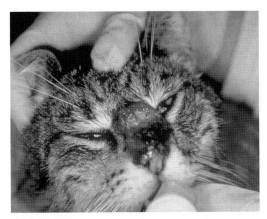

Fig. 11. Ulcerative dorsal muzzle lesion with marked hemorrhagic crusting and extension to involve the nasal planum in a cat. Lesion location and appearance is typical for the ulcerative dermatitis seen secondary to feline herpes virus 1 ulcerative dermatitis. Intranuclear inclusion bodies were seen on histopathology of a skin biopsy, and PCR from the biopsied skin sample was positive for feline herpes virus 1. (*Courtesy of* University of California Davis, Veterinary Dermatology Service.)

presence of eosinophilic inflammation and the clinical appearance of the lesions make it difficult to differentiate from mosquito bite hypersensitivity or other feline eosinophilic ulcerative lesions. Unless intranuclear viral inclusions can be identified, it is not possible to definitively diagnose the virus as the etiologic agent for the ulcerative dermatitis. PCR has been shown to be a sensitive test to detect the presence of the virus within skin biopsies.[32] Treatment can include subcutaneous administration of α-interferon (1,000,000 units/m^2, 3 times a week), oral famciclovir (Famvir, Novartis Pharmaceuticals Corp, East Hanover, NJ, USA) (90 mg/kg),[33] or lysine.

AUTOIMMUNE SKIN DISEASES ASSOCIATED WITH SYSTEMIC DISEASE

Canine autoimmune skin diseases are uncommon skin disorders and are reported to account for less than 2% of all skin diseases seen in small-animal practice.[3] They often are clinically impressive and can even be life threatening. Definitive diagnosis requires timely biopsy of appropriate representative skin lesions and cannot be based solely on clinical impression or appearance.

Systemic Lupus Erythematosus

Systemic lupus erythematosus (SLE) is a multisystemic autoimmune disease. The collie, Shetland sheepdog, German shepherd dog, spitz, and poodle are reported to be at increased risk.[3] Skin disease occurs in less than 20% of SLE cases. Fever, polyarthritis, protein-losing nephropathy, anemia, and thrombocytopenia are more common clinical signs seen with SLE. Organ-specific and non–organ-specific autoantibodies target a variety of tissue antigens in SLE. Resultant tissue damage occurs when there is immune complex deposition (as occurs in glomerulonephritis) or can occur because of direct cytotoxic effects or cell-mediated immunity.

Cutaneous lesions are variable and can include erythema, scaling, crusting, depigmentation, alopecia, and ulcerations. Lesions often involve the face, pinnae, and distal extremities. Lesions may be present on mucocutaneous junctions and within the oral cavity. Ulcers and erosions are rarely diagnostic lesions to biopsy, because an intact epidermis is needed to make a definitive diagnosis. The histopathologic findings are variable, but classic lesions include apoptosis of basal cells and basal cell vacuolation, which lead to dermo-epidermal separation and consequent ulceration.

Diagnosis of SLE requires demonstration of concurrent autoimmune disease in 2 organ systems in addition to the presence of antinuclear antibodies (ANAs). There are published criteria for the diagnosis of SLE in dogs, and diagnosis requires the presence of at least 3 or more criteria.[3] SLE is a progressive disease, and evidence of immunologic involvement in multiple organ systems may not always be evident on the initial presentation. A thorough systemic evaluation, including a complete blood cell count, serum biochemistry, urinalysis with and without protein-to-creatinine ratio, ANA, arthrocentesis, and evaluation of joint fluid cytologically may be indicated in patients suspected of having SLE. Most patients with SLE have an elevated ANA level, although this may not always be present. Prognosis depends in large part on the organ systems involved. Immunosuppressive therapy with corticosteroids with or without other immunosuppressive drugs (azathioprine, chlorambucil, cyclosporine) is used.

Erythema Multiforme

Erythema multiforme (EM) terminology has been confusing. More recent nomenclature categorizes EM clinically based on severity of lesions. In EM minor, characteristic lesions involve only one mucosal surface and affect less than 10% of body surface. EM major has clinically similar lesions with more than one mucosal surface affected,

10%–50% of body surface affected, and less than 10% epithelial detachment.[2] It has been documented that the cell-mediated immune response in EM has a Th1 cytokine pattern.[34] The T cell–mediated response is directed at keratinocytes that may express antigens in a novel way because of drug administration, infection, or neoplasia resulting in apoptosis (single cell necrosis) of keratinocytes. The more severe the clinical presentation of EM, the more likely it is to be related to adverse drug reaction.[35] There is a report of EM associated with parvovirus in a dog,[36] and herpes virus has been implicated in the cat.[37]

Lesions are often pleomorphic with an acute onset of erythematous plaques and macules that often become annular or serpiginous as they coalesce or they may appear targetoid. Progression to ulcerations is common, and lesions may become variably crusted (**Fig. 12**). Lesions often are generalized but are most commonly found on the ventrum, axillae, inguinal region, mucocutaneous junctions, oral cavity, and pinnae. Biopsies should be obtained from areas of erythema without ulceration or crusting because an intact epidermis is needed for the diagnosis. Histologically, apoptosis with lymphocyte satellitosis is the characteristic microscopic lesion of EM.

Prognosis for EM depends on the severity of the disease and identification of underlying triggers. In about 50% of canine cases, an underlying trigger cannot be found. Use of immunosuppressive drugs in human medicine is controversial because EM often is induced by herpes simplex virus.[34] In veterinary medicine, EM patients should be evaluated for underlying triggers: drugs, infection, or neoplasia. EM is often treated with immunosuppressive therapy using glucocorticoids with or without concurrent azathioprine (Imuran). Severe generalized mucocutaneous EM (EM major) often requires aggressive supportive care in addition to removal of underlying triggers and immunosuppressive therapy.

Sterile Nodular Panniculitis

Sterile nodular panniculitis typically presents with ulcerated or draining nodular lesions or nonulcerative subcutaneous nodules (**Fig. 13**). Dogs often are febrile when lesions

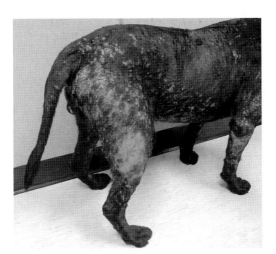

Fig. 12. Multifocal coalescing discrete erosions and ulcerations create large geographic erosive lesions. There are also generalized, multifocal crusting lesions evident in this dog with erythema multiforme. (*Courtesy of* University of California Davis, Veterinary Dermatology Service.)

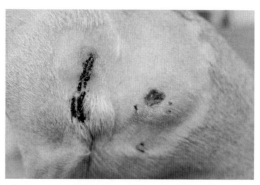

Fig. 13. A dog with discrete nodular lesions, lesions progress in size and then ulcerate and drain. Histopathology of a skin biopsy confirmed sterile nodular panniculitis. (*Courtesy of University of California Davis, Veterinary Dermatology Service.*)

are present, and a peripheral neutrophilia may be present. Lesions most commonly are seen on the trunk but can be present on the head, cervical area, or perineum or can be generalized (see **Fig. 11**). Diagnosis is made based on appropriate clinical history, compatible histology of deep tissue biopsies with negative special stains, and negative cultures for any infectious organisms. In some cases, concurrent pancreatic disease (pancreatitis and pancreatic neoplasia) or immune-mediated disease in other organ systems (polyarthritis, SLE, rheumatoid arthritis) have been identified.[38] Sterile nodular panniculitis, if associated with pancreatitis, often resolves when the underlying pancreatic disease is managed successfully. Often, sterile nodular panniculitis requires a tapering course of immunosuppressive therapy, most often glucocorticoids, unless underlying or concurrent diseases make this contraindicated.

REFERENCES

1. Credille KM, Slater MR, Moriello KA, et al. The effects of thyroid hormones on the skin of beagle dogs. J Vet Intern Med 2001;15:539–46.
2. Gross TL, Ihrke PJ, Walder EJ, et al. Skin diseases of the dog and cat. Clinical and histopathologic diagnosis. 2nd edition. Ames (IA): Blackwell Science Ltd; 2005.
3. Scott DW, Miller WH, Griffin DE. Muller and Kirk's small animal dermatology. 6th edition. Philadelphia: Elsevier Health; 2001.
4. Turek MM. Cutaneous paraneoplastic syndromes in dogs and cats: a review of the literature. Vet Dermatol 2003;14:279–96.
5. Tasker S, Griffon DJ, Nuttal TJ, et al. Resolution of paraneoplastic alopecia following surgical removal of a pancreatic carcinoma in a cat. J Small Anim Pract 1999;40:16–9.
6. Forster-Van Hijfte MA, Curtis CF, White RN. Resolution of exfoliative dermatitis and Malassezia pachydermatis overgrowth in a cat after surgical thymoma resection. J Small Anim Pract 1997;38:451–4.
7. Rivierre C, Olivry T. Dermatite exfoliative paraneoplasique associee a un thymoma chez unchat: resolution des symptoms après thymectomie. Pract Med Chir Anim Comp 1999;34:533–7.
8. Lium B, Moe L. Hereditary multifocal renal cystadenocarcinomas and nodular dermatofibrosis in the German shepherd dog: macroscopic and histologic changes. Vet Pathol 1985;22:447–55.

9. Moe L, Lium B. Hereditary multifocal renal cystadenocarcinomas and nodular dermatofibrosis in 51 German shepherd dogs. J Small Anim Pract 1997;38:498–505.
10. Olivry T, Linder KE. Dermatoses affecting desmosomes in animals: a mechanistic review of acantholytic blistering skin diseases. Vet Dermatol 2009;20:313–26.
11. Elmore SA, Basseches J, Anhalt G, et al. Paraneoplastic pemphigus in a dog with splenic hematopoietic neoplasia. Vet Pathol 2003;40:609.
12. Lansdown AB, Sampson B. Trace metals in keratinizing epithelia in beagle dogs. Vet Rec 1997;141:571–2.
13. White SD, Bourdeau P, Rosychuk RA, et al. Zinc-responsive dermatosis in dogs: 41 cases and literature review. Vet Dermatol 2001;12:101–9.
14. Cambell GA, Crow D. Zinc responsive dermatosis in a litter of pharaoh hounds. J Vet Diagn Invest 2010;22:663–6.
15. Sousa C, Ihrke P, Reinke S, et al. Generic dog food and skin disease. J Am Vet Med Assoc 1983;182:198–9.
16. Sousa CA, Stannard AA, Ihrke PJ, et al. Dermatosis associated with feeding generic dog food 13 cases (1981-1982). J Am Vet Med Assoc 1988;192:676–80.
17. Jezyk PF, Haskins MF, MacKay-Smith WE, et al. Lethal acrodermatitis in bull terriers. J Am Vet Med Assoc 1986;188:833–9.
18. Grider A, Mouat MF, Mauldin EA, et al. Analysis of the liver soluble proteome from bull terriers affected with inherited lethal acrodermatitis. Mol Genet Metab 2007; 92:249–57.
19. McEwan NA, McNeil PE, Thompson H, et al. Diagnostic features, confirmation and disease progression in 28 cases of lethal acrodermatitis of bull terriers. J Small Anim Pract 2000;41:501–7.
20. McEwan NA, Huang HP, Mellon DJ. Immunoglobulin levels in bull terriers suffering from lethal acrodermatitis. Vet Immunol Immunopathol 2003;96:235–8.
21. Outerbridge CA. Hepatocutaneous syndrome. In: Ettinger SJ, Feldman EC, editors. Textbook of veterinary internal medicine, vol. 1, 7th edition. St Louis (MO): Saunders Elsevier; 2010. p. 112–5.
22. Outerbridge CA, Marks S, Rogers Q. Plasma amino acid concentrations in 36 dogs with histologically confirmed superficial necrolytic dermatitis (SND). Vet Dermatol 2002;13:177–87.
23. Gross TL, Song MD, Havel PJ, et al. Superficial necrolytic dermatitis (necrolytic migratory erythema) in dogs. Vet Pathol 1993;30:75–81.
24. Byrne KP. Metabolic epidermal necrosis-hepatocutaneous syndrome. Vet Clin North Am Small Anim Pract 1999;29:1337–55.
25. Oberkirchner U, Linder KE, Zadrozny L, et al. Successful treatment of canine necrolytic migratory erythema (superficial necrolytic dermatitis) due to metastatic glucagonoma with octreotide. Vet Dermatol 2010;21:510–6.
26. Chastain CB, Graham CL. Xanthomatosis secondary to diabetes mellitus in a dog. J Am Vet Med Assoc 1978;172:1209–11.
27. Duprey ZH, Steurer FJ, Rooney JA, et al. Canine visceral leishmaniasis, United States and Canada, 2000-2003. Emerg Infect Dis 2006;12:440–6.
28. Maia C, Campino L. Methods for diagnosis of canine leishmaniasis and immune response to infection. Vet Parasitol 2008;158:274–87.
29. Denerolle P, Bourdoiseau G. Combination allopurinol and antimony treatment versus antimony alone and allopurinol alone in the treatment of canine leishmaniasis (96 cases). J Vet Intern Med 1999;13:413–5.
30. Haines DM, Martin KM, Chelack BJ, et al. Immunohistochemical detection of canine distemper virus in haired skin, nasal mucosa, and footpad epithelium: a method for antemortem diagnosis of infection. J Vet Diagn Invest 1999;11:396–9.

31. Favrot C, Wilhelm S, Grest P, et al. Two cases of FeLV-associated dermatoses. Vet Dermatol 2005;16:407–12.
32. Holland JL, Outerbridge CA, Affolter VK, et al. Detection of feline herpes virus 1 DNA in skin biopsy specimens from cats with or without dermatitis. Am J Vet Res 2006;229:1442–6.
33. Thomasy SM, Lim CC, Reilly CM, et al. Evaluation of orally administered famciclovir in cats experimentally infected with feline herpesvirus type-1. Am J Vet Res 2011;72:85–95.
34. Caproni M, Torchia D, Schincaglia E, et al. Expression of cytokines and chemokine receptors in the cutaneous lesions of erythema multiforme and Stevens–Johnson syndrome/toxic epidermal necrolysis. Br J Dermatol 2006;155:722–8.
35. Hinn A, Olivry T, Luther P, et al. Erythema multiforme, Stevens-Johnson syndrome, and toxic epidermal necrolysis in the dog: clinical classification, drug exposure, and histopathological correlations. J Vet Allergy Clin Immunol 1998;6:13–20.
36. Favrot C, Olivry T, Dunstan SM, et al. Parvovirus infection of keratinocytes as a cause of canine erythema multiforme. Vet Pathol 2000;37:647–9.
37. Scott D, Miller W. Erythema multiforme in dogs and cats: literature review and case material from the Cornell University College of Veterinary Medicine (1988–1996). Vet Dermatol 1999;10:297–309.
38. O'Kell AL, Inteeworn N, Diaz SF, et al. Canine sterile nodular panniculitis: a retrospective study of 14 cases. J Vet Intern Med 2010;24:278–84.

Cyclosporine in Veterinary Dermatology

Brian S. Palmeiro, VMD

KEYWORDS

- Cyclosporine • Atopic dermatitis • Immune-mediated skin disease • Perianal fistula
- Sebaceous adenitis

KEY POINTS

- Cyclosporine is an immunomodulatory medication that is approved for atopic dermatitis in dogs and allergic dermatitis in cats.
- Cyclosporine has been used to manage a variety of immune-mediated skin diseases including perianal fistulas and sebaceous adenitis.
- Drug interactions with cyclosporine are commonly reported caused by the shared metabolic pathways involving cytochrome P450 and/or competition with P-glycoprotein.
- The most commonly reported side effects caused by cyclosporine are gastrointestinal in nature; other reported side effects are typically reversible with discontinuation of cyclosporine.

INTRODUCTION

Cyclosporine A (CsA) is an immunomodulatory medication that was initially isolated from the fungus *Tolypocladium inflatum*.[1] It has been successfully used in the treatment of a variety of inflammatory and immune-mediated skin diseases. This article reviews the use of CsA in veterinary dermatology, including its mechanism of action, pharmacokinetics, drug interactions, side effects, and relevant clinical updates. Dermatologic indications including atopic/allergic dermatitis, perianal fistulas, sebaceous adenitis, and other immune-mediated skin diseases are discussed.

FORMULATIONS OF CYCLOSPORINE

In humans, CsA was first developed as a vegetable oil formulation (Sandimmune; Novartis Pharmaceuticals) that is highly dependent on biliary excretion for absorption.[2] A newer microemulsified (ME; ie modified) CsA product (Neoral; Novartis Pharmaceuticals) was developed that improves oral bioavailability, decreases individual variability

Funding sources: None.
Conflicts of interest: None.
Lehigh Valley Veterinary Dermatology & Fish Hospital, 4580 Crackersport Road, Allentown, PA 18104, USA
E-mail address: skin@lehighvetderm.com

in absorption, and decreases the effect of bile secretion on absorption; approved generic preparations of modified CsA are available for use in humans.[2] In humans, the bioavailability of the ME form of CsA is 30% to 40%, compared with 20% to 30% for the nonmodified formulation.[3] In canine patients, the ME form offers an approximate 35% bioavailability, compared with 20% to 25% with the vegetable oil formulation.[2,4] In veterinary medicine, modified CsA (Atopica, Novartis Animal Health) is approved for use in dogs for atopic dermatitis; this product is available in 10, 25, 50, and 100 mg soft gelatin capsules.[5] ME CsA (Atopica for Cats, Novartis Animal Health) was recently approved for the treatment of allergic dermatitis in cats; this product is available as an oral solution with a concentration of 100 mg/mL.[6]

MECHANISM OF ACTION

CsA, a calcineurin inhibitor, is an immunosuppressive medication that inhibits T-cell activation.[1] CsA binds to the intracellular protein cyclophilin-1; the cyclophilin-CsA complex inhibits calcineurin, preventing the dephosphorylation/activation of nuclear factor of activated T cells (NFAT).[2] NFAT helps regulate the production of several important proinflammatory cytokines including interleukin (IL)-2, IL-4, interferon (IFN)-γ, and tumor necrosis factor (TNF)-α.[7] Inhibition of IL-2, a potent T-cell growth promoter and activator, is most commonly implicated as the main mechanism of immunosuppression.[7,8] In feline lymphocytes in vitro, CsA has been shown to decrease IL-2, IL-10, IFN-γ, and granulocyte-macrophage colony-stimulating factor production.[9] A recent article used flow cytometry to assess the pharmacyodynamic effect of CsA on the production of various cytokines in dogs.[10] High-dosage CsA (10 mg/kg twice daily) resulted in significant decreases in IL-2 and IFN-γ expression, but not IL-4 expression.[10] Low-dosage CsA was associated with a significant decrease in IFN-γ expression, whereas IL-2 expression was not affected.[10] CsA affects several cells in the skin, including T cells, dendritic cells, Langerhans cells, keratinocytes, mast cells, and eosinophils.[2,11] It impairs the ability of dendritic cells to stimulate proliferation of T cells, decreases the number and activity of Langerhans cells in the epidermis, decreases cytokine secretion by keratinocytes, and decreases the functions of mast cells and eosinophils.[11–13] CsA inhibits eosinophil survival, cytokine secretion and recruitment of eosinophils to the sites of allergic inflammation.[11–13] It also inhibits mast cell survival, secretory response, histamine release, prostaglandin production, and cytokine secretion.[13,14]

CsA has been shown to inhibit canine and murine keratinocyte proliferation, reduce lipopolysaccharide-induced prostaglandin-E2 synthesis in canine and murine keratinocytes, and inhibit the production of chemokines (CXC chemokine KC and CCL2) in the murine keratinocytes.[15] It has also been shown to significantly reduce the IFN-γ–induced production of IFN-γ–inducible protein 10 in human keratinocytes.[15] All of these properties contribute to the antiinflammatory and immunomodulatory action of CsA in the treatment of allergic skin disease.[15]

PHARMACOKINETICS

The absolute oral bioavailability of CsA in dogs and cats is low and highly variable.[2] Oral bioavailability is higher in cats than in dogs, with a lower clearance and a slightly longer elimination half-life.[16] The low bioavailability of CsA can be explained by the high molecular weight of the drug, its low water solubility, the effect of the P-glycoprotein efflux pump at the intestinal level, and metabolism by cytochrome P450 3A enzymes located in the small intestinal mucosa and liver.[17–19] In dogs, the veterinary-labeled oral CsA is rapidly absorbed, but bioavailability is variable and can range from

23% to 45%.[20] Based on pharmacokinetic data in dogs, administration of CsA is recommended 2 hours before or after feeding, because its bioavailability decreases when given with food.[18] The mean bioavailability of an ME CsA was reduced by 22% when administered to dogs with food, whereas the individual variability in drug absorption increased.[18] Therefore, it is recommended that dogs be dosed on an empty stomach to optimize the drug's bioavailability. Even though there is an obvious effect of feeding on oral bioavailability, a small-scale study found that administration of CsA with food did not influence the clinical response in dogs.[21] In cats, a pharmacokinetic study showed no consistent difference in the mean extent of drug absorption when administered orally to fed or starved cats or mixed in with food.[6]

Being lipophilic, CsA distributes widely in the tissues. The drug concentration in epidermis and dermis is about 10-fold higher than in the blood.[22]

CsA is metabolized primarily by cytochrome P450, in particular CYP3A4, in the liver and small intestine.[23] P-glycoprotein is also associated with excretion of CsA, acting as a drug efflux pump that actively transports CsA back into the intestinal lumen.[23] The same cytochrome P450 enzymes (CYP3A4) are involved in both intestinal and hepatic metabolism.[24] As much as 50% of oral CsA metabolism may be attributed to intestinal metabolism.[23] Elimination is mainly biliary with minimal renal excretion in all species.[25]

When applied epicutaneously, CsA has a poor skin penetration despite being lipid soluble; presumably this is related to the large molecular weight of the compound.[2,26] In an abstract evaluating transdermal CsA, only 1/6 cats had blood levels that were considered to be therapeutic.[27]

Effect of Bodyweight on Dosing

Because CsA is hydrophobic and concentrates in fat, some have proposed dosing patients based on their ideal body weight.[28] In humans, obesity does not significantly affect CsA pharmacokinetics.[29] In dogs weighing greater than 15 kg, a reduced CsA dosage (mean 4.4 mg/kg/d) was required to control symptoms when compared to dogs less than 15 kg.[30] A mean decrease of 0.04 mg/kg/d was found for every kilogram increase in body weight.[30]

MONITORING BLOOD LEVELS OF CYCLOSPORINE

The most commonly used methods for measuring blood CsA levels include high-pressure liquid chromatography (HPLC), fluorescent polarization immunoassay (FPIA), and radioimmunoassay (RIA).[2] HPLC is time consuming and not cost-effective for routine practice. RIA and FPIA use antibodies that may cross-react with CsA metabolites, resulting in higher blood concentrations compared with HPLC.[2,18] In dogs, CsA blood levels using FPIA were 1.5 to 1.7 times higher than when using HPLC.[18] A trough concentration of 600 ng/mL has previously been established to attain sufficient immunosuppression to prevent organ rejection in canine transplant recipients.[31,32] A study evaluating the pharmacodynamic effects of CsA using flow cytometry and cytokine expression concluded that T-cell function is suppressed at trough blood drug concentrations exceeding 600 ng/mL, and is at least partially suppressed in some dogs at lower dosages.[10]

Interpretation of CsA levels for treatment of atopic dermatitis is difficult because there is limited data correlating positive clinical responses with CsA blood levels. Clinical response to therapy is often the most reliable method of assessing efficacy with CsA therapy. Considering the large margin of safety of CsA in dogs, the variability of bioavailability, and the lack of correlation between blood concentrations and clinical response, routine monitoring of blood CsA is not currently recommended in dogs with atopic dermatitis.[18] The author typically only performs trough CsA levels if there is a lack of clinical response (before increasing dose) or if there is a concern for toxicity or superabsorption.

In cats, blood levels of CsA in field studies were highly variable, even among cats with similar clinical response, suggesting that correlations could not be generalized between cats with regard to blood CsA levels and clinical response.[6] CsA levels pertaining to toxoplasmosis are discussed later.

DRUG INTERACTIONS

Numerous interactions have been reported between CsA and other drugs, mainly caused by the shared metabolic pathways involving cytochrome P450 (CYP3A4) and/or competition with P-glycoprotein.[18] Drugs that inhibit cytochrone P450 decrease hepatic clearance of CsA, resulting in increased serum levels of CsA, whereas drugs that induce P450 activity can result in decreased blood concentrations of CsA.[18] Common medications/treatments that may interact with CsA that have been studied in veterinary medicine are reviewed here.

Azole Antifungals

Azole antifungals are commonly used in veterinary dermatology to increase blood levels of CsA and save on associated costs. Ketoconazole is most commonly used for this purpose. Ketoconazole inhibits CYP3A and results in increased blood levels of CsA. Ketoconazole also inhibits P-glycoprotein, resulting in decreased transport of CsA into the intestinal lumen and higher bioavailability. Depending on the dose of ketoconazole administered, the total dose of CsA may be decreased by up to 75% to 90% in dogs.[33,34] The extent of the interaction between ketoconazole and CsA is variable, and CsA blood concentrations are not predictable.[2] Individual dose adjustments may therefore be required. The author commonly uses a starting dosage of ketoconazole 5 to 10 mg/kg once daily combined with modified CsA 2.5 mg/kg once daily.

Unlike ketoconazole, which is mainly metabolized in the liver, fluconazole is primarily excreted unchanged in the urine.[20] Although fluconazole inhibits hepatic CYP3A in vitro, it seems to have no inhibitory effect on the P-glycoprotein encoded by MDR1.[35] Fluconazole has been shown to significantly increase the oral bioavailability of CsA and increase its blood concentration in healthy beagles.[36] Increased oral bioavailability of CsA after fluconazole administration in dogs is likely achieved by decreasing the first-pass effect that is associated with CYP3A, rather than P-glycoprotein activity during intestinal absorption of CsA.[36] The effect of fluconazole on the CsA dosage has also been investigated in renal-transplanted and normal dogs receiving CsA-based immunosuppressive therapy.[37] At first, CsA was administered orally twice daily to increase the blood trough level between 400 and 600 ng/mL. After the addition of fluconazole (5 mg/kg once daily), the CsA dosage was adjusted to maintain its therapeutic blood concentration.[37] Fluconazole significantly decreased CsA dosage in both normal and renal-transplanted dogs, but a higher dosage of CsA was needed in renal-transplanted dogs.[37] In normal dogs, the CsA requirements significantly decreased by 29% to 51% compared with initial CsA doses.[37]

Metoclopramide

A recent article showed no effect of metoclopramide (0.3–0.5 mg/kg) on the pharmacokinetic parameters of CsA in healthy dogs.[38] An adjustment of the CsA dose may not be needed when metoclopramide is coadministered orally to prevent common adverse effects of CsA.[38]

Cimetidine

Cimetidine is a potent inhibitor of hepatic microsomal enzymes.[39] In dogs, cimetidine may delay (but not decrease) absorption of orally administered CsA with no overall effect on the pharmacokinetics of CsA.[39]

Grapefruit Juice

In human studies, grapefruit juice administered before oral administration of CsA enhances the blood concentration of CsA by 45% to 62%.[40,41] Grapefruit juice contains furanocoumarins, which are inhibitors of intestinal (but not hepatic) CYP3A enzymes.[42,43] Inhibition of CYP3A-mediated metabolism of CsA is the proposed main mechanism by which grapefruit juice increases CsA bioavailability.[40,41] Powdered whole grapefruit (PWG) had the potential to reduce the required oral administered dose of CsA in dogs, but only when PWG was used in an amount of at least 10 g; this is currently not a cost-effective option.[38]

St. John's Wort

St. John's Wort (SJW) is a herb that is known to induce cytochrome P450, and, in humans, is associated with decreased blood levels of CsA.[42] In dogs, repeated administration of SJW affected the pharmacokinetic profiles (decreased maximum concentration and area under the curve) of CsA, presumably secondary to an increase in metabolism of CsA caused by upregulation of cytochrome P450 enzymes.[42]

SIDE EFFECTS IN DOGS

In dogs, vomiting, diarrhea, and anorexia are the most commonly seen side effects. In a review of prospective clinical trials with CsA, vomiting (25% overall prevalence) and soft stools or diarrhea (15% overall prevalence) were the most commonly reported side effects.[44] Decreased appetite or anorexia was reported in 2% of the total adverse reactions.[44] In a different study, vomiting was reported in 31% of dogs receiving CsA at 5 mg/kg/d.[45] Of the dogs that vomited, 73% had less than 3 vomiting episodes during the 16-week trial; 10% had 4 to 7 episodes and 6% vomited once to twice weekly.[45] Diarrhea was reported in 20% of dogs, with most dogs only having a single episode.[45] Most gastrointestinal (GI) disturbances with CsA in dogs are observed early in the course of treatment and abate with time.[44]

To help alleviate GI symptoms, the author commonly has owners freeze the CsA capsule for 30 to 60 minutes before administration and recommends administering the medication with a small amount of food. If this does not improve the vomiting, metoclopramide can be given 30 to 60 minutes before administration of CsA. Another medication that can be helpful in decreasing CsA-associated GI side effects is maropitant citrate (Cerenia; Pfizer Animal Health). The author has had good success using high-fiber supplements such as canned pumpkin and probiotics in dogs that develop diarrhea/soft stools on CsA. Zinc-carnosine and vitamin E supplementation (Gastri-Calm; Teva Animal Health) did not ameliorate GI side effects associated with CsA therapy.[46] In a small-scale study, giving CsA with food did not decrease the frequency of adverse events/side effects.[21]

Other adverse reactions reported in dogs with CsA therapy include:

- Gingival hyperplasia[2,19,47]
- Cutaneous papillomatosis[2,19]
- Hypertrichosis[2,19]
- Psoriasiform lichenoid dermatosis[48]

- Excessive shedding, increase in nail growth[2,19]
- Hyperkeratosis of the footpads[19,47]
- Seizures[47]
- Shaking, trembling, or convulsions[47]
- Urinary tract infections[47,49]
- Behavioral changes including lethargy, hyperactivitiy, nervousness, restlessness, irritability, and light sensitivity[47]
- Polyuria/polydipsia[47]
- Pruritus after administration[47]
- Cutaneous flushing[47]
- Weight loss[47]
- Lymphadenopathy[47]
- Neoplasia: histiocytoma, lymphoma, mast cell tumor[47]
- Disseminated nocardiosis in a dog with neurologic disease receiving CsA/ketoconazole for atopic dermatitis[50]
- Multiple papillomavirus-associated epidermal hamartomas and squamous cell carcinomas in situ in a dog following chronic treatment with prednisone and CsA[51]

Most of these reported side effects are reversible with discontinuation of the CsA.

In a review of 9 dogs that developed hyperplastic skin growths on CsA, most dogs (7/9) had lesions that clinically and histopathologically were compatible with psoriasiform lichenoid dermatosis and 2/9 were positive for papillomavirus.[48] Psoriasiform lichenoid dermatosis is thought to be a reaction secondary to staphylococcal pyoderma; these cases typically completely respond to antimicrobial therapy.[48]

Gingival hyperplasia (**Fig. 1**) is presumed to be secondary to CsA-mediated inhibition of collagen degradation and stimulation of fibroblast proliferation.[44]

Based on evidence in humans, the author has used azithromycin-containing toothpaste to help control CsA-induced gingival hyperplasia in dogs.[52] More severe cases may require dental treatments and surgical debulking.

Cutaneous papillomas in dogs receiving CsA are typically self-limiting once CsA is discontinued. Azithromycin 10 mg/kg once daily for 10 days can be prescribed to hasten resolution of the papillomas.[53] In the author's experience, CsA can often be restarted in these cases at a decreased dosing frequency without recurrence of papillomas.

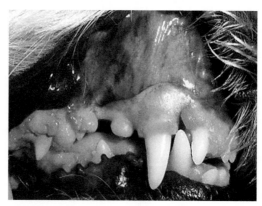

Fig. 1. Gingival hyperplasia in a West Highland white terrier receiving CsA for atopic dermatitis.

Nephrotoxicity and hypertension are commonly reported in humans treated with CsA; however, this has not been shown in dogs, even when given at a dosage of 30 mg/kg/d for 90 days.[43,46] Hepatotoxicity has also been reported in humans receiving CsA; safety studies have not reported this side effect in dogs.[44]

Clinicopathologic Changes

Clinicopathologic abnormalities are reported in up to 25% of patients receiving long-term CsA.[54] Reported changes (with frequencies when available) include increased alkaline phosphatase, alanine aminotransferase, gamma-glutamyl transpeptidase, aspartate aminotransferase, creatinine (7.8%), hyperglobulinemia (6.4%), hyperphosphatemia (5.3%), hyperproteinemia (3.4%), hypercholesterolemia (2.6%), hypoalbuminemia (2.3%), hypocalcemia (2.3%), increased blood urea nitrogen (2.3%), hypernatremia, hyperkalemia, hypercalcemia and hyperchloremia; these changes were not typically associated with clinical signs of disease.[47,54] Proteinuria has rarely been reported in dogs receiving CsA,[47] and urinary tract infections and hypertension should be ruled out in these cases.

A retrospective analysis of 87 dogs receiving CsA for greater than 5 months found that dogs in the CsA treatment group were significantly more likely to have a positive urine culture.[49] CsA-treated cases were divided into dogs receiving concurrent glucocorticoids and those receiving CsA alone. Dogs receiving CsA and glucocorticoids concurrently were significantly more likely than those on CsA alone to have a positive urine culture.[49] A prospective study is needed to further evaluate the risk of developing urinary tract infections in dogs treated with CsA.

Cautions/Contraindications

The safety and efficacy of CsA in dogs less than 6 months old or less than 1.8 kg are unknown.[5] The drug is contraindicated for use in dogs with a history of malignant neoplasia and should not be given to breeding dogs and pregnant or lactating bitches.[5] The long-term concurrent use of CsA with glucocorticoids should be avoided to prevent the development of potentially severe opportunistic infections.[55]

Effect of CsA on Glucose Metabolism

After 3 weeks of CsA administration at 20 mg/kg, dogs remained normoglycemic, but retrieved islet tissue showed a significantly lower total insulin output than that of control animals.[56] In an article evaluating the effects of modified CsA at the labeled dose for atopic dermatitis, a disturbance of glucose metabolism was shown.[57] The fructosamine levels were significantly increased after treatment with CsA, although the disturbances were mild because no dogs had a fructosamine concentration after treatment that was more than the reference range.[57] Peak glucose concentrations were increased 20 and 30 minutes after a glucagon stimulation tests and the overall plasma glucose concentrations (based on areas under concentration-time curves before and after CsA treatment) were increased with CsA therapy.[57] Serum insulin levels were significantly lower following CsA treatment.[57] The mechanism for alteration in glucose metabolism is not fully understood, but has been theorized to involve reduced ability of islets to secrete insulin in response to a secretagogue stimulus.[57] The clinical significance of these findings is unclear because CsA is commonly used for the treatment of atopic dermatitis in dogs with diabetes mellitus.

In a study evaluating the effect of diabetes/hyperglycemia on CsA pharmacokinetics, diabetic dogs showed a significant increase in total body clearance of CsA compared with healthy dogs and a decrease in its biologic half-life (9.32 hours vs 22.56 hours).[58]

SIDE EFFECTS IN CATS

Commonly reported adverse reactions in cats receiving CsA from 2 large field studies (total 205 cats) included[59]:

- Vomiting, retching, regurgitation (35%)
- Weight loss (20%)
- Diarrhea (15%)
- Anorexia/decreased appetite (14%)
- Lethargy/malaise (14%)
- Hypersalivation (11%)
- Behavioral changes including hiding, hyperactivity, aggression (9%)
- Ocular discharge/epiphora/conjunctivitis (7%)
- Sneezing/rhinitis (5%)
- Gingivitis/gingival hyperplasia (4%)
- Polydipsia (3%)

Persistent, progressive weight loss that resulted in hepatic lipidosis occurred in 2 of 205 cats in field studies.[59] Close monitoring of body weight is recommended in cats during treatment with CsA.

CsA may increase the susceptibility to infection and the development of neoplasia.[6] One of 205 field study cats died of the effusive form of feline infectious peritonitis.[59] In CsA safety studies, 1 cat receiving 5 times the approved dose developed lymphoma that was present in the kidneys and mesenteric lymph nodes on necropsy.[59] Cats treated with CsA after receiving kidney transplants had more than 6 times higher odds of developing posttransplant metastatic neoplasia (most commonly lymphoma) compared with control cats.[60]

In a article evaluating side effects of 50 allergic cats receiving CsA, adverse events occurred in 66% of cats.[61] Adverse events likely to be associated with CsA included vomiting or diarrhea within 1 to 8 weeks of receiving CsA (24%), weight loss (16%), anorexia and subsequent hepatic lipidosis (2%), and gingival hyperplasia (2%).[61]

Toxoplasmosis

Seropositivity for toxoplasmosis is widespread in the United States, with 31.6% of clinically ill cats being positive on immunoglobulin (Ig) M or IgG.[62] Toxoplasmosis in association with CsA for feline atopic dermatitis has been previously reported in case reports.[63,64] The reported clinical signs included respiratory symptoms and hepatic failure.[63,64] The effect of CsA (label dose) on the *Toxoplasma gondii* status of cats when administered before and after infection with *T gondii* or only after infection with *T gondii* was recently evaluated.[59,65] In the group that was treated with CsA before and after infection with *T gondii*, 2 cats developed disseminated toxoplasmosis.[59] Clinical signs typical for toxoplasmosis (GI symptoms, lethargy) were seen in most cats in the study, but resolved within 6 weeks following infection; clinical signs were more severe and lasted the longest in the group that was treated with CsA before and after infection.[59] CsA did not reactivate oocyst shedding or clinical disease/illness in cats previously exposed (seropositive) to *T gondii*.[59,65,66] CsA increased the severity of *T gondii* infection in naive cats, but not in seropositive cats.[59,65] Recrudescence of toxoplasmosis in seropositive cats receiving the labeled dose of CsA for atopic dermatitis is unlikely, but further data are needed to determine the risk; it is likely that potential for *T gondii* activation relates to CsA concentrations in individual cats.[66] *T gondii* is not cleared from the tissues of cats treated with clindamycin, potentiated sulfonamides, or azithromycin; therefore, the benefit of treating *T gondii*–seropositive cats before administration of CsA is unknown.[66]

Seronegative cats with high CsA levels (typically >1000 ng/mL) are at the highest risk of developing acute fatal toxoplasmosis if they are newly exposed to the parasite.[66] Therefore it is critical that *T gondii*–negative cats treated with CsA avoid exposure. Methods to decrease exposure include keeping cats indoors, restricting any hunting behavior, and avoiding raw meats. If CsA is administered to cats that go outdoors (which the author does not recommend), monitoring CsA levels is strongly recommended.

Feline Herpesvirus 1 Infection

A recent abstract evaluated the effect of CsA and methylprednisolone on recrudescence of feline herpesvirus 1 (FHV-1) infection in cats with chronic herpesvirus infection.[67] Although clinical signs of activated FHV-1 occurred in some cats administered methylprednisolone or CsA, disease was mild/self-limiting and there was no significant difference in development of clinical signs between the treatment groups.[67]

Clinicopathologic Changes

Reported clinicopathologic changes in cats receiving CsA at 3 times the label dose included mild increases of cholesterol, glucose, total protein, blood urea nitrogen, creatinine, and lymphopenia.[6] Glucosuria was noted in 3 treated animals that also had hyperglycemia.[6]

Cautions/Contraindications

CsA should not be used in cats with a history of malignant disorders, suspected malignancy, and cats infected with feline leukemia virus (FeLV) or feline immunodeficiency virus (FIV).[6] The safety and effectiveness has not been established in cats less than 6 months of age or less than 1.4 kg body weight.[6] CsA is not labeled for use in breeding cats and pregnant or lactating queens.[6] CsA is not labeled for use with other immunosuppressive agents.[6]

EFFECT OF CYCLOSPORINE ON VACCINATION

In a small study, 16 dogs received either 20 mg/kg daily of CsA or placebo for 56 days and were vaccinated on day 27 with a killed rabies vaccine and a multivalent distemper, hepatitis, leptospirosis, parainfluenza, parvovirus (DHLPP) vaccine (including modified live parvovirus).[47] Results revealed no antibody titer increase in any dog (including placebo/control dogs) to any of the components of the multivalent DHLPP vaccine, but appropriate antibody titer response in all dogs to the killed rabies vaccine by day 42.[47] Studies have not been performed at the therapeutic/approved dosing and it is unclear why dogs in the control group did not develop an increase in antibody titer.[47] Because of the drug's mechanism of action, the manufacturer recommends the use of killed vaccines in patients receiving CsA.[5]

Fully vaccinated (feline viral rhinitis, calicivirus, and parvovirus [FVRCP], rabies, FeLV) cats were administered CsA at 3 times the labeled dose.[59] Twenty-eight days into treatment, cats received booster vaccines for FVRCP, FeLV, and rabies, and were vaccinated for the first time with FIV.[59] Vaccine titers for previously administered vaccinations were decreased in the CsA-treated cats compared with controls, but remained adequate.[59] However, cats on CsA failed to develop titers to FIV vaccine.[59] Titer response to cats receiving 3 times the labeled dose of CsA depended on vaccination status before treatment; vaccine naive cats failed to develop titers when they were vaccinated while being treated with CsA.[59] Studies have not been performed at the labeled dose. The long-term effects of CsA on vaccine titers in dogs and cats remain unclear.

EFFECT OF CSA ON ALLERGY TESTING

CsA was found to have no significant effect on serum allergen-specific IgE levels and intradermal tests when administered at 5 mg/kg for 21 days to dogs with experimentally induced flea allergy dermatitis.[68] No significant effect was found on moderate and strong intradermal allergy test results in dogs before and after 42 days of treatment with CsA.[69] In a double-blinded, placebo-controlled study evaluating the effect of CsA (5 mg/kg once daily for 30 days) on intradermal and serum IgE allergy testing, CsA did not have a statistically significant effect on intradermal reactivity or serology results.[70]

CSA AND ALLERGEN-SPECIFIC IMMUNOTHERAPY

The effect of CsA on allergen-specific immunotherapy (ASIT) has not been studied in dogs and cats. In the author's practice, CsA is commonly used both during the induction and maintenance phases of ASIT, with no perceived decrease in efficacy. In humans with atopic dermatitis, low-dose CsA has been shown to significantly increase the T-regulatory cell population.[71] Success of allergen-specific immunotherapy in dogs has recently been shown to be associated with an increase in T-regulatory cell population, which regulates immune system homeostasis via production of cytokines such as IL-10.[72] It is possible that the CsA may be synergistic with ASIT, but the interaction between CsA and ASIT requires further investigation.

DERMATOLOGIC USES/INDICATIONS

CsA has been used to treat a variety of inflammatory and immune-mediated dermatoses in dogs and cats.

Atopic Dermatitis in Dogs

The main indication for CsA in veterinary dermatology is for the treatment of atopic dermatitis. CsA is approved for use in dogs for the treatment of atopic dermatitis at the dosage of 5 mg/kg once daily.[5] The International Task force on Canine Atopic Dermatitis 2010 practice guidelines concluded that there is good evidence for high efficacy of CsA at 5 mg/kg once daily in the treatment of dogs with atopic dermatitis.[55] Clinical improvement takes a minimum of 4 to 6 weeks, so no adjustment in dosing is recommended before 30 days of therapy.[55] In a systematic review and meta-analysis, 799 dogs in 10 studies had been treated with CsA (n = 622), placebo (n = 160), oral glucocorticoids (n = 24), or antihistamines (n = 23).[44] Dogs were treated from 2 weeks to 6 months and doses ranged from 2.5 to 5 mg/kg.[44] After 4 to 6 weeks of CsA (5 mg/kg once daily), a 40% decrease in skin lesions and at least a 30% decrease in pruritus were noted.[44] The percentage of dogs showing at least a 50% improvement in clinical signs increased from 20% to 60%, after 4 weeks of treatment and from 63% to 87% after 12 to 16 weeks of therapy.[44]

In most of the evaluated studies, 40% to 50% of patients were able to have their dosage decreased to every other day; in 20% to 26% of dogs the dosage could be decreased to twice weekly after 14 to 16 weeks, and the remainder of dogs (approximately 25%) required once-daily treatment.[44] A significant difference in efficacy was noted in CsA compared with placebo; however; no significant difference was noted in CsA compared with glucocorticoids.[44] Overall, CsA had a good to excellent response in 65% to 76% of patients, with better responses noted in dogs receiving longer treatment regimens.[44]

Using Generic Modified CsA for Atopic Dermatitis in Dogs

A recent article evaluated the efficacy of a commercially available human generic CsA product (Equoral; Teva Pharmaceuticals) for canine atopic dermatitis.[73] Lesion and pruritus scores were reduced similarly to prednisone, with a reduction of lesion scores of greater than or equal to 50% in 85% (generic CsA) and 100% (prednisone) of dogs, and a reduction in pruritus scores of greater than or equal to 50% in 77% and 86% of dogs treated with generic CsA and prednisone, respectively.[73]

Allergic Dermatitis and Eosinophilic Granuloma Complex in Cats

CsA in cats is labeled for the control of feline allergic dermatitis as manifested by excoriations (including facial and neck), miliary dermatitis, eosinophilic plaques, and self-induced alopecia in cats.[6] The approved dosage is 7 mg/kg once daily for a minimum of 4 to 6 weeks or until resolution of clinical signs.[6] The author most commonly starts cats on 5 mg/kg once daily with good success.

Various studies have reported efficacy of CsA for cats with allergic skin disease, eosinophilic granuloma complex, and stomatitis.[59,74,75] A placebo-controlled field study was performed in 217 client-owned cats with allergic dermatitis.[59] Cats in the treatment group had a 65% improvement in lesional score and a perceived owner success rate of 79%.[59] Following initial daily treatment period, the dose of CsA may be tapered by decreasing the frequency of dosing to every other day or twice weekly to maintain the desired therapeutic effect.[59] Frequency of administration was reduced to every other day in 70% of cats, and, after 4 additional weeks, 57% of cats could be reduced from every other day to twice-weekly administration.[59] In a controlled double-blinded study comparing the efficacy of CsA and prednisolone in feline atopic dermatitis, it was shown that CsA is an effective alternative to prednisolone therapy in cats with atopic dermatitis.[76]

IMMUNE-MEDIATED SKIN DISEASES

CsA is a safe and effective immunosuppressive therapy for many immune-mediated skin diseases. Immune-mediated skin diseases for which CsA has been used include:

- Perianal fistulas[34,77–81]
- Sebaceous adenitis[82–85]
- Pemphigus foliaceus and erythematosus[86–90]
- Juvenile cellulitis[91]
- Vesicular cutaneous lupus erythematosus[92]
- Erythema multiforme[2,19]
- Discoid lupus erythematosus
- Sterile nodular panniculitis[93]
- Metatarsal fistulae[19]
- Granulomatous folliculitis and furunculosis[82]
- Nasal arteritis/ulcerative dermatosis of nasal philtrum[19]
- Facial dermatitis in Persian cats[94]
- Sterile granuloma/pyogranuloma syndrome[19]
- Immune-mediated adnexal targeting including mural folliculitis, alopecia areata in a dog,[82] and pseudopelade in a cat[19]
- Cutaneous reactive histiocytosis[95]
- Feline plasma cell pododermatitis
- Vasculitis and ischemic dermatopathy (See articles by Innera and Morris elsewhere in this issue)

Perianal Fistula

Many publications have documented the efficacy of CsA for the treatment of perianal fistulas.[34,77–81] In a randomized placebo-controlled study of dogs with perianal fistulas, lesions of all CsA-treated dogs, but none of the placebo dogs, improved after 4 weeks.[77] Mean total surface area and mean depth decreased 78% and 62%, respectively, in the CsA group but increased 29% and 11%, respectively, in the control group.[77]

The most effective therapeutic dosing regimen for perianal fistulas has yet to be established. In many studies, CsA was given twice daily but data from recent studies suggest that once-daily administration may be equally beneficial.[34,78,79] In a study evaluating once-daily treatment of perianal fistulas, various dosages (1.5, 3.0, 5.0, or 7.5 mg/kg once daily) were compared.[78] After 13 weeks of treatment 6/24 dogs were in complete remission, 11/24 were controlled or improved, and 7/24 had failed to respond.[78] The response of the dogs given the highest dosage (7.5 mg/kg once daily) was significantly better than the response of the other groups.[78] Relapses were common after discontinuation of treatment.[78] In a similar study, CsA 5 mg/kg once daily was more effective at reducing the surface area and severity of perianal fistula lesions than 2 mg/kg once daily.[79]

Concurrent use of ketoconazole and CsA has also been evaluated for the management of perianal fistulas.[34,61] One study evaluated ketoconazole (10 mg/kg once daily) and CsA (1 mg/kg twice daily) for 16 weeks to treat dogs with perianal fistulas.[34] Ninety-three percent of dogs showed complete resolution of fistulas during the treatment period and 50% had no recurrence after 12 months.[34] A similar study evaluated oral CsA (initial dosage of 2.5 mg/kg twice daily in 8 dogs and 4 mg/kg once daily in 4 dogs) and ketoconazole (8 mg/kg once daily).[80] Clinical signs resolved in all dogs within 9 weeks and recurred in 5/8 dogs.[80] The cost savings with combination CsA/ketoconazole therapy varied between 36% and 71%.[80] Preoperative therapy with CsA or CsA/ketoconazole in dogs undergoing surgical correction of their perianal fistulas has also been shown to be beneficial at minimizing recurrence.[81]

The author most commonly uses CsA 5 mg/kg once daily as a monotherapy or CsA 2 to 4 mg/kg/d combined with ketoconazole 5 to 10 mg/kg once daily when treating perianal fistulas in dogs. Given the high recurrence rates when treatment is discontinued, the dosing interval is decreased to the lowest frequency that controls the symptoms. The author does not commonly perform CsA levels in patients with perianal fistulas receiving CsA because serum CsA concentrations have been shown to be unpredictable and do not correlate with clinical response in many cases.[79]

Sebaceous Adenitis

CsA was first reported to be effective for granulomatous sebaceous adenitis in a miniature pinscher.[83] CsA (5 mg/kg once daily) significantly decreased clinical scores in dogs with sebaceous adenitis after 4 months of treatment and remained low after 8 and 12 months.[84] On histology, the severity of inflammation was significantly decreased with CsA treatment.[83] The percentage of hair follicles with sebaceous glands increased, suggesting regeneration of sebaceous glands.[83] Clinical signs recurred when CsA administration was discontinued.[84]

A recent article compared the efficacy of CsA alone or combined with topical therapy with conventional topical therapy for sebaceous adenitis.[85] Topical treatment, both alone and in combination with CsA, reduced scaling more effectively than CsA alone.[85] Both therapies reduced alopecia. There was evidence of a synergistic benefit on both scaling and alopecia if both treatment options were combined.[85] Inflammation of the sebaceous glands was also best reduced by a combination of both CsA and topical therapy.[85] Regeneration of sebaceous glands was best achieved by CsA, either given alone or in combination with topical treatment.[85]

Pemphigus Foliaceus

CsA at a dosage of 5 and 10 mg/kg once daily was evaluated in 5 dogs with PF.[88] No cases achieved complete remission, and 4/5 dogs had to be withdrawn from the trial because of exacerbation of lesional scores.[88] CsA as a monotherapy at 5 to 10 mg/kg once daily cannot be recommended for the treatment of pemphigus foliaceus in dogs; however, higher doses have not been studied.[88] No studies exist on using CsA to manage feline pemphigus foliaceus, but the author has used CsA to manage several cases both as a steroid-sparing agent and as sole therapy.

CsA is more effective for canine pemphigus foliaceus when used in combination with other therapies.[87] In 3 dogs with pemphigus foliaceus already receiving azathioprine and glucocorticoids, oral CsA at 7.5 to 10 mg/kg/d was used with oral ketoconazole at 2.5 to 5 mg/kg/d to successfully induce remission.[89] CsA was used successfully with prednisone alone to induce remission of pemphigus foliaceus in 5 dogs.[90] Initial dosages ranged from 1 to 2.6 mg/kg/d for prednisone and 5 to 18 mg/kg/d for the CsA.[90] Although the initial CsA dosage was maintained in each patient, the prednisone dosage was then tapered to 0.5 mg/kg every other day with no relapse of signs.[90] The CsA was continued and eventually tapered to 3 to 4 mg/kg every other day.

MISCELLANEOUS DERMATOLOGIC CONDITIONS

Other dermatologic conditions reported to respond to CsA include:

- Follicular hyperkeratosis of cocker spaniels[19]
- German shepherd deep pyoderma[19]
- Primary seborrhea in springer spaniels, cairn terriers, and West Highland white terriers[96]
- Chronic pedal furunculosis[19]
- End-stage proliferative external otitis in cocker spaniels and golden retrievers[97]
- Feline urticaria pigmentosa[98]

Table 1
Patient monitoring during cyclosporine therapy

Time	Recommended Monitoring
Before starting therapy	CBC, serum chemistry, urinalysis ± urine culture Physical and dermatologic examinations Body weight FeLV/FIV test (cats)
3 mo after starting therapy	CBC, serum chemistry, urinalysis ± urine culture Physical and dermatologic examinations Body weight
Every 6 mo during treatment	CBC, serum chemistry, urinalysis ± urine culture Physical and dermatologic examinations Body weight

Abbreviation: CBC, complete blood count.

PATIENT MONITORING DURING CYCLOSPORINE THERAPY

Table 1 shows the author's recommended patient monitoring during CsA therapy.

SUMMARY

CsA is a calcineurin inhibitor that is efficacious and approved for atopic dermatitis in dogs and allergic dermatitis in cats; it has also been used to successfully manage a variety of immune-mediated dermatoses. Drug interactions are commonly reported because of the shared metabolic pathways involving cytochrome P450 and/or competition with P-glycoprotein; ketoconazole can be used in clinical cases to reduce the oral required dosage and associated costs of CsA. Given the lack of correlation between blood concentrations and clinical response, CsA levels are not typically performed. The most commonly reported side effects caused by CsA are GI in nature; other reported side effects are typically reversible with discontinuation of CsA.

REFERENCES

1. Marsella R. Calcineurin inhibitors: a novel approach to canine atopic dermatitis. J Am Anim Hosp Assoc 2005;41:92–7.
2. Guaguére E, Steffan J, Olivry T, et al. Cyclosporine A: a new drug in the field of canine dermatology. Vet Dermatol 2004;15:61–74.
3. Choc ML. Bioavailability and pharmacokinetics of cyclosporine formulations: Neoral vs Sandimmune. Int J Dermatol 1997;36:1–6.
4. Gridelli B, Scanlon L, Pellicci R, et al. Cyclosporine metabolism and pharmacokinetics following intravenous and oral administration in the dog. Transplantation 1986;41:388–91.
5. Atopica [product insert]. Greensboro (NC): Novartis Animal Health; 2007.
6. Atopica for cats [product insert]. Greensboro (NC): Novartis Animal Health; 2011.
7. Taylor AL, Watson CJE, Bradley JA. Immunosuppressive agents in solid organ transplantation: mechanisms of action and therapeutic efficacy. Crit Rev Oncol Hematol 2005;56:23–46.
8. Shibasaki F, Hallin U, Uchino H. Calcineurin as a multifunctional regulator. J Biochem 2002;131:1–15.
9. Aronson LR, Stumhofer JS, Drobatz KJ, et al. Effect of cyclosporine, dexamethasone, and human CTLA4-Ig on production of cytokines in lymphocytes of clinically normal cats and cats undergoing renal transplantation. Am J Vet Res 2011;72(4):541–9.
10. Fellman CL, Stokes JV, Archer TM, et al. Cyclosporine A affects the in vitro expression of T cell activation-related molecules and cytokines in dogs. Vet Immunol Immunopathol 2011;140(3–4):175–80.
11. Marsella R, Olivry T. The ACVD task force on canine atopic dermatitis (XXII): nonsteroidal anti-inflammatory pharmacotherapy. Vet Immunol Immunopathol 2001;81:331–4.
12. Ciesek S, Ringe BP, Strassburg CP, et al. Effects of cyclosporine on human dendritic cell subsets. Transplant Proc 2005;37:20–4.
13. Al-Dajari WI, Grant KR, Ryan K, et al. Localization of calcineurin/NFAT in human skin and psoriasis and inhibition of calcineurin/ NFAT activation in human keratinocytes by cyclosporine A. J Invest Dermatol 2002;118:779–88.
14. Matsuda S, Koyasu S. Mechanisms of action of cyclosporine. Immunopharmacology 2000;47:119–25.

15. Bäumer W, Kietzmann M. Effects of cyclosporin A and cilomilast on activated canine, murine and human keratinocytes. Vet Dermatol 2007;18(2):107–14.
16. Latimer KS, Rakich PM, Purswell BJ, et al. Effects of cyclosporine A administration in cats. Vet Immunol Immunopathol 1986;11:161–73.
17. Wacher VJ, Silverman JA, Zhang Y, et al. Role of P-glycoprotein and cytochrome P450 3A in limiting oral absorption of peptides and peptidomimetics. J Pharm Sci 1998;87:1322–9.
18. Steffan J, Strehlau G, Maurer M, et al. Cyclosporine A pharmacokinetics and efficacy in the treatment of atopic dermatitis in dogs. J Vet Pharmacol Ther 2004;27: 231–8.
19. Robson DC, Burton GG. Cyclosporin: applications in small animal dermatology. Vet Dermatol 2003;14(1):1–9.
20. Plumb DC. Plumb's veterinary drug handbook. 6th edition. Ames (IA): PharmaVet; 2008.
21. Thelen A, Mueller RS, Linek M, et al. Influence of food intake on the clinical response to cyclosporin A in canine atopic dermatitis. Vet Rec 2006;159(25): 854–6.
22. Ellis CN, Fradin MS, Messena JM, et al. Cyclosporine for plaque-type psoriasis: result of a multidose, double blind trial. N Engl J Med 1991;324:277–84.
23. Hebert MF. Contributions of hepatic and intestinal metabolism and P-glycoprotein to cyclosporine and tacrolimus oral drug delivery. Adv Drug Deliv Rev 1997;27: 201–14.
24. Whalen RD, Tata PN, Burckart GJ, et al. Species differences in the hepatic and intestinal metabolism of cyclosporine. Xenobiotica 1999;29:3–9.
25. Venkataramanan R, Wang CP, Habucky K, et al. Species specific cyclosporine metabolism. Transplant Proc 1988;20:680.
26. Lauerma AI, Surber C, Maibach HI. Absorption of topical tacrolimus (FK506) in vitro through human skin: comparison with cyclosporin A. Skin Pharmacol 1997;10:230–4.
27. Miller A, Schick A, Booth D, et al. Absorption of transdermal cyclosporine versus orally administered cyclosporine in six healthy cats. In: Proceedings North American Veterinary Dermatology Forum. Galveston (TX); 2011. p. 198.
28. Diesel A, Moriello K. A busy clinician's review of cyclosporine. Vet Med 2008; 103(5):266–8.
29. Lindholm A. Factors influencing the pharmacokinetics of cyclosporine in man. Ther Drug Monit 1991;13(6):465–77.
30. Cohen LB, Zabel S, Olea-Poekla FO, et al. Relationship of bodyweight to cyclosporin dose in canine atopic dermatitis. In: Proceedings North American Veterinary Dermatology Forum. Galveston (TX); 2011. p. 197.
31. Nam HS, McAnulty JF, Kwak HH, et al. Gingival overgrowth in dogs associated with clinically relevant cyclosporine blood levels: observations in a canine renal transplantation model. Vet Surg 2008;37:247–53.
32. Mathews KA, Holmberg DL. Kidney transplantation in dogs with naturally occurring end-stage renal disease. J Am Anim Hosp Assoc 2000;36:475.
33. Dahlinger J, Gregory C, Bea J. Effect of ketoconazole on cyclosporine in healthy dogs. Vet Surg 1998;27:64–8.
34. Mouatt JG. Cyclosporine and ketoconazole interaction for treatment of perianal fistulas in the dog. Aust Vet J 2002;80:207–11.
35. Sakaeda T, Iwaki K, Kakumoto M, et al. Effect of micafungin on cytochrome P450 3A4 and multidrug resistance protein 1 activities, and its comparison with azole antifungal drugs. J Pharm Pharmacol 2005;57:759–64.

36. Katayama M, Igarashi H, Tani K, et al. Effect of multiple oral dosing of fluconazole on the pharmacokinetics of cyclosporine in healthy beagles. J Vet Med Sci 2008; 70(1):85–8.

37. Katayama M, Igarashi H, Fukai K, et al. Fluconazole decreases cyclosporine dosage in renal transplanted dogs. Res Vet Sci 2010;89(1):124–5.

38. Radwanski NE, Cerundolo R, Shofer FS, et al. Effects of powdered whole grapefruit and metoclopramide on the pharmacokinetics of cyclosporine in dogs. Am J Vet Res 2011;72(5):687–93.

39. Daigle JC, Hosgood G, Foil CS, et al. Effect of cimetidine on pharmacokinetics of orally administered cyclosporine in healthy dogs. Am J Vet Res 2001;7:1046–50.

40. Ducharme MP, Warbasse LH, Edwards DJ. Disposition of intravenous and oral cyclosporine after the administration with grapefruit juice. Clin Pharmacol Ther 1995;57:485–91.

41. Ku YM, Min DI, Flanigan M. Effect of grapefruit juice on the pharmacokinetics of microemulsion cyclosporine and its metabolite in healthy volunteers: does formulation differences matter? J Clin Pharmacol 1998;38:959–65.

42. Schmiedlin-Ren P, Edwards DJ, Fitzsimmons ME, et al. Mechanisms of enhanced oral availability of CYP3A4 substrates by grapefruit constituents. Decreased enterocyte CYP 3A4 concentrations and mechanism-based inactivation by furanocoumarins. Drug Metab Dispos 1997;11:1228–33.

43. Fukunaga K, Orito K. Time-course effects of St John's wort on the pharmacokinetics of cyclosporine in dogs. J Vet Pharmacol Ther 2011;1365–2885.

44. Steffan J, Favrot C, Mueller R. A systematic review and metaanalysis of the efficacy and safety of cyclosporine for the treatment of atopic dermatitis in dogs. Vet Dermatol 2006;17:3–16.

45. Steffan J, Parks C, Seewald W, et al. Clinical trial evaluating the efficacy and safety of cyclosporine in dogs with atopic dermatitis. J Am Vet Med Assoc 2005;226(11):1855–63.

46. Wilson LS, Rosenkrantz WS, Roycroft LM. Zinc-carnosine and vitamin E supplementation does not ameliorate gastrointestinal side effects associated with ciclosporin therapy of canine atopic dermatitis. Vet Dermatol 2011;(1):53–60.

47. Novartis. Freedom of information summary. Greensboro (NC): Novartis Animal Health; 2003. Atopica, NADA 141–218.

48. Favrot C, Olivry T, Werner AH, et al. Evaluation of papillomaviruses associated with cyclosporine-induced hyperplastic verrucous lesions in dogs. Am J Vet Res 2005;66(10):1764–9.

49. Peterson AL, Torres SM, Rendahl A, et al. Frequency of urinary tract infection in dogs with inflammatory skin disorders treated with ciclosporin alone or in combination with glucocorticoid therapy: a retrospective study. Vet Dermatol 2012;23: 240–3.

50. Paul AE, Mansfield CS, Thompson M. Presumptive *Nocardia* spp. infection in a dog treated with cyclosporin and ketoconazole. N Z Vet J 2010;58(5):265–8.

51. Callan MB, Preziosi D, Mauldin E. Multiple papillomavirus-associated epidermal hamartomas and squamous cell carcinomas in situ in a dog following chronic treatment with prednisone and cyclosporine. Vet Dermatol 2005;16(5):338–45.

52. Argani H, Pourabbas R, Hassanzadeh D, et al. Treatment of cyclosporine-induced gingival overgrowth with azithromycin-containing toothpaste. Exp Clin Transplant 2006;4(1):420–4.

53. Yağci BB, Ural K, Ocal N, et al. Azithromycin therapy of papillomatosis in dogs: a prospective, randomized, double-blinded, placebo-controlled clinical trial. Vet Dermatol 2008;19(4):194.

54. Radowicz SN, Power HT. Long term use of cyclosporine therapy in the treatment of canine atopic dermatitis. Vet Dermatol 2005;16(2):81–6.
55. Olivry T, DeBoer DJ, Favrot C, et al. Treatment of canine atopic dermatitis: 2010 clinical practice guidelines from the International Task Force on Canine Atopic Dermatitis. Vet Dermatol 2010;21(3):233–48.
56. Basadonna G, Montorsi F, Kakizaki K, et al. Cyclosporin-A and islet function. Am J Surg 1988;156:191–3.
57. Kovalik M, Thoday KL, Handel IG, et al. Ciclosporin A therapy is associated with disturbances in glucose metabolism in dogs with atopic dermatitis. Vet Dermatol 2011;(2):173–80.
58. Alkharfy KM. Influence of overt diabetes mellitus on cyclosporine pharmacokinetics in a canine model. Exp Diabetes Res 2009;2009:363–9.
59. Novartis. Freedom of information summary. Novartis Animal Health; 2001. Atopica for Cats, NADA 141–329.
60. Schmiedt CW, Grimes JA, Holzman G, et al. Incidence and risk factors for development of malignant neoplasia after feline renal transplantation and cyclosporine-based immunosuppression. Vet Comp Oncol 2009;7:45–53.
61. Heinrich NA, McKeever PJ, Eisenschenk MC. Adverse events in 50 cats with allergic dermatitis receiving ciclosporin. Vet Dermatol 2011;6:511–20.
62. Vollaire MR, Radecki SV, Lappin MR. Seroprevalence of *Toxoplasma gondii* antibodies in clinically ill cats in the United States. Am J Vet Res 2005;66(5):874–7.
63. Barrs VR, Martin P, Beatty JA. Antemortem diagnosis and treatment of toxoplasmosis in two cats on cyclosporine therapy. Aust Vet J 2006;84:30–5.
64. Last RD, Suzuki Y, Manning T, et al. A case of fatal systemic toxoplasmosis in a cat being treated with cyclosporine A for feline atopy. Vet Dermatol 2004;15:194–8.
65. Lappin MR, Scorza V. *Toxoplasma gondii* oocyst shedding in normal cats and cats treated with cyclosproine. J Vet Intern Med 2011;2011(3):632–767.
66. Lappin MR. Infectious disease complications of cyclosporine use in cats. In: Proceedings North American Veterinary Dermatology Forum. Galveston (TX); 2011. p. 16.
67. Lappin MR, Roycroft L. Effect of cyclosporine and methylprednisolone acetate on cats with chronic feline herpesvirus 1 infection. J Vet Intern Med 2011;25(3):632–767.
68. Clarke K, McCall C, Steffan J, et al. The effects of cyclosporine A and oral prednisolone on flea allergen specific serum IgE and intradermal tests in experimentally sensitized laboratory beagles. Proceedings of the 18th European Society of Veterinary Dermatology- European College Veterinary Dermatology. 2002. p. 223.
69. Burton G, Robson D, Bassett R, et al. A pilot trial on the effect of cyclosporin A on intradermal skin test reactions in dogs with atopic dermatitis. Vet Dermatol 2002; 13(4):211–29.
70. Goldman C, Rosser E Jr, Petersen A, et al. Investigation on the effects of ciclosporin (Atopica) on intradermal test reactivity and allergen-specific immunoglobulin (IgE) serology in atopic dogs. Vet Dermatol 2010;21(4):393–9.
71. Brandt C, Pavlovic V, Radbruch A, et al. Low-dose cyclosporine A therapy increases the regulatory T cell population in patients with atopic dermatitis. Allergy 2009;64(11):1588–96.
72. Keppel KE, Campbell KL, Zuckermann FA, et al. Quantitation of canine regulatory T cell populations, serum interleukin-10 and allergen-specific IgE concentrations in healthy control dogs and canine atopic dermatitis patients receiving allergen-specific immunotherapy. Vet Immunol Immunopathol 2008;123(3–4):337–44.

73. Kovalik M, Taszkun I, Pomorski Z, et al. Evaluation of a human generic formulation of ciclosporin in the treatment of canine atopic dermatitis with in vitro assessment of the functional capacity of phagocytic cells. Vet Rec 2011;168(20):537.

74. Noli C, Scarampella F. Prospective open pilot study on the use of ciclosporin for feline allergic skin disease. J Small Anim Pract 2006;47(8):434–8.

75. Vercelli A, Raviri G, Cornegliani L. The use of oral cyclosporin to treat feline dermatoses: a retrospective analysis of 23 cases. Vet Dermatol 2006;17(3): 201–6.

76. Wisselink MA, Willemse T. The efficacy of cyclosporine A in cats with presumed atopic dermatitis: a double blind, randomised prednisolone-controlled study. Vet J 2009;180(1):55–9.

77. Mathews KA, Sukhiani HR. Randomised controlled trial of cyclosporine for the treatment of perianal fistulas in dogs. J Am Vet Med Assoc 1997;211:1249–53.

78. Doust R, Griffiths LG, Sullivan M. Evaluation of once daily treatment with cyclosporine for anal furunculosis in dogs. Vet Rec 2003;152(8):225–9.

79. House AK, Guitian J, Gregory SP, et al. Evaluation of the effect of two dose rates of cyclosporine on the severity of perianal fistulae lesions and associated clinical signs in dogs. Vet Surg 2006;35(6):543–9.

80. Patricelli A, Hardie RJ, McAnulty JE. Cyclosporine and ketoconazole for the treatment of perianal fistulas in dogs. J Am Vet Med Assoc 2002;220:1009–16.

81. Klein A, Deneuche A, Fayolle P, et al. Preoperative immunosuppressive therapy and surgery as a treatment for anal furunculosis. Vet Surg 2006;35(8):759–68.

82. Noli C, Toma S. Three cases of immune-mediated adnexal skin disease treated with cyclosporin. Vet Dermatol 2006;17(1):85–92.

83. Carothers MA, Kwochka KW, Rojko JL. Cyclosporine-responsive granulomatous sebaceous adenitis in a dog. J Am Vet Med Assoc 1991;198(9):1645–8.

84. Linek M, Boss C, Haemmerling R, et al. Effects of cyclosporine A on clinical and histologic abnormalities in dogs with sebaceous adenitis. J Am Vet Med Assoc 2005;226(1):59–64.

85. Lortz J, Favrot C, Mecklenburg L, et al. A multicentre placebo-controlled clinical trial on the efficacy of oral ciclosporin A in the treatment of canine idiopathic sebaceous adenitis in comparison with conventional topical treatment. Vet Dermatol 2010;6:593–601.

86. Rosenkrantz WS, Griffin CE, Barr RJ. Clinical evaluation of cyclosporine in animal models with cutaneous immune mediated disease and epitheliotropic lymphoma. J Am Anim Hosp Assoc 1989;25:377–84.

87. Tater K, Olivry T. Canine and feline pemphigus foliaceus: improving your chances of a successful outcome. Vet Med 2010;18–32.

88. Olivry T, Rivierre C, Murphy KM. Efficacy of cyclosporine for treatment induction of canine pemphigus foliaceus. Vet Rec 2003;152:53–4.

89. Rosenkrantz WS, Aniya JS. Cyclosporine, ketoconazole and azathioprine combination therapy in three cases of refractory canine pemphigus foliaceus. Vet Dermatol 2007;18:192.

90. Maeda H, Takahashi M, Nakashima K, et al. Treatment of five dogs with pemphigus foliaceus with cyclosporine and prednisone. Vet Dermatol 2008;19:51.

91. Park C, Yoo JH, Kim HJ, et al. Combination of cyclosporin A and prednisolone for juvenile cellulitis concurrent with hindlimb paresis in 3 English cocker spaniel puppies. Can Vet J 2010;51(11):1265–8.

92. Font A, Bardagi M, Mascort J. Treatment with oral cyclosporin A of a case of vesicular cutaneous lupus erythematosus in a rough collie. Vet Dermatol 2006; 17(6):440–2.

93. Guaguere E. Efficacy of cyclosporin in the treatment of idiopathic sterile nodular panniculitis in two dogs [abstract]. Vet Dermatol 2000;11(1):22.
94. Fontaine J, Heimann M. Idiopathic facial dermatitis of the Persian cat: three cases controlled with cyclosporine. Vet Dermatol 2004;15:64.
95. Palmeiro BS, Morris DO, Goldschmidt MH, et al. Cutaneous reactive histiocytosis in dogs: a retrospective evaluation of 32 cases. Vet Dermatol 2007;18:332–40.
96. Kwochka KW. Therapy of cornification and keratinization disorders. In: Proceedings of North American Veterinary Dermatology Forum. Monterey (CA); 2003. p. 93–7.
97. Hall JA, Waiglass SE, Mathiews KA, et al. Oral cyclosporine in the treatment of end stage ear disease: a pilot study. Proceedings of North American Veterinary Dermatology Forum. Monterey (CA); 2003. p. 217.
98. Guaguere E, Fontaine J. Efficacy of cyclosporin in the treatment of feline urticaria pigmentosa: two cases. Vet Dermatol 2004;15:63.

Nonsteroidal, Nonimmunosuppressive Therapies for Pruritus

Paul Bloom, DVM[a,b,*]

KEYWORDS

- Pruritus • Dog • Barrier dysfunction • Epidermal lipids • Atopic dermatitis
- Topical therapy • Antihistamines • Essential fatty acids

KEY POINTS

- Pruritus is a symptom associated with a wide variety of causes and treatment options.
- There is no single therapy that is effective in every case of pruritus (no magic solution).
- Treatment frequently involves a multimodal approach.
- Atopic dermatitis is a common cause of pruritus in the dog.
- Percutaneous absorption of antigen and barrier dysfunction are now recognized as important components of pruritus associated with atopic dermatitis.
- Topical therapy is becoming the new target for the treatment of pruritus.
- Systemic therapy, other than with immunosuppressive agents, is becoming a less important treatment of pruritus.

INTRODUCTION

Pruritus, or itch, is defined as "a sensation that, if sufficiently strong, will provoke scratching or the desire to scratch."[1,2] Pruritus does serve a useful purpose. It has a self-protective mechanism that helps defend the skin against harmful external agents. Pruritus can be evoked in the skin directly by mechanical and thermal stimuli or indirectly through chemical mediators. Chemical mediators include histamine, catecholamines, acetylcholine, neuropeptides (eg, substance P , calcitonin gene-related peptide , vasoactive intestinal polypeptide, serotonin, corticotropin-releasing hormone, opioids, cannabinoids , neurotrophins (nerve growth factor, neurotrophin-4), bradykinin, proteases (chymases, tryptases, and carboxypeptidase), lipid mediators (leukotriene B4), cytokines, and interleukins (IL-2, IL-4, IL-6, IL-8, and most recently IL-31).[3–7]

Dr Bloom has had lectures or meetings sponsored by Virbac; their products include Resicort, Allermyl, and Allerderm Spot On.
[a] Allergy, Skin, and Ear Clinic for Pets, 31205 Five Mile, Livonia, MI 48154, USA; [b] Small Animal Clinical Sciences, Department of Dermatology, Michigan State University Veterinary Teaching Hospital, 736 Wilson Road, East Lansing, MI 48824, USA
* Allergy, Skin, and Ear Clinic for Pets, 31205 Five Mile, Livonia, MI 48154.
E-mail address: dermdoc@cvm.msu.edu

Vet Clin Small Anim 43 (2013) 173–187
http://dx.doi.org/10.1016/j.cvsm.2012.09.001
0195-5616/13/$ – see front matter © 2013 Published by Elsevier Inc.

CAUSES OF PRURITUS

There are many different classification schemes for pruritus described in human medicine. One method divides pruritus into 4 categories.[8] These categories help dictate the treatment of the patient. They are as follows:

1. Dermatologic (associated with skin diseases, eg, psoriasis, atopic dermatitis [AD])
2. Systemic disease (eg, primary cholestatic liver disease, renal failure)
3. Neuropathic causes by diseases of the central or peripheral nervous system (eg, brain tumor)
4. Psychogenic

Pruritus is regulated by a large number of neurotransmitters that transmit information between the skin, nervous system, endocrine system, and immune system.[9] The wide array of causes, as demonstrated by the different categories of pruritus along with the numerous neurotransmitters, explains why the symptomatic treatment of pruritus can be difficult and why there is no magic solution for treating the pruritus.

TREATMENT OVERVIEW

Treatment of pruritus involves both identifying and treating the primary cause. Although the primary cause is addressed, adjunctive supportive therapy may be needed. Symptomatic treatment of pruritus can be broken down into 2 categories: topical treatment and systemic therapy.

In human medicine, a suggested therapeutic ladder[10] for generalized pruritus is described:

1. Topical medications
2. Sedating antihistamines
3. Narrow-band ultraviolet B rays
4. Combination treatments
5. Mirtazapine or thalidomide
6. Butorphanol

For the purpose of this article, only therapies that have been used in dogs or cats are discussed in depth. Allergen-specific immunotherapy, sublingual immunotherapy, systemic glucocorticoid therapy, and cyclosporine therapy are beyond the scope of this article and are discussed in other articles in this issue.

TOPICAL THERAPY OVERVIEW

A ladder approach to pruritus is appropriate in veterinary medicine. It is important that the treatment is not worse than the disease (eg, side effects being worse than the pruritus). Treatment must also take into account the owner's ability to comply with the recommended treatment and to be able to afford the prescribe treatments. Symptomatic treatment of pruritus can be similar to eating at a buffet in which you can eat whatever you want, just not everything. Our goal is to select the items that are most "palatable" for that patient.

The first step in the ladder is topical therapy. Evidence-based medicine supporting the effectiveness of any of the following topical therapies will be presented. Unfortunately, there are no controlled studies supporting the efficacy of one topical therapy over another. Until then, anecdotal evidence must suffice.

Topical therapy has a few advantages over systemic treatment. Topical therapy can access the diseased tissue directly, allowing for higher concentrations of the drug at the site of the problem with fewer side effects. Topical therapy may also be effective enough that systemic therapy either is not needed or can be used at a lower dose.

There are some disadvantages associated with topical therapy. Topical therapy, even if limited to a localized area, may be more time-consuming and labor-intensive. It may be easier depending on the patient and the location of the lesion to administer an oral medication rather than washing, drying, and then applying a topical residual acting product to the affected area. Because shampoos are rinsed off the skin, residual ingredients that are included in shampoos are of limited effectiveness. Therefore, moisturizers, emollients, and antipruritic agents have limited to no effect when used in a shampoo formulation.

Cost can be an advantage or a disadvantage of using topical therapy. If a small area needs to be treated, topical therapy is usually less expensive than systemic treatment. However, if large areas or costly topical medication needs to be used, topical therapy may be prohibitive.

Before applying topical medication, it is important to consider what will happen to the drug once it is applied. In some cases, the goal is to obtain therapeutic blood levels ("transdermal" medication), whereas in other cases the goal is to obtain therapeutic local tissue levels ("topical" medication). In cases of pruritus, medication will be most effective when it stays locally rather than being systemically absorbed. Both chemical factors (drug's properties) and physical factors (host factors) affect whether a medication that is applied to the skin (or mucous membrane) stays on the surface of the skin or penetrates it. These same factors also determine how much of the drug remains in the epidermis and how much is absorbed into the systemic circulation. To be most effective, ingredients for residual effects should be applied as a leave-on product.

TOPICAL THERAPY—MECHANISM OF ACTION

Five different mechanisms in which topical therapy may control pruritus are listed.[7,11]

1. *Mechanically substituting another sensation for pruritus.* This substitution involves cooling (baths, ice packs), heating, or counter irritation, which may be accomplished with ingredients such as menthol (0.12%–1%), camphor (0.12–5.0%), or thymol (0.5%–1%). There are a variety of products available for veterinary use. Anecdotal evidence has demonstrated that this therapy is largely ineffective in controlling pruritus in the moderately to severely pruritic patient.
2. *Anesthetizing sensory nerve endings.* Pramoxine and lidocaine work by this mechanism. Limitations with these products include unpredictability of effectiveness, short duration of activity, and the development of tachyphylaxis. A crossover study[12] applying a pramoxine-containing cream rinse (Relief or Dermal-Soothe) was performed. In this study, bathing with a baby shampoo was followed by one of the products, twice weekly for 2 weeks. After 2 weeks, the treatment with the cream rinse was reversed between the 2 groups. Based on the owner's evaluation, a good reduction (51%–75%) in pruritus in 41% of the dogs was reported. This antipruritic effect remained for approximately 48 hours. Be aware that in human beings allergic sensitization or contact dermatitis may occur with lidocaine or pramoxine.[8] Anecdotal clinical response to this therapy is ineffective in the moderately to severely pruritic patient.
3. *Blocking pruritogenic mediators.* Because of the diversity of mediators involved in pruritus, this therapy is of limited value. Capsaicin has been used in human medicine and canine medicine.[9,13] Capsaicin is the active component derived from the fruit of capsicum (cayenne pepper). It is thought that capsaicin works by temporarily depleting substance P, a neurotransmitter involved in transmitting pruritus

to the brain. However, it has been reported to be frequently ineffective for pruritus associated with AD in humans.[9] In dogs, a blinded randomized placebo-controlled crossover study evaluating the efficacy of 0.025% capsaicin treatment was reported.[13] There was a significant decrease in pruritus (>50%) in 25% of the dogs as reported by the owners. This observation was reported in only 8% of the dogs by the investigators. In addition, 8% of the dog owners reported a 90% decrease in their dog's pruritus by the end of the study (6 weeks). A meta-analysis report concluded there was fair evidence of low-to-medium efficacy of topical capsaicin in the treatment of pruritus in dogs.[14] Human patients frequently report a burning sensation associated with capsaicin application. It has been suggested to minimize this effect by gradually increasing the capsaicin concentration from 0.025 to 0.05, 0.075, and finally 0.1% or to the highest concentration that is tolerated.[15] It was noted, in the previously mentioned dog study, that owners observed an increase in pruritus in the first week of treatment; however, this worsening was not statistically significant.

   a. Topical over-the-counter antipruritic products containing antihistamines have been used for many years in human medicine with the goal of avoiding the sedation associated with orally administered agents. Despite being one of the most commonly used topical antihistamines, there has only been one study performed evaluating the antipruritic effectiveness in human patients. In this study, topical diphenylhydramine failed to demonstrate any effective antipruritic activity.[16] In canine patients, a study evaluating interferon-gamma in the treatment of atopic dogs used diphenhydramine spray in the control group. The spray was applied every 12 hours for 4 weeks in 1 group and for 8 weeks in the other group of dogs. A good-to-excellent response for reduction of skin lesions or pruritus was reported in 23% (6/26) to 39% (10/26) of treated dogs depending on the clinical signs or symptoms assessed.[17] This therapy is relatively ineffective in treating the moderately to severely pruritic canine patient.

4. *The fourth method is reducing inflammation of the skin.* Topical glucocorticoids are currently the "best in class" in regards to effectiveness of topical therapies for treating pruritic dogs. Topical steroids are divided based on their strengths into 4 groups/7 classes, ranging from class I/high potency to class VII/low potency. The strength of a steroid is determined by measuring vasoconstriction of vessels in the upper dermis. The most potent steroids are in group I and the least potent steroids are in group VII.[18] The quickest and most effective way to get positive results with topical steroids is to start with one of the more potent steroid-containing products when clinical improvement is noted: either discontinue the use of topical glucocorticoids altogether or switch to one with lower potency. The use of low-potency steroids decreases the likelihood of cutaneous reactions such as cutaneous atrophy, ulceration, telangectasia, alopecia, comedones, and calcinosis cutis. Topical steroids can cause systemic effects, such as adrenal suppression, polyuria and polydypsia, elevated liver enzymes, and suppression of thyroid levels.[19,20] To help combat this problem, newly developed topical steroids have been introduced that are metabolized in the skin. These metabolites are largely inactive molecules that tend to limit the systemic or topical side effects of topical steroids. Hydrocortisone aceponate (Cortavance) is one such glucocorticoid. It is available in many parts of the world including Europe as a veterinary spray product. Unfortunately, it is not currently available in the United States. Hydrocortisone aceponate is a diester, which because of its lipophilic properties readily penetrates an intact stratum corneum. It accumulates in the skin while obtaining a low plasma concentration, providing for local effectiveness with

minimal systemic effects. It is a prodrug, which after absorption is deesterified by esterases present in the skin into hydrocortisone 17 (HC 17) propionate. This latter molecule's potency is equivalent to dexamethasone. While in the skin, HC 17 propionate is converted to HC 21 propionate and then to HC. HC is conjugated with glucoronic acid and excreted primarily in the feces. This therapy is extremely effective at decreasing pruritus and inflammation except when microbial infection or ectoparasites are present. In those cases, antimicrobial/parasiticidal therapy is more effective. A recommended protocol may include the application of a moderately potent topical steroid (containing triamcinolone, 0.1%; dexamethasone, 0.1%; or prednisolone, 0.5% twice a day for 7 days then every day for 7 days. Assuming the dog's symptoms are in remission, therapy is then changed to 1% hydrocortisone lotion (ResiCort Leave-On Lotion). This product is selected because a study[21] showed that applying it twice weekly over the entire body of dogs for 6 weeks did not result in clinically evident adverse effects and only minor, clinically insignificant changes in blood parameters. Personal experience with this product has demonstrated that there are limited cutaneous long-term side effects with the application of this lotion if applied to limited areas of the body. Calcinosis cutis has been observed from the chronic use of low-dose (0.015%) triamcinolone spray (Genesis) and, therefore, as with the more potent steroid-containing products, should not be used long term.

Other topical anti-inflammatories/immunomodulators that are sometimes effective for treating pruritus in human patients and dogs belong to the family of calcineurin inhibitors.[22–25] In human medicine, it has been reported that drugs such as tacrolimus and other calcineurin inhibitors block sensory nerve fibers that may have direct antipruritic activity in addition to its anti-inflammatory activity.[22] Because of the delay in effectiveness associated with topical tacrolimus, it may be best reserved for proactive applications as part of a preventive maintenance. Because of the high cost and the availability of other effective, less costly topical therapies, it is not a commonly prescribed treatment. The fifth mechanism of treating pruritus includes addressing any microbial overgrowth/infection or ectoparasite infestation. Bacterial (most commonly *Staphylococcus pseudintermedius*) and *Malassezia pachydermatis* overgrowth can contribute significantly to pruritus in dogs or humans.[26–28] It has been shown that dogs and human beings with AD have an increased incidence of cutaneous bacterial and/or *Malassezia* overgrowth/infection.[26,29] In humans this may be partially explained by the observation that *Staphylococcus aureus* colonizes 80% to 100% of patients with AD as opposed to 5% to 30% of healthy controls.[30] In dogs, there are studies that demonstrate that *Staphylococcus intermedius* (now recognized as *S pseudintermedius*) adheres more readily to canine corneocytes of dogs with AD than healthy dogs. Treating these secondary bacterial or fungal infections and/or ectoparasite infestation is an important part of treating pruritus. The response to this treatment varies from partial to complete, depending on how much the organism is contributing to the pruritus. Topical antibiotics (mupricin, fusidic acid, and chloroxylenol), antiseptics (chlorhexidine, benzoyl peroxide, acetic acid/boric acid), and antifungal agents (3% or higher chlorhexidine, azoles) are effective antimicrobials that will decrease pruritus associated with bacterial pyoderma or *Malassezia* dermatitis. It is generally recommended to treat the secondary infections with both topical and systemic therapy. Because many dogs will at some point develop a bacterial infection or *Malassezia* dermatitis, a common recommendation is to dispense a product that contains both an antibacterial and an antifungal agent. Systemic antibacterial or antifungal therapy and antiparasitic therapy are beyond the scope of this article.

PRURITUS AND ATOPIC DERMATITIS

In addition to topical or systemic medication, good skin care may help control pruritus. There are a number of studies demonstrating the persistence of antigens on the skin and its involvement in cutaneous pathologic abnormalities. These studies help support the importance of good skin care (clipping, bathing, and topical therapy) in regard to managing pruritus in dogs. In 1 study,[31] a group of house dust mite (HDM) allergic research beagles were exposed to house dust mites by 3 different methods—oral, percutaneous, and inhalation. In the percutaneous group clinical signs peaked at 72 hours after the first exposure to the HDM, even though no new exposure occurred after 48 hours. This peak was suspected to be caused by continued exposure to HDM antigen that persisted on the skin of the beagle dogs. This persistence of antigen on the skin and coat of the dogs was also documented in a study of 29 pet dogs of various breeds. In this study, skin and coat dust samples were obtained via vacuuming. HDM antigen (Der f 1) was then measured in the collected samples. Der f 1 was detected in skin and coat dust samples from 6 of 29 (21%) dogs.[32] In 2 subsequent studies HDM antigen was found on 11.7% and 35.5% of the hair coat samples, respectively.[33,34] It stands to reason that good skin care includes bathing that mechanically removes irritants and antigens. Removing these substances will decrease the load of allergens that the skin is exposed to and thereby help control pruritus.

BATHING

Bathing is routinely used as a part of the management of pruritic dogs. The frequency of bathing needs to be individualized for each case. Factors that should be taken into consideration include the owners' ability and desire to bathe the dog, the dog's acceptance of the baths, and the effectiveness (or lack thereof) of the baths in that individual dog. It is usually recommended to initially bathe the dog semiweekly to weekly. This recommendation is based on a couple of different studies. In 1 study, a double-blinded randomized controlled trial (RCT), dogs were bathed weekly with a shampoo containing lipids, complex sugars, and antiseptics (Allermyl). This bathing led to a 50% decrease in pruritus for 24 hours in 25% of the dogs and >90% decrease in pruritus in 6.3% of the bathed dogs.[35] In a separate study published as an abstract, 35 dogs with AD were treated with Allermyl shampoo or lotion. One of the products was applied, alternating every 3 days. They evaluated the response to therapy based on lesional score and pruritus scores. Within 3 weeks, both the lesional and the pruritus scores had decreased significantly (55% and 58%, respectively). More than 48% of the dogs had a >50% improvement and 75.9% had obvious clinical improvement (defined as 30% reduction).[36] Even though these studies support the effectiveness of bathing based on an analysis of all available published reports, selection of ingredients for the treatment of pruritus has not been performed. The American College of Veterinary Dermatology task force on AD stated that, "There is currently no evidence of any benefit from using other shampoos or conditioners containing ingredients such as oatmeal, pramoxine, antihistamine, lipids or glucocorticoids." Please note that lack of evidence does not mean that the benefits are not present, only that the studies could not support that statement.[37]

COMPONENTS OF GOOD SKIN CARE

In addition to bathing, clipping medium-haired to long-haired dogs is also a component of good skin care. It has been shown that dogs with long hair have more HDM antigen on their skin/hair coat than short-coated dogs. By clipping the hair, there is a decrease in the amount of antigen present on the surface of the skin that can cause an increase in antigen contact. It also allows for more effective drying of the hair, coat, and skin. Excessive moisture or drying can lead to an increase in clinical signs. Water evaporating off the skin dries it out and can lead to an increase in pruritus. This evaporation has been demonstrated in people[38] and probably occurs in dogs as well. Maintaining a shorter hair coat will help to ensure that the skin and coat will be thoroughly dried after each bath. It has been suggested that all atopic dogs have their coats clipped to less than 5 cm.

EPIDERMAL BARRIER DYSFUNCTION

Epidermal barrier dysfunction has been recognized as a key component of the pathogenesis of pruritus in cases of human AD.[39] Recently, barrier dysfunction has been reported to be involved with the pathogenesis of AD in dogs.[40]

In people, there are many different causes of barrier dysfunction associated with AD.[41] These defects include deficiencies of intercellular lipids, especially ceramides, such as ceramide-1 (in dogs ceramides-1 and ceramides-9 are deficient),[42] loss-of-function mutations in the filaggrin gene, mutations in the genes encoding for proteases (gain of function) and protease inhibitors (loss of function), and impaired expression of cornified cell envelope proteins.[40,41] Decreased ceramides may be due to a decrease in epidermal sphingomyelinase activity, a decrease in the biosynthesis of free glucosylceramides and ceramides in the skin, or an excess of sphingomyelin glucosylceramide deacylase (a sphingolipid-metabolizing enzyme).[40] A decrease in ceramides, an important water-retaining intercellular lipid, is one of the defects that has been identified in the skin of dogs with AD.[42,43]

CONSEQUENCES OF BARRIER DYSFUNCTION

When epidermal barrier dysfunction occurs, regardless as to the cause, there is an increase in percutaneous absorption of antigen. If this occurs in a genetically predisposed individual, an abnormal immunologic response (production of antigen-specific Immunoglobulin E [IgE]) occurs. On subsequent exposure, crosslinking of 2 IgE molecules on the surface of the mast cells is followed by the degranulation of the mast cell and the release of preformed inflammatory chemical mediators, such as histamine and proteases, de novo production, and release of eicosanoids and cytokines.[44,45] In addition, in atopic individuals, Langerhan cells in the epidermis will capture and then present, via their high-affinity IgE receptor (Fc epsilonRI), antigens to allergen-specific T cells inducing an immunologic response.[41,46,47] Emollients and moisturizers help restore skin hydration and barrier function. By repairing/restoring the barrier function, this cascading of events will become less frequent.[48,49] There are a variety of barrier repair products available; some are general moisturizers, whereas others are specific lipid replacement therapy. Topical emollient and moisturizers containing ceramides have been reported to be more effective at repairing the barrier than those without such lipids.[50,51] Children with AD improve clinically and need less topical steroids when an emollient is a component of their treatment.[52,53] In fact, even when asymptomatic, continued emollient application to the previously affected areas can be beneficial in delaying recurrence of the pruritic lesions.[54]

In contrast to allergic contact dermatitis, irritant contact dermatitis may occur when the skin comes in contact with a substance that directly damages the skin. Human patients with AD are at risk because of the barrier dysfunction. Whether this occurs in dogs with AD has not been investigated. It is reasonable to assume that this occurs because of the many similarities between humans with AD and dogs with AD. To help address this potential contributor to pruritus, it is recommended to the owners that they wipe the dog off with a wet cloth after coming in from outdoors. Another recommendation is to purchase breathable socks (Power paws dog socks) to apply to the patient's feet before going outdoors. The breathable socks may help to decrease contact with allergens. Another option is to use clothing to protect the skin. The author has owners use t-shirts or a dog body suit (Medical Pet Shirt [**Fig. 1**] or K9 TOP COAT Lycra bodysuit). These t-shirts or dog body suits are left on the dog all the time, other than when they are being bathed.

TREATMENT OF BARRIER DYSFUNCTION AND PRURITUS

Because of all the evidence in human medicine and the evolving evidence in veterinary medicine that treatment of the epidermal barrier dysfunction is critical in the successful management of pruritus in atopic patients, it is rational to consider topical moisturizers/emollients as adjunct therapy. Because bathing, in addition to cleansing, also hydrates the stratum corneum, it is valuable to retain some of this moisturizer. It is important in people to obey the 3-minute rule. The rule states that after bathing/showering, the skin should be patted dry. Patting dry should be followed by the application of a moisturizer. By applying the moisturizer within 3 minutes of exiting the bath, the water has not had a chance to evaporate and thus prevents drying out of the skin. There are numerous veterinary products that claim to moisturize the skin. There are currently no quality studies suggesting which products might be more efficacious for an atopic canine patient. It may be prudent to try several products to see which might work best for the individual dog.

LIPID REPLACEMENT LOTIONS

There are now lipid replacement lotions available for dogs and cats. They are Dermoscent Essential 6 Spot-on Skin Care, Douxo Calm Micro-emulsion Spray, and Allerderm Spot-On. They may contain essential fatty acids (EFA), essential oils, and/or complex lipid mixtures. Only 3 studies evaluating their effectiveness in repairing barrier function have been published to date.[55–57]

The study using Dermoscent Essential 6 Spot-on involved 5 normal dogs and 14 dogs with AD. They used either the spot-on or a spray that had similar but different ingredients than the spot-on. The spot-on was applied weekly, whereas the spray

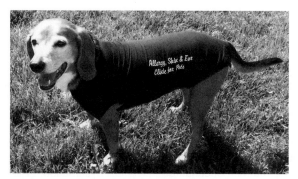

Fig. 1. Medical pet shirt.

was used daily. The results did demonstrate a decrease in scale and odor along with improvement in the quality of the hair coat. The effects on pruritus and barrier repair were inconsistent.

The next study investigated phytosphingosine, which is a pro-ceramide included in Douxo Calm Micro-emulsion Spray. In this study, 47 dogs were assigned to 1 of 3 groups: a control group, a group that was bathed with a phytosphingosine-containing shampoo, and a group that would have phytosphingosine shampoo used initially but then the last 4 baths were replaced by a phytosphingosine spray. The dogs were bathed every 3 days. None of the dogs had more than a 50% decrease in pruritus. As a point of reference, most clinical studies use a threshold of 50% improvement or more to define effectiveness.

The last study investigated Allerderm Spot-On. This lotion contains ceramides, free fatty acids, and cholesterol that mimic the composition and structure of the lipids in the canine epidermal barrier. It was demonstrated that treatment stimulated the production and secretion of endogenous stratum corneum lipids, improved the quality and quantity of epidermal intercellular lipids, and helped to repair the lipid layer of the stratum corneum. Improvement in clinical signs (pruritus, excoriation, etc) was not evaluated in this study.

CLiNICAL APPLICATION OF LOTIONS

Many dogs have their "favorite" spots to itch when symptoms occur. Of the 3 lipid replacement products, only the Allerderm Spot-On evaluated how far its product diffuses (10 cm halo) when applied to the back of a dog. None diffused to the ventrum of the extremities, which are common problem areas. Based on the concern that the products do not diffuse as extensively as desired, these products are best reserved for treating focal lesions. It is currently recommended to have the owners apply the lotions to the affected areas once daily, even though the instructions recommend less frequent application. This daily application of lotion is based on the recommendation for these types of lotions in human patients with AD, where daily applications of barrier repair products are recommended.[58] When using the spot-on product for dogs, any remaining product can be capped and refrigerated for use the next day. This spot-on treatment is administered for 30 days and then the dog is reevaluated. If the symptoms have not improved or have recurred, then one of the other products is tried. A key point is that these products should be used for prevention or maintenance of the pruritic atopic dog.

SYSTEMIC TREATMENT OF PRURITUS

Various systemic treatments for pruritus associated with canine AD have been reported. A review of all published RCTs was published in 2010.[59] These RCTs will be summarized by category.

ANTIHISTAMINES THERAPY

Effectiveness of antihistamine therapy in dogs was recently reviewed.[59] Based on 6 RCTs, there was inadequate conclusive evidence to demonstrate the efficacy of oral antihistamines in reducing clinical signs. This conclusion is consistent with the reports in human medicine. In fact, although antihistamines are often used in the treatment of human AD, there is limited objective evidence to demonstrate relief of pruritus.[60] The American College of Veterinary Dermatology AD task force states that first-generation and second-generation type 1 antihistamines are unlikely to be

of clinical benefit in dogs with chronic AD-associated skin lesions.[37] There is anecdotal evidence that first-generation antihistamines are effective at decreasing pruritus
in canine atopic patients. Perhaps this discrepancy can be explained by the fact that
pruritic dogs are a heterogeneous group. Those without chronic skin changes may
respond better to antihistamines compared with those with chronic changes. Antihistamines can be effective in dogs that are mildly pruritic and without chronic changes.
They seem to work better if given consistently and prophylactically rather than after
the dog has become moderately pruritic. They also seem to be synergistic with
EFA. Unfortunately, there is no antihistamine clinically proven to be the most effective.
Recommended products and the dosages are listed in **Table 1**. Each antihistamine
should be tried for at least 2 weeks before evaluating their effectiveness. Interestingly,
there is clinical evidence of steroid sparing when using a combination of the antihistamine trimeprazine and prednisolone (Temaril-P).[61] Other antihistamines do not seem
to be synergistic with glucocorticoid medications.

TRICYCLIC ANTIDEPRESSANTS AND MISCELLANEOUS OTHER MEDICATIONS

Tricyclic antidepressants are used to treat behavioral diseases (eg, obsessive/compul-
sive disorder) of dogs and people. They have also been used to treat pruritus even
though studies show that they are ineffective.[14] Anecdotal reports have shown that
these drugs will occasionally be effective at reducing pruritus in canine atopic patients.
It is unclear whether the response is due to the behavioral effects, sedating properties, or
the antihistamine effects (eg, doxepin is 800 times more potent than diphenhydramine as
a histamine receptor antagonist).[62] These drugs may be synergistic with EFA in a manner
similar to the antihistamines. Doxepin or amitriptyline should be considered in an antihistamine trial. Both are dosed for dogs at 0.5 to 1 mg/lb every 12 hours. They should be
used for at least 21 days before evaluating their effectiveness. Sedation is a common
side effect. In the review article, it was stated that leukotriene inhibitors or a phosphodi-
esterase inhibitor (pentoxifylline) had poor efficacy in controlling pruritus. In contrast,
others report that oral pentoxifylline[63] or misoprostol (Cytotec)[64] may have some effect

Table 1		
Antihistamines and tricyclic antidepressants		
Drug	**Dose**	**Frequency**
Amitriptyline[a,b]	0.5–1 mg/lb	q12h
Cetirizine	0.2–0.5 mg/lb	q24h
Chlorpheniramine[c,d]	0.2–0.25 mg/# Maximum 0.5 mg/#/d	q12h
Cyproheptadine[e]	0.1–0.5 mg/lb	q8–12h
Diphenhydramine	0.5–1 mg/lb	q8–12h
Doxepin[a]	0.5–1 mg/lb	q12h
Hydroxyzine	0.5–1 mg/lb	q8–12h
Loratadine	0.2–0.5 mg/lb	q24h

[a] Do not administer concurrently with amitraz or phenylpropanolamine.
[b] Use for 21 days.
[c] Bitter tasting if cut.
[d] Do not exceed 0.5 mg/lb/d; sudden death has occurred.
[e] In some dogs, agitation or restlessness may occur at higher doses.

on pruritus. These products are generally regarded as ineffective in controlling pruritus in canine atopic patients.

FATTY ACIDS THERAPY

EFA have been used for many years in the management of canine AD. The mechanisms of action of EFAs may be due to their anti-inflammatory and immunomodulatory properties or an improvement of barrier function. The latter is evaluated by measuring the transepidermal water loss. A decrease in transepidermal water loss correlates to an improvement in barrier function. The anti-inflammatory properties of EFA include the following: production of anti-inflammatory eicosanoids (prostaglandin and leukotriene) and inhibition of inflammatory cytokine production. There are many studies evaluating the effectiveness of EFA (omega 3, omega 6) in the treatment of canine AD. From 19 RCTs there were only 2 that were rated as high quality.[59] In one of the studies[65] that used a specific EFA liquid supplement (Viacutan Plus), there was a statistically significant reduction in prednisolone dosage needed to control pruritus after approximately 2 months of administration. In the other study,[66] the efficacy of an EFA-containing supplement (Megaderm) combined with an antipruritic shampoo (Allermyl) was as effective in treating the pruritus as prednisolone. It is unclear whether the bathing, the specific shampoo, the EFA, or some combination of these therapies was responsible for the result. The question that needs to be answered is whether these results are product dependent. The overall conclusion from the RCTs was that there is limited improvement with EFA whether used as a supplement or fed as an EFA-enhanced diet. In addition, there was no evidence that any particular formation or ratio of omega 3 and omega 6 was effective. Because of the 2 previous studies, the low cost and the very mild side effects (diarrhea), EFA should be considered as a part of the therapy for canine AD. Omega 3 series fatty acids do not form the inflammatory eicosanoid, arachidonic acid, and therefore, a product containing only omega 3 should be used. Based on a study,[67] the recommended amount of EFA that is administered should be18 mg/lb of eicosapentaenoic acid, administered for a minimum of 60 days.[37] Sixty days should allow enough time for the anti-inflammatory EFAs to be incorporated into the phospholipid layer of cell membranes of keratinocytes, replacing some of the inflammatory arachidonic acid. Omega 6, specifically linoleic acid, is the most important epidermal lipid in regard to barrier function. Because omega 6s are converted to arachidonic acid when administered systemically, it might be best to use them as topical agents.

ANTIMICROBIAL THERAPY

Dogs with atopic dermatitis frequently have overcolonization and/or infection from S pseudintermedius and/or M pachydermatis. Many times the infection is generalized and therefore not amendable to topical monotherapy. Systemic antibiotics (beta-lactams, clindamycin, and potentiated sulfas) and antifungals (ketoconazole, itraconazole, or fluconazole) are frequently needed. Because infections can contribute a significant amount to the dog's pruritus, it is important to identify (via cytology and physical examination) and treat the secondary infections. If the infections are generalized, it is better to withhold glucocorticoids or cyclosporine until the infection has resolved. This will allow the evaluation of how much pruritus is due to the infection and how much is due to the underlying disease. Giving steroids concurrently will only complicate this assessment. In cases of generalized pruritus and localized infection, judicious administration of short-acting oral glucocorticoids could be considered.

SUMMARY

The treatment of pruritus in the dog must be approached in a systematic manner and should include the search and resolution of the primary causes. Identifying and treating the primary cause of pruritus greatly increase the rate of success of any therapy for pruritus. In addition to identifying and treating the underlying cause, symptomatic therapy for pruritus is frequently needed. Successful treatment usually involves a multimodal approach that encompasses both topical and systemic therapy. Atopic dermatitis is a frequent cause of pruritus in both human beings and dogs. In recent years, the importance of barrier dysfunction as a major contributor to pruritus in atopic dermatitis has been recognized in both species. Restoration of barrier function is the foundation of treatment in those cases of human AD and is becoming recognized as an important component in the treatment of pruritus in canine atopic dermatitis. Recognizing and treating secondary bacterial and *Malassezia* overgrowth/infection is essential to treating the pruritic dog successfully.

REFERENCES

1. Savin JA. How should we define itching? J Am Acad Dermatol 1998;38:268–9.
2. Winkelmann RK, Muller SA. Pruritus. Annu Rev Med 1964;15:53–64.
3. Sonkoly E, Muller A, Lauerma AI, et al. IL-31: a new link between T cells and pruritus in atopic skin inflammation. J Allergy Clin Immunol 2006;117(2):411–7.
4. Steinhoff M, Bienenstock J, Schmelz M, et al. Neurophysiological, neuroimmunological, and neuroendocrine basis of pruritus. J Invest Dermatol 2006;126: 1705–18.
5. Lerner EA. Chemical mediators of itching. In: Bernhardt JD, editor. Itch: mechanisms and management of pruritus. New York: McGraw-Hill; 1994. p. 27–36.
6. Hägermark O. Itch mediators. Semin Dermatol 1995;14(4):271–6.
7. Hercogová J. Topical anti-itch therapy. Dermatol Ther 2005;18(4):341–3.
8. Twycross R, Greaves MW, Handwerker H, et al. Itch: scratching more than the surface. QJM 2003;96:7–26.
9. Birò T, Ko MC, Bromm B, et al. How best to fight that nasty itch—from new insights into the neuroimmunological neuroendocrine and neurophysiological bases of pruritus to novel therapeutic approaches. Exp Dermatol 2005;14:225–40.
10. Yosipovitch G, Dawn A, Greaves MW. Pathophysiology and clinical aspects of pruritus. In: Wolff K, Goldsmith LA, Katz SI, et al, editors. Fitzpatrick's dermatology in general medicine, vol. 1, 7th edition. New York: McGraw-Hill; 2008. p. 908–11.
11. Scott DW, Miller WE, Griffin CE. Dermatologic therapy. In: Scott DW, Miller WE, Griffin CE, editors. Muller & Kirk's small animal dermatology. 6th edition. Philadelphia: WB Saunders Company; 2001. p. 207–73.
12. Scott DW, Rothstein E, Miller WH. A clinical study on the efficacy of two commercial veterinary pramoxine cream rinses in the management of pruritus in atopic dogs. Canine Practice 2000;25:15–7.
13. Marsella R, Nicklin CF, Melloy C. The effects of capsaicin topical therapy in dogs with atopic dermatitis: a randomized, double-blinded, placebo-controlled, crossover clinical trial. Vet Dermatol 2002;13:131–9.
14. Olivry T, Mueller RS, The International Task Force On Canine Atopic Dermatitis. Evidence-based veterinary dermatology: a systematic review of the pharmacotherapy of canine atopic dermatitis. Vet Dermatol 2003;14:121–46.
15. Metz M, Grundmann S, Ständer S. Pruritus: an overview of current concepts. Vet Dermatol 2011;22:121–31.

16. Eschler DC, Klein PA. An evidence-based review of the efficacy of topical antihistamines in the relief of pruritus. J Drugs Dermatol 2010;9(8):992–7.
17. Iwasaki T, Hasegawa A. A randomized comparative clinical trial of recombinant canine interferon-gamma (KT-100) in atopic dogs using antihistamine as control. Vet Dermatol 2006;17:195–200.
18. Buys LM. Treatment options for atopic dermatitis. Am Fam Physician 2007;15(75): 523–8.
19. Gottschalk J, Einspanier A, Ungemach FR, et al. Influence of topical dexamethasone applications on insulin, glucose, thyroid hormone and cortisol levels in dogs. Res Vet Sci 2011;90:491–7.
20. Behrend EN. Can I diagnose anything with an animal on glucocorticoids? In: ACVIM Proceedings 2003. Available at: http://www.vin.com/Members/Proceedings/Proceedings.plx?CID=acvim2003&PID=pr04114&O=VIN. Accessed May 14, 2012.
21. Thomas RC, Logas D, Radosta L, et al. Effects of a 1% hydrocortisone conditioner on haematological and biochemical parameters, adrenal function testing and cutaneous reactivity to histamine in normal and pruritic dogs. Vet Dermatol 1999;10:109–16.
22. Ständer S, Schürmeyer-Horst F, Luger TA, et al. Treatment of pruritic diseases with topical calcineurin inhibitors. Ther Clin Risk Manag 2006;2:213–8.
23. Marsella R, Nicklin CF, Saglio S, et al. Investigation on the clinical efficacy and safety of 0.1% tacrolimus ointment (protopic) in canine atopic dermatitis: a randomized, double-blinded, placebo controlled, cross-over study. Vet Dermatol 2004;15:294–303.
24. Bensignor E, Olivry T. Treatment of localized lesions of canine atopic dermatitis with tacrolimus ointment: a blinded randomized controlled trial. Vet Dermatol 2005;16:52–60.
25. Marsella R. Calcineurin inhibitors: a novel approach to canine atopic dermatitis. J Am Anim Hosp Assoc 2005;41:92–7.
26. DeBoer D, Marsella R. The ACVD task force on canine atopic dermatitis (XII): the relationship of cutaneous infections to the pathogenesis and clinical course of canine atopic dermatitis. Vet Immunol Immunopathol 2001;81:239–49.
27. Boguniewicz M, Schmid-Grendelmeier P, Leung DY. Atopic dermatitis. J Allergy Clin Immunol 2006;118:40–3.
28. Ramirez de Knott HM, McCormick TS, Kalka K, et al. Cutaneous hypersensitivity to Malassezia sympodialis and dust mite in adult atopic dermatitis with a textile pattern. Contact Dermatitis 2006;54:92–9.
29. Elias PM, Hatano Y, Williams ML. Basis for the barrier abnormality in atopic dermatitis: outside-inside-outside pathogenic mechanisms. J Allergy Clin Immunol 2008;121:1337–43.
30. De Benedetto A, Agnihothri R, McGirt LY, et al. Atopic dermatitis: a disease caused by innate immune defects? J Invest Dermatol 2009;129:14–30.
31. Marsella R, Nicklin C, Lopez J. Studies on the role of various routes of allergen exposure in high IgE producing Beagle dogs sensitized to house dust mites. Vet Dermatol 2006;17:306–12.
32. Glass EV, Reid RA, Hillier A, et al. Use of an amplified ELISA technique for detection of a house dust mite allergen (Derf 1) in the skin and coat dust samples from dogs. Am J Vet Res 2003;64:162–5.
33. Jackson AP, Foster AP, Hart BJ, et al. Prevalence of house dust mites and dermatophagoides group 1 antigens collected from bedding, skin and hair coat of dogs in south-west England. Vet Dermatol 2005;16:32–8.

34. Randal A, Hillier A, Cole LK, et al. Quantitation of house dust mite allergens (Der f 1 and group 2) on the skin and hair of dogs. Am J Vet Res 2005;66:143–9.

35. Loeflath A, von Voigts-Rhetz A, Jaeger K, et al. The use of a whirlpool in topical antipruritic therapy–a double-blinded, randomized, cross-over study. Vet Dermatol 2007 Dec;18(6):427–31.

36. Reme CA, Mondon A, Calmon JP, et al. Efficacy of combined topical therapy with antiallergic shampoo and lotion for the control of signs associated with atopic dermatitis in dogs. Vet Dermatol 2004;15:S33.

37. Olivry T, DeBoer DJ, Favrot C, et al. Treatment of canine atopic dermatitis: 2010 clinical practice guidelines from the International Task Force on Canine Atopic Dermatitis. Vet Dermatol 2010;21:233–8.

38. Nojima H, Carstens MI, Carstens E. c-fos expression in superficial dorsal horn of cervical spinal cord associated with spontaneous scratching in rats with dry skin. Neurosci Lett 2003;14:62–4.

39. Proksch E, Fölster-Holst R, Jensen JM. Skin barrier function, epidermal proliferation and differentiation in eczema. J Dermatol Sci 2006;43(3):159–69.

40. Marsella R, Olivry T, Carlotti DN, et al. Current evidence of skin barrier dysfunction in human and canine atopic dermatitis. Vet Dermatol 2011;22:239–48.

41. Novak N, Simon D. Atopic dermatitis—from new pathophysiologic insights to individualized therapy. Allergy 2011;66:830–9.

42. Reiter LV, Torres SM, Wertz PW. Characterization and quantification of ceramides in the nonlesional skin of canine patients with atopic dermatitis compared with controls. Vet Dermatol 2009;20:260–6.

43. Shimada K, Yoon JS, Yoshihara T, et al. Increased transepidermal water loss and decreased ceramide content in lesional and non-lesional skin of dogs with atopic dermatitis. Vet Dermatol 2009;20:541–6.

44. Kunder CA, St John AL, Abraham SN. Mast cell modulation of the vascular and lymphatic endothelium. Blood 2011;118:5383–93.

45. Prussin C, Metcalfe DD. IgE, mast cells, basophils, and eosinophils. J Allergy Clin Immunol 2003;111:S486–94.

46. Stingl G, Maurer D. IgE-mediated allergen presentation via Fc epsilon RI on antigen-presenting cells. Int Arch Allergy Immunol 1997;13:24–9.

47. Mudde GC, van Reijsen FC, Bruijnzeel-Koomen CA. Ige-positive Langerhans cells and TH2 allergen-specific T cells in atopic dermatitis. J Invest Dermatol 1992;99:103S.

48. Ainley-Walker PF, Patel L, David TJ. Side to side comparison of topical treatment in atopic dermatitis. Arch Dis Child 1998;79:149–52.

49. Chamlin SL, Frieden IJ, Fowler A, et al. Ceramide-dominant, barrier-repair lipids improve childhood atopic dermatitis. Arch Dermatol 2001;137:1110–2.

50. Chamlin SL, Kao J, Freiden IJ, et al. Ceramide-dominant barrier repair lipids alleviate childhood atopic dermatitis: changes in barrier function provide a sensitive indicator of disease activity. J Am Acad Dermatol 2002;47:198–208.

51. Loden M, Andersson AC, Lindberg M. Improvement in skin barrier function in patients with atopic dermatitis after treatment with a moisturizing cream (Canoderm). Br J Dermatol 1999;140:264–7.

52. Hanifin JM, Hebert AA, Mays SR, et al. Effects of a low potency corticosteroid lotion plus a moisturizing regimen in the treatment of atopic dermatitis. Curr Ther Res Clin Exp 1998;59:227–33.

53. Lucky AW, Leach AD, Laskarzewski P, et al. Use of an emollient as a steroid-sparing agent in the treatment of mild to moderate atopic dermatitis in children. Pediatr Dermatol 1997;14:321–4.

54. Wirén K, Nohlgård C, Nyberg F, et al. Treatment with a barrier-strengthening moisturizing cream delays relapse of atopic dermatitis: a prospective and randomized controlled clinical trial. J Eur Acad Dermatol Venereol 2009;23:1267–72.

55. Tretter S, Mueller RS. The influence of topical unsaturated fatty acids and essential oils on normal and atopic dogs—a pilot study. Vet Dermatol 2010;21:311–28.

56. Bourdeau P, Bruet V, Gremillet C. Evaluation of phytosphingosine containing shampoo and micro-emulsion spray in the clinical control of allergic dermatosis in dogs: preliminary results of a multicentric study. In: Proceedings from the North American Veterinary Dermatology Forum. Hawaii; April 2007. p. 221.

57. Piekutowska A, Pin D, Rème CA, et al. Effects of a topically applied preparation of epidermal lipids on the stratum corneum barrier of atopic dogs. J Comp Pathol 2008;138:197–203.

58. Boguniewicz M, Nicol N, Kelsay K, et al. A multidisciplinary approach to evaluation and treatment of atopic dermatitis. Semin Cutan Med Surg 2008;27:115–27.

59. Olivry T, Foster AP, Mueller RS, et al. Interventions for atopic dermatitis in dogs: a systematic review of randomized controlled trials. Vet Dermatol 2010;21:4–22.

60. Klein PA, Clark RA. An evidence-based review of the efficacy of antihistamines in relieving pruritus in atopic dermatitis. Arch Dermatol 1999;135:1522–5.

61. Paradis M, Scott DW, Giroux D. Further investigations on the use of nonsteroidal and steroidal antiinflammatory agents in the management of canine pruritus. J Am Anim Hosp Assoc 1991;27:44–8.

62. Gupta M, Gupta A. The use of antidepressant drugs in dermatology. J Eur Acad Dermatol Venereol 2001;15:512–8.

63. Marsella R, Nicklin CF. Double-blinded cross-over study on the efficacy of pentoxifylline for canine atopy. Vet Dermatol 2000;11:255–60.

64. Olivry T, Dunston SM, Rivierre C, et al. A randomized controlled trial of misoprostol monotherapy for canine atopic dermatitis: effects on dermal cellularity and cutaneous tumor necrosis factor-alpha. Vet Dermatol 2003;14:37–46.

65. Saevik BK, Bergvall K, Holm BR, et al. A randomized, controlled study to evaluate the steroid sparing effect of essential fatty acid supplementation in the treatment of canine atopic dermatitis. Vet Dermatol 2004;15:137–45.

66. Reme CA, Lloyd DH, Burrows A, et al. Anti-allergic shampoo and oral essential fatty acid combination therapy to relieve signs of canine atopic dermatitis: a blinded, prednisolone-controlled trial. Vet Dermatol 2003;14:355.

67. Logas D, Kunkle GA. Double-blinded crossover study with marine oil supplementation containing high-dose for the treatment of canine pruritic skin disease. Vet Dermatol 1994;5:99–104.

Alternative Therapies in Veterinary Dermatology

Jeanne B. Budgin, DVM[a],*, Molly J. Flaherty, DVM[b]

KEYWORDS

- Alternative • Veterinary • Dermatology • Acupuncture • Chinese herbs
- Homeopathy • Western herbs • Plant extracts

KEY POINTS

- Interest in complementary and alternative veterinary medicine (CAVM) by veterinarians and pet owners has increased in recent years.
- There is a need for additional safe and effective treatments for canine atopic dermatitis.
- Acupuncture, Chinese herbs, homeopathy, and Western herbs and plant extracts all have potential therapeutic benefits in veterinary dermatology; however, there are limited well-designed studies to support their use in both people and animals.
- It is important for veterinarians to familiarize themselves with the common uses, potential benefits, and adverse effects of alternative therapies.

INTRODUCTION

The practice of complementary and alternative medicine (CAM) is described by various terms, including integrative, holistic, and Eastern medicine. These modalities are often used in conjunction with, or as a complement to, more conventional treatments. Conventional, allopathic, or Western medicine involves managing symptoms, treating disease, and maintaining health through the use of pharmaceutical and surgical interventions. Complementary and alternative approaches address the "whole" individual: the energy of the body and its influence on health and disease, the mobilization of the body's own resources to heal itself, and treatment of the underlying causes, not symptoms, of disease. Patients with chronic conditions for which clinical signs are not sufficiently relieved by conventional treatments often seek alternative therapies.

Interest and acceptance of complementary and alternative veterinary medicine (CAVM) within the veterinary profession has continued to increase over the past decade. The American Veterinary Medical Association's (AVMA) *Guidelines for Complementary and Alternative Medicine* were approved in 2001 and state that the AVMA "recognizes the interest in and use of these modalities and is open to their

Disclosures: None declared.
[a] Department of Dermatology and Allergy, Animal Specialty Center, 9 Odell Plaza, Yonkers, NY 10701, USA; [b] Integrative Pet Care, 2520 West Armitage, Chicago, IL 60647, USA
* Corresponding author.
E-mail address: Jeanne.Budgin@vcahospitals.com

consideration."[1] The definition was modified in 2012 as a result of "the increasing scientific information available about these modalities as well as increasing inclusion of these modalities in the curriculum at accredited veterinary schools."[2] A survey published in 2011 indicated that 12 accredited veterinary schools in North America offered programs in CAVM[3] versus 7 veterinary schools reported in a survey conducted 11 years earlier.[4] The American Holistic Veterinary Medical Association was established in 1982 with 30 veterinary members. Interest in this organization has continued to grow with approximately 900 members at the time of this writing (Nancy Scanlan, DVM, personal communication, 2012).

Graduate veterinarians are seeking additional training in CAVM, particularly in acupuncture and Chinese herbs. This is in part because of increasing client demand, but also a desire by veterinarians to offer additional therapeutic options to improve treatment outcome and quality of life for their patients. In 1974, the International Veterinary Acupuncture Society offered the first comprehensive veterinary acupuncture program in the United States, with an enrollment of 30 students. Interest in this program has steadily increased and currently there are between 100 and 110 registrants per year, as well as courses offered in several countries. At the time of this writing, 6000 veterinarians throughout the world have completed the training (Vikki Weber, personal communication, 2012). The Chi Institute of Chinese Medicine, an organization based in Reddick, Florida, has reported similar trends. Their veterinary herbal medicine course, a 165-hour program that may be completed online, has documented an increase in enrollment from 74 to 226 students over the past 10 years (Zhen Zhao, personal communication, 2012).

Atopic dermatitis (AD) is estimated to affect 10% to 15% of the canine population.[5–7] Pruritus is the most common clinical sign associated with allergic skin disease and results in significant distress for both client and patient.[8–10] Because of the complex underlying pathomechanism of pruritus, relief from skin itch and inflammation remains a common therapeutic challenge for veterinary practitioners. Many atopic dogs require long-term anti-inflammatory medications. Antihistamines and essential fatty acids may be of benefit in mild to moderate cases; however, effective control of pruritus is often not achieved.[7] Allergen-specific immunotherapy may be administered, but clinical improvement may be slow in onset (6–9 months) and delivery via subcutaneous injection may challenge owner compliance. Although previous evidence-based studies have supported the efficacy of oral glucocorticoids and cyclosporine,[11,12] owners may be reluctant to administer these therapies because of cost and/or concern with side effects. Adverse effects have been reported in 10% to 81% of animals receiving glucocorticoids[12–14] and 14% to 81% of those receiving cyclosporine.[12,14] It is beyond the scope of this article to review conventional management strategies for pruritic skin disease; however, it is evident that both pet owners and veterinarians recognize a need for safe and efficacious complementary and alternative therapies.

Alternative therapies for skin disorders encompass many treatment modalities, including, but not limited to, traditional Chinese medicine (acupuncture and Chinese herbs), homeopathy, Western herbs, and plant extracts. This article reviews the human and veterinary literature on the aforementioned modalities with a focus on reduction of inflammation and pruritus of the skin and ear canal in the canine species. Clinical application and potential adverse effects will also be included when available.

TRADITIONAL CHINESE MEDICINE

Traditional Chinese medical (TCM) theories have been documented in existence for more than 4000 years. In TCM, which includes acupuncture and Chinese herbs, health is considered to be a state of balance or equilibrium within the body. Treatment involves the identification of patterns followed by the selection of acupuncture points and herbal formulas. Traditional Chinese veterinary medicine (TCVM) is derived from human TCM. Veterinary herbal formulas, as well as the location of acupuncture points and meridians, are extrapolated from prescriptions and anatomic locations recognized in human medicine. Although the awareness and development of TCVM has increased during the past 20 to 30 years, historical evidence indicates that this modality has been practiced in ancient China for more than 2000 years. *The Yellow Emperor's Classic of Internal Medicine* was written during 475 to 221 BC and described medical problems of humans and animals treated with acupuncture and herbal remedies.[15]

The classification of patterns is based on states of excess or deficiency, heat or cold, and internal or external factors. For example, internal factors may be correlated with immunologic or endocrine dysfunction, whereas external factors may involve season change, pollen, or contact allergens and ectoparasites.[16] Common patterns in dermatology patients include dampness, heat, wind invasion, and blood deficiency. These terms may be considered metaphorically, but also in relation to conventional manifestations of disease. Dampness may be involved in conditions such as pyoderma, pododermatitis, and otitis externa. Lesions involving dampness are often moist, exudative, purulent, or greasy. Clinical signs of heat include erythema and/or inflammation. Wind invasion may be used to describe an acute onset of pruritus, or pruritus associated with weather changes. Blood deficiency may manifest as a chronic condition involving reduced skin immunity or barrier function. Clinical signs may include dry skin and hair coat with dander, low-level pruritus, and brittle claws.

ACUPUNCTURE

Acupuncture involves the insertion of needles into acupoints along meridians near the body surface. It is theorized that Qi, a form of energy, travels along these meridians and may be influenced by needle placement and stimulation. Qi may be further defined as the energetic life force that, when imbalanced or misdirected, creates physiologic disturbance. Yin and Yang merge to generate Qi; thus, an imbalance between Yin and Yang results in a disruption of Qi and, consequently, a state of disease.

Various acupuncture techniques exist, including acupressure, aquapuncture, electro-acupuncture, moxibustion, and laser application. Finger pressure is used to stimulate points during acupressure. Aquapuncture involves the injection of substances (often vitamin B12) into acupuncture points, electro-acupuncture uses low electrical stimulation applied to needles, moxibustion involves heated moxa (mugwort) for stimulation, and laser acupuncture uses low-energy laser light for point stimulation. Cupping, or the placement of cups on the skin with vacuum suction, is also described, but not commonly used in veterinary medicine.

Much of the research on both the mechanism of action and the efficacy of acupuncture has focused on analgesia. Acupuncture for the treatment of chronic pain has been demonstrated to be comparable to morphine without the risk of drug dependence and other adverse side effects.[17–19] It has been postulated that pruritus may be alleviated by acupuncture along a similar neural pathway to that of pain. Acupuncture involves the stimulation of A delta nerve fibers during treatment. Once stimulated, interneurons are activated in the dorsal horn of the spinal cord, produce enkephalins, and inhibit C fiber activity at the level of the dorsal horn. Needling close to the area where C fiber pain originates may have an effect via segmental acupuncture, influencing areas supplied by the same segment of the spinal cord.[20] Pruritus and pain are both transmitted along C fibers, although it remains unclear if different types of fibers are involved.[21] Repeated pinpricks in areas surrounding cowage-induced pruritus blocked intense pruritus in an experimental human study. These findings suggest that stimulation of adjacent acupuncture points, in addition to points along the involved dermatome, may be effective in the management of pruritus.[22] In controlled studies involving healthy volunteers, acupuncture has been shown to inhibit histamine-induced itch and flare; this is most effective when needling is applied in the same segment as experimentally induced itch created via intradermal injection of histamine.[23,24] The influence of acupuncture on type I hypersensitivity pruritus, as well as wheal and flare response, has been evaluated in atopic adults with promising results.[25–27]

Acupuncture, specifically points for stimulating Qi and blood, has also been postulated to have an effect on immune system function, which may be clinically relevant in veterinary dermatology. A commonly used acupuncture point, ST 36, has been documented in research studies to increase the phagocytic function of neutrophils.[28] Promotion of both humoral and cellular immunity, as well as natural killer cell activity, was also demonstrated in the peripheral blood of healthy volunteers following acupuncture treatment.[29]

The effects of acupuncture on canine otitis externa have been investigated. In a comparative, randomized, placebo-controlled study of 25 dogs with acute otitis externa, patients receiving acupuncture combined with conventional therapy (n = 13) demonstrated greater than 50% reduction in recovery time and pain, as compared with patients receiving placebo acupuncture and conventional therapy (n = 12). Dogs included in this study had at least one prior episode of otitis externa.[30] It is important to note that complete recovery was based on resolution of clinical signs without cytologic or cultural analysis. After 1 year, reevaluation was performed to determine if improvement was sustained and if treatment had an influence on recurrence of otitis. With the inclusion of data from 6 additional cases, 93% of the dogs that received acupuncture treatment did not have recurrent disease compared with 50% that received placebo acupuncture.[31]

Acral lick dermatitis is one of the most widely recognized conditions in veterinary dermatology that may benefit from acupuncture treatment. The initial therapeutic approach is aimed at managing secondary pyoderma with oral antibiotics, deterring licking and self-trauma with the application of topical agents and barriers (Elizabethan collar, leg wrap), and evaluating for underlying causes, such as allergic skin disease, musculoskeletal or neurologic disease, and behavioral disorders. Environmental evaluation/enrichment and behavioral modifying therapies may also be indicated. According to TCVM, and depending on the presentation, acral lick dermatitis may be classified as involving wind, heat, and damp, but more commonly as an obstruction of the flow of energy or Qi along the acupuncture channel or meridian underlying the lesion.[32] Acupuncture treatment points selected locally, proximally, and distally to the lesion will facilitate clearing the obstruction. "Surrounding the dragon" involves inserting needles obliquely or transversely along the border forming a circular pattern directed toward the center the lesion. This technique provides analgesia and assists in the reduction of tissue edema and inflammation. Additional local, proximal, and distal points will vary according to the underlying TCVM diagnosis. In the author's (M.J.F.) experience, heat-clearing points and points along the Large Intestine or Triple Heater meridians to move Qi are generally useful for forelimb lesions. These may include LI-4, LI-11, LI-15, TH-4, TH-5, TH-14, and GV-14. Needles should not be placed directly into the lesion, thus acupuncture points should be avoided if they are located deep to the lick granuloma.

Few adverse effects are reported with acupuncture treatment. A low risk of infection exists with the use of sterile needles and proper technique. Hematomas and hemorrhage may occur in patients with coagulopathies. Although extremely rare, serious complications, such as pneumothorax, as well as organ and nerve injuries, are reported in the human literature.[33] Acupuncture should be used with caution during pregnancy.[34] Veterinary acupuncturists working with pregnant animals should have knowledge of points that may stimulate abortion or labor. Needling in the thoracic region must be closely monitored to avoid penetration of the chest cavity. This is particularly important with animals, as they may change position during treatment. Needle placement around or near tumors or masses, especially malignancies, should be avoided, as this may promote growth and metastasis. Electro-acupuncture is contraindicated for patients with pacemakers or a history of seizures. Acupuncture is well tolerated by most animals; some may experience transient relaxation and somnolence for 24 hours following treatment.

CHINESE HERBS

The beneficial effects of traditional Chinese herbal formulations for severe atopic dermatitis (AD) have been described in double-blind, placebo-controlled, crossover human studies.[35–37] The combination of herbs, *Glycyrrhiza uralensis*, *Paeonia lactiflora*, and *Rehmannia glutinosa*, has also been studied in atopic dogs. Interest in evaluating this preparation for veterinary use was based on the selection of 3 of the original 10 herbs in Zemaphyte (Phytopharm, Godmanchester, UK), a product with demonstrated clinical efficacy in atopic human patients.[35–37] Nagel and colleagues[38] conducted a randomized, double-blind, placebo-controlled study to evaluate the use of this formula (P07P, consisting of the 3 aforementioned botanicals) for the control of AD in dogs. A total of 50 dogs with year-round pruritus, a diagnosis of AD based on standard criteria, and exclusion of other pruritic skin diseases, were included in the study. Patients received oral P07P at 200 mg/kg per day or placebo for 8 weeks. The primary outcome measure was the owners' assessment of response to treatment at the end of the study period. Nine (37.5%) of the 24 dogs in the P07P group and 3 (13%) of the 23 dogs in the placebo group were considered to have improved, but this difference did not reach statistical significance. Significant changes in erythema and a reduction in pruritus compared with placebo were also reported. The study concluded that P07P may be of benefit as a nonsteroidal therapy for dogs with AD.

The results of a subsequent trial by Ferguson and colleagues[39] evaluated the same herbal combination (designated PYM00217) and were in agreement with the aforementioned study. A total of 120 dogs with perennial AD and a minimum canine AD extent and severity index (CADESI) were enrolled in the study. Patients received PYM00217 at 100 mg/kg, 200 mg/kg, or 400 mg/kg per day or placebo for a total of 12 weeks. The primary outcome measure was a reduction in CADESI evaluated at 4, 8, and 12 weeks following initiation of treatment. After completion of treatment, dogs that received the 200 mg/kg dose had a statistically significant reduction (23.4%) in CADESI compared with baseline. Upon further analysis of data from a subgroup of 14 dogs with more severe disease, those receiving PYM00217 at 200 mg/kg had a 29.3% reduction in CADESI, as compared with a 10.6% increase in CADESI for the placebo group. The investigators concluded that the efficacy of this herbal combination was comparable, if not superior to, that of other steroid-sparing agents.

The glucocorticoid-sparing effects of the previously mentioned herbal combination (*G uralensis*, *P lactiflora*, and *R glutinosa*) have also been studied.[40] In a randomized, double-blind, placebo-controlled trial, Phytopica (Intervet-Schering Plow Animal Health UK Ltd, Milton Keynes, UK) at 200 mg/kg per day or placebo was administered to 22 dogs with perennial AD for an 8-week duration. Oral methylprednisolone was provided concurrently with dosage adjustments based on a daily pruritus score. Results indicated that 80% of dogs treated with Phytopica had a greater than 50% reduction in the required dose of methylprednisolone to maintain remission, compared with 36% in the placebo group. The Phytopica treatment group also had significantly lower pruritus scores during the trial. The investigators concluded that Phytopica may provide a significant steroid-sparing effect when used in combination with methylprednisolone.

No serious adverse effects were reported in the aforementioned studies. Dose-dependent, intermittent, and often self-limited vomiting, soft feces, diarrhea, and flatulence resulted in withdrawal of therapy for 5 dogs in 1 study; however, 2 were from the placebo group.[39] Reports of toxicity and adverse effects have increased with more widespread use of Chinese herbs.[41–44] Chinese herbal medicines are not regulated by governmental agencies and there are no quality control measures in the United States to ensure purity, concentration, or safety.[45] Adverse reactions may result from the administration of known toxic herbs, as well as accidental substitution, inappropriate combination, use, and dosage of herbal formulas. Individual patient sensitivity, interactions with conventional pharmaceutical medications, and the misdiagnosis of TCVM patterns are also important considerations.[46] Some herbal formulas have been determined to be carcinogenic or hepatotoxic.[47] Perharic and colleagues[48] documented 11 human cases of liver damage following the use of a Chinese herbal medicine for skin disease. The formulas varied in composition, so a single causative ingredient could not be isolated. Contaminants, such as pharmaceutical medications, heavy metals, and glucocorticoids, have been identified in herbal preparations from China.[49] To ensure patient safety, veterinarians prescribing herbal therapies should be aware of potential toxicities and contaminants and obtain formulas only from reliable sources with established processing standards. Routine laboratory monitoring, especially of liver values, may be warranted in select cases. The American Association of Traditional Chinese Veterinary Medicine (AATCVM), http://www.aatcvm.org, collects data on adverse effects and drug interactions involving Chinese herbal medicines.

HOMEOPATHY

Samuel Hahnemann, a German botanist, chemist and physician, formulated the theoretical principles of homeopathy approximately 200 years ago.[50] Homeopathic medicine is based on the law of similars or the theory that "like cures like." Substances have the ability to cure diseased individuals who exhibit signs similar to those generated if extremely dilute forms of the substance are administered to healthy individuals. The principle of potentization involves a series of dilutions and shaking (or succussion) of the original compounds, which are derived from plant, mineral, or animal sources. Following dilution, no pharmacologic effect remains; however, exposure to the dilution, or remedy, is believed to stimulate natural healing in the body. The treatment approach is individualized and based on the totality of clinical signs that are uniquely expressed. Remedies are selected and influenced by answers to a series of questions about general health and personality traits, as well as physical examination.

A systemic review of controlled clinical trials investigating homeopathic remedies in human dermatology was recently published.[51] A limited number of studies were identified with 9 of 12 trials indicating no positive effect from treatment and the remaining 3 being of low methodological quality. Several studies have evaluated homeopathic treatment for the management of acute otitis media in children. Findings suggest that homeopathy may contribute to a rapid reduction in symptoms, shorter duration of pain, and less recurrence of disease and antibiotic use.[52,53]

Few studies have evaluated the efficacy of homeopathy in veterinary dermatology. Hill and colleagues[54] performed a pilot study of the effect of individualized remedies on pruritus associated with atopic dermatitis (AD) in dogs. Twenty dogs with confirmed AD were initially treated by a veterinary homeopath based on cutaneous signs and constitutional characteristics. Owners assessed the response to treatment using a validated pruritus scoring system. In 15 cases, owners reported no improvement following homeopathic treatment. For 5 of 20 cases, a reduction in pruritus ranging from 64% to 100% was described. Complete resolution in one dog's skin condition, allowing for the discontinuation of conventional treatments (immunotherapy and glucocorticoids administered for 2 years before study enrollment), was also documented. Three cases were then entered into a second randomized, blinded, placebo-controlled trial during which owners could correctly distinguish between active remedy administration and placebo. Sixteen different homeopathic remedies were prescribed throughout the study; the most common therapies included Pulsatilla 200C, Sulfur 30C, and Phosphorus 200C.

The management of canine AD with a homeopathic remedy has also been evaluated in a single, blinded, placebo-controlled study.[55] Eighteen dogs with AD and moderate to severe pruritus were treated with a commercially available homeopathic remedy (Skin and Seborrhea Remedy; HomeoPet, West Hampton Beach, NY) containing sulfur, staphysagria, psorinum, graphites, and arsenicum album. The remedy was administered orally during the first 3 weeks of the trial, followed by placebo (ethanol containing vehicle only) for a similar duration. Owners evaluated a reduction in pruritus by classifying the observed change as poor, fair, good, or excellent. Only 1 dog each in both treatment and placebo groups had a repeated and sustained "fair" response (<50% reduction in pruritus). Homeopathic practitioners were critical of the study design and claimed the investigators disregarded the importance of individualization of remedies.[56–60] A study performed by veterinary homeopathic practitioners reported a moderate or major improvement in 56% of dogs with AD; however, the study design was noncontrolled and failed to use standardized methods of diagnosis, monitoring, and assessment.[61]

Owing to the dilute nature of homeopathic remedies, they are generally considered to have little to no risk of adverse effects. Aggravation of symptoms for several hours after remedy administration is reported in 10% to 20% of human patients.[62] Arsenic toxicity, manifesting as melanosis and keratosis, acute gastrointestinal disease, leukopenia, thrombocytopenia, and polyneuropathy is also described in 3 human cases with improper use of homeopathic remedies.[63]

WESTERN HERBS AND PLANT EXTRACTS

The provision of Western herbs is similar to conventional drug therapy. Herbs that have a proven, or empiric beneficial effect, are prescribed based on clinical signs and/or a conventional diagnosis. Western herbs are often applied topically as single agents or in combination with oral therapies. Many botanic compounds, including, but not limited to, bromelain, honey, propolis, arnica, grape seed extract, green tea, lavender oil, gotu kola, feverfew, rosemary, and turmeric, may be of potential benefit in various human skin conditions. The most commonly used Western herbs and plant extracts, as well as those that have been studied in veterinary medicine, are reviewed.

CAPSAICIN

Capsaicin is derived from the seeds and membranes of plants in the nightshade family and is the main capsaicinoid in chili peppers. A number of pruritic skin conditions in people, particularly of neuropathic origin, have been managed with topical capsaicin. Two randomized, placebo-controlled trials have evaluated capsaicin cream in the treatment of human psoriasis with significant improvement in scaling, erythema, skin thickness, and pruritus reported over the study period.[64,65] Although the mechanism of action has not been fully elucidated, it may involve depletion of substance P (SP) in type C sensory nerve endings[66–68] and modulation of inflammatory mediators through inhibition of nuclear factor kB activation.[69] SP is a neuropeptide that is involved in the pathogenesis of human AD[70–72] and may serve as a mediator of neurogenic inflammation in dogs.[73] Marsella and colleagues[74] evaluated topical capsaicin therapy for canine AD in a randomized, double-blind, placebo-controlled, crossover clinical trial. Twelve dogs with AD received 0.25% capsaicin or vehicle lotion applied twice daily for 6 weeks, followed by a wash-out period, after which treatments were crossed over. Owners recorded weekly pruritus scores; the investigator evaluated and scored pruritus before and after each treatment period. Skin biopsies to assay SP were also collected from both normal and lesional skin at the beginning and end of each treatment. Significant improvement in pruritus was reported by owners, but not by the investigator; pruritus scores in 11 of the 12 dogs either improved or remained the same during treatment. SP concentrations in the skin did not correlate with the degree of pruritus and did not change significantly throughout the study. Possible adverse effects included a slight increase in pruritus following the first week of capsaicin application. A transient intense burning sensation that resolves after several days is reported in humans, especially at higher concentrations.[75] It was concluded that topical capsaicin should be further evaluated as an antipruritic agent in dogs with AD.

HARDY KIWI

Actinidia arguta (hardy kiwi) is a perennial vine that is similar, but slightly smaller and sweeter than the true kiwi, *Actinidia deliciosa*. A native plant of East Asian countries, preparations of hardy kiwi are claimed to have multiple health benefits. PG 102, a water-soluble extract prepared from hardy kiwi, has been demonstrated to reduce clinical signs, decrease immunoglobulin (Ig)E and interleukin (IL)-4, and increase levels of IgG2 and IL-12 in a mouse model of AD.[76,77] More recently, 90 asymptomatic atopic human subjects were enrolled in a randomized, double-blind, placebo-controlled exploratory clinical study. After 8 weeks of oral treatment with PG102, total IgE levels were effectively reduced when compared with placebo.[78]

The efficacy of an *Actinidia arguta* preparation (EFF1001) on CADESI and pruritus in dogs with mild to moderate nonseasonal AD has been investigated in a randomized, double-blind, placebo-controlled study.[79] After a 2-week course of oral prednisolone, responsive dogs were maintained on 0.2 mg/kg every 48 hours of prednisolone and assigned to either EFF1001 (30 mg/kg per day) or a placebo treatment group for 4 weeks (stage 1). Investigators used the CADESI for assessment, whereas owners were asked to provide a weekly pruritus score using a visual analog scale. Dogs that responded in stage 1 were advanced to stage 2, which involved the administration of EFF1001 only. At the end of stage 1, improvement was noted in 35 (61%) of 57 dogs (18 in the EFF1001 and 17 in the placebo treatment group). CADESI scores did not differ significantly between groups; however, pruritus decreased in the EFF1001 group and approached statistical significance. At the conclusion of stage 2, there was a total response rate of 54% (19/35) with 79% of these cases having received EFF1001 and 21% placebo. Longer treatment durations with EF1001 were more likely to result in improvement of clinical signs. The investigators concluded that EFF1001 was a beneficial adjunctive therapy for AD when administered for at least 8 weeks. No adverse effects or clinical laboratory abnormalities were reported.

TEA TREE OIL

Tea tree oil (TTO) is a volatile oil extracted from the leaves of *Melaleuca alternifolia*, a tree native to Australia. Melaleuca oil is marketed for use in dogs, cats, ferrets, and horses in various over-the-counter skin care products. Many indications for this essential oil are reported in the human literature, including acne, psoriasis, fungal infection, and pediculosis. TTO contains more than 100 chemical compounds, most being monoterpene and sesquiterpene hydrocarbons and their alcohols. Terpinen-4-ol, one of the main terpenes in TTO, has well-documented antibacterial and antifungal properties.[80,81] Susceptibility studies have been performed for many pathogens of clinical relevance in veterinary medicine, including methicillin-resistant *Staphylococcus aureus*,[82,83] *Pseudomonas aeruginosa*,[83] and *Malassezia pachydermatis*.[84]

A 10% TTO cream has been evaluated in 2 veterinary studies. Reichling and colleagues[85] investigated topical TTO compared with a commercial skin care cream for the management of localized pruritic dermatitis in a randomized, double-blind, controlled clinical trial. The 57 dogs enrolled in this study had skin disease of mixed etiology. After 10 days of twice-daily application, a significant improvement in both pruritus and alopecia was reported in the treatment versus placebo group. In an open multicenter study, 53 dogs with various forms of chronic localized dermatitis were treated with 10% TTO cream (Bogaskin, Bogar AG, Zurich, Switzerland) twice daily for 4 weeks.[86] Exclusion criteria included corticosteroids, antibiotics, and other oral and topical treatments administered 2 weeks before or during the study period. Efficacy was determined by investigators and judged to be "good" to "very good" in 82% of the dogs. At the conclusion of the study, pruritus, erythema, and erosive/ exudative lesions had resolved in 72%, 79%, and 94% of the dogs, respectively. Adverse effects related to the study medication were reported in 2 dogs and included local irritation, erythema, and pruritus at the site of application.

A high incidence of contact allergy has been reported in people following the use of topical TTO.[87] Less commonly, immediate systemic hypersensitivity reactions may also occur.[88] Similar adverse effects have been documented in both dogs and cats, especially when applied at inappropriately high concentrations. Clinical signs of toxicity may include depression, weakness, incoordination, and tremors that often develop within 2 to 8 hours after exposure. Bathing and supportive care have been sufficient for full recovery within 2 to 3 days in most cases.[89] Cats may be more susceptible to TTO toxicosis; death has been reported following the application of concentrated (100%) essential oil. The terpenes contained in TTO are highly lipophilic and rapidly absorbed through the skin and digestive tract; oral ingestion may be more important in cats because of their inherent grooming behavior.[90]

CHAMOMILE

German chamomile (*Matricaria chamomilla*) is one of the most commonly used medicinal herbs. Multiple therapeutic properties, including improvement in skin texture and elasticity, as well as reduction of pruritus and inflammation, have long been recognized.[91] The influence of chamomile oil on AD-like immune alterations has been studied in an experimental mouse model. After 2 to 4 weeks of application, the treatment group demonstrated significantly lower scratching frequency, serum histamine, and IgG1 and IgE levels when compared with placebo.[92] Allergic contact dermatitis to the essential oil, as well as anaphylaxis following tea ingestion, has been reported in people.[93,94] As chamomile may cross react with other pollens, patients sensitized to mugwort and giant ragweed may be at increased risk for adverse effects. The relevancy of this in veterinary patients is unknown.

CALENDULA

Calendula officinalis (pot marigold), an herbaceous plant in the daisy family Asteraceae, may be contained in cosmetics and personal care products. The anti-inflammatory activity of calendula is attributed to its constituent triterpene flavonoids and saponins.[95] In human medicine, calendula is beneficial in the management of skin toxicity during radiation therapy.[96] Side effects from topical application are infrequently reported; however, contact sensitization has been documented.[97]

OATMEAL

The use of wild oats (*Avena sativa*) for skin care dates back to ancient Egypt and the Arabian peninsula when oats were used in various forms to treat eczema, burns, and other inflammatory conditions.[98] Colloidal oatmeal, a complex fraction containing lipids, carbohydrates, and beta-glucan is derived from the grinding of oat grain. Avenanthramides are phenolic compounds present in oats that exhibit antioxidant, antipruritic, and anti-inflammatory properties.[99] Oatmeal extract may decrease arachidonic acid, cytosolic phospholipase A2, and tumor necrosis factor-alpha. The activity of nuclear factor kB in keratinocytes, as well as the release of proinflammatory cytokines and histamine, may also be inhibited.[100] Colloidal grain suspensions of oatmeal are often recommended as adjunctive therapies in human AD to improve cutaneous barrier function and reduce the use of corticosteroids and calcineurin inhibitors.[101,102] High concentrations of starch and beta-glucan in oat provide protective and hydrating properties that aid in skin barrier restoration.[99] Many topical formulations containing colloidal oatmeal, often combined with aloe vera, are available in veterinary medicine.

ALOE VERA

Aloe vera is one of about 400 species of the genus *Aloe*, a succulent plant native to northern Africa. Fresh aloe gel, obtained from the inner part of the leaf, has been used for thousands of years to assist in wound healing and treat burns in both humans and animals. The active component is a polysaccharide that forms a protective and soothing layer when applied to the skin. The gel has antibacterial, antifungal, and anti-prostaglandin effects, as well as inhibitory effects on bradykinin and thromboxane.[47,103] The beneficial effects of aloe vera in the treatment of psoriasis and wound healing have been documented in human studies.[104,105] Sixty human patients with mild to moderate chronic plaque-type psoriasis were randomized to apply a 5% aloe cream or placebo 3 times daily. At the end of the 16-week study period, 83% of the patients in the aloe vera group showed significant improvement in desquamation, erythema, and PASI (psoriasis area severity index) score, compared with only 6.6% in the placebo group. Additionally, aloe vera cream has been demonstrated to be more effective than 0.1% triamcinolone acetonide in the management of mild to moderate plaque psoriasis.[106] A recent review of randomized, controlled clinical trials evaluating aloe vera for the treatment of acute and chronic wounds in human patients found little evidence to support its use.[107] Adverse effects from topical preparations are not reported.

SUMMARY

The popularity of and interest in complementary and alternative medicine is expected to continue in the future. Pet owners seek more "natural" therapies for themselves and their companions when conventional treatments are ineffective, too costly, or associated with unacceptable side effects. It is important for veterinarians to familiarize themselves with the common uses, potential benefits, and complications of these therapies, as many are available over the counter and are perceived to be less toxic. Well-tolerated and cost-effective treatment options, even with low to moderate efficacy, may be beneficial in combination with other medications, such as systemic glucocorticoids or cyclosporine, to reduce dose and potential adverse effects. In both human and veterinary medicine, there is a need for randomized controlled studies of higher design quality, as currently insufficient evidence exists to support the use of most therapies reviewed herein. The development and implementation of quality control measures and surveillance programs will generate more information on the composition and safety of herbal and homeopathic preparations, which, in turn, will result in increased confidence among practitioners and better treatment outcomes.

REFERENCES

1. AVMA Executive Board and House of Delegates. AVMA guidelines for complimentary and alternative veterinary medicine. In: AVMA Policy. 2007. Available at: http://www.avma.org/issues/policy/comp_alt_medicine.asp. Accessed May 30, 2012.
2. AVMA Executive Board and House of Delegates. Model Veterinary Practice Act. In: AVMA Policy. 2012. Available at: http://www.avma.org/issues/policy/mvpa. asp. Accessed May 30, 2012.
3. Memon MA, Sprunger LK. Survey of colleges and schools of veterinary medicine regarding education in complementary and alternative veterinary medicine. J Am Vet Med Assoc 2011;239:619–23.
4. Schoen AM. Results of a survey on educational and research programs in complementary and alternative veterinary medicine at veterinary medical schools in the United States. J Am Vet Med Assoc 2000;216:502–9.
5. Bevier DE. Long term management of atopic dermatitis in the dog. Vet Clin North Am Small Anim Pract 1990;20:1487–507.
6. Scott DW, Paradis M. A survey of canine and feline skin disorders seen in a university practice: small animal clinic, University of Montreal, Saint-Hyacinthe, Quebec (1997–98). Can Vet J 1990;31:830–5.
7. Scott DW, Miller WH, Griffin CE. Skin immune system and allergic skin disease. In: Muller and Kirk's small animal dermatology. Philadelphia: WB Saunders; 2001. p. 543–666.
8. Scott DW. Observations on canine atopy. J Am Anim Hosp Assoc 1981;17: 91–100.
9. Halliwell RE, Schwartzman RM. Atopic disease in the dog. Vet Rec 1971;89: 209–14.
10. Nesbitt GH. Canine allergic inhalant dermatitis: a review of 230 cases. J Am Vet Med Assoc 1978;172:55–60.

11. Olivry T, Mueller RS. Evidence-based veterinary dermatology: a systematic review of the pharmacology of canine atopic dermatitis. Vet Dermatol 2003; 14:121–46.

12. Olivry T, Foster AP, Mueller RS, et al. Interventions for atopic dermatitis in dogs: a systemic review of randomized controlled trials. Vet Dermatol 2010;21:4–22.

13. Paradis M, Scott DW, Giroux D. Further investigations on the use of nonsteroidal and steroidal anti-inflammatory agents in the management of canine pruritus. J Am Anim Hosp Assoc 1991;27:44–8.

14. Steffan J, Alexander D, Brovedani F, et al. Comparison of cyclosporine A with methylprednisolone for treatment of canine atopic dermatitis: a parallel blinded randomized controlled trial. Vet Dermatol 2003;14:11–22.

15. Hunley S, Xie H. Veterinary acupuncture: current use, trends and opinions. American Journal of Traditional Chinese Veterinary Medicine 2011;6:55–62.

16. Waters KC. Acupuncture for dermatologic disorders. Probl Vet Med 1992;4: 194–9.

17. Lewith GT, Machin D. On the evaluation of the clinical effects of acupuncture. Pain 1983;16:111–27.

18. Pomeranz B. Acupuncture analgesia for chronic pain: brief survey of clinical trials. In: Pomeranz B, Stux G, editors. Scientific basis of acupuncture. Berlin, Heidelberg (Germany): Springer-Verlag; 1989. p. 197–9.

19. Richardson PH, Vincent CA. Acupuncture for the treatment of pain: a review of evaluative research. Pain 1986;24:15–40.

20. Lindley S, Cummings M. Acupuncture—what is it and how does it work?. In: Lindley S, Cummings M, editors. Essentials of western veterinary acupuncture. 1st edition. Ames (IA): Blackwell Publishing; 2006. p. 33–43.

21. Lindley S, Cummings M. Acupuncture for the treatment of non-painful conditions. In: Lindley S, Cummings M, editors. Essentials of western veterinary acupuncture. 1st edition. Ames (IA): Blackwell Publishing; 2006. p. 129–50.

22. Lorinez AL. Neurophysiologic reactions of the skin: pathophysiology of pruritus. In: Fitzpatrick TB, editor. Dermatology in general medicine. New York: McGraw-Hill; 1979.

23. Belgrade MJ, Solomon LM, Lichter EA. Effect of acupuncture on experimentally induced itch. Acta Derm Venereol 1984;64:129–33.

24. Lundeberg T, Bondesson L, Thomas M. Effect of acupuncture on experimentally induced itch. Br J Dermatol 1987;117:771–7.

25. Lee KC, Keyes A, Hensley JR. Effectiveness of acupressure on pruritus and lichenification associated with atopic dermatitis: a pilot study. Acupunct Med 2012;30:8–11.

26. Pfab F, Athanasiadis GI, Huss-Marp J, et al. Effect of acupuncture on allergen-induced basophil activation in patients with atopic eczema: a pilot trial. J Altern Complement Med 2001;17:309–14.

27. Pfab F, Huss-Marp J, Gatti A, et al. Influence of acupuncture on type I hypersensitivity itch and the wheal and flare response in adults with atopic eczema—a blinded, randomized, placebo-controlled, crossover trial. Allergy 2010;65:803–10.

28. Shanghai College of Traditional Medicine. Acupuncture: a comprehensive text. Seattle (WA): Eastland Press; 1981.

29. Yamaguchi N, Takahashi T, Sakuma M, et al. Acupuncture regulates leukocyte subpopulations in human peripheral blood. Evid Based Complement Alternat Med 2007;4:447–53.

30. Sánchez-Araujo M, Puchi A. Acupuncture enhances the efficacy of antibiotic treatment for canine otitis crises. Acupunct Electrother Res 1997;22:191–206.

31. Sánchez-Araujo M, Puchi A. Acupuncture prevents relapses of recurrent otitis in dogs: a 1-year follow-up of a randomised controlled trial. Acupunct Med 2011; 29:21–6.
32. Bierman N. Acupuncture for dermatological disorders. In: Schoen AM, editor. Veterinary acupuncture: ancient art to modern medicine. 2nd edition. St Louis (MO): Mosby; 2001. p. 281–94.
33. White A. A cumulative review of the range and incidence of significant adverse events associated with acupuncture. Acupunct Med 2004;22:122–33.
34. Baker DJ. Getting to the point: the potential for modern medical acupuncture in dermatological therapy. Clin Dermatol 2008;26:309–11.
35. Sheehan MP, Atherton DJ. A controlled trial of traditional Chinese medicinal plants in widespread non-exudative atopic eczema. Br J Dermatol 1992;126: 179–84.
36. Sheehan MP, Rustin MH, Atherton DJ, et al. Efficacy of a traditional Chinese herbal therapy in adult atopic dermatitis. Lancet 1992;340:13–7.
37. Sheehan MP, Atherton DJ. One year follow up of children treated with Chinese medicinal herbs for eczema. Br J Dermatol 1994;130:488–93.
38. Nagel TM, Torres SM, Horne KL, et al. A randomized, double-blind, placebo-controlled trial to investigate the efficacy and safety of a Chinese herbal product (P07P) for the treatment of canine atopic dermatitis. Vet Dermatol 2001;12: 265–74.
39. Ferguson EA, Littlewood JD, Carlotti DN, et al. Management of canine atopic dermatitis using the plant extract PYM00217: a randomized, double-blind, placebo-controlled clinical study. Vet Dermatol 2006;17:236–43.
40. Schmidt V, McEwan N, Volk A, et al. The glucocorticoid sparing efficacy of Phytopica™ in the management of canine atopic dermatitis. Vet Dermatol 2010;21:97–105.
41. Ward T. Safety concerns involving Chinese herbal medicine. In: Mills S, Bone K, editors. The essential guide to herbal safety. St Louis (MO): Elsevier Churchill Livingston; 2005. p. 119–27.
42. Poppenga RH. Herbal medicine: potential for intoxication and interactions with conventional drugs. In: Wynn SG, Fougere B, editors. Veterinary herbal medicine. St Louis (MO): Mosby; 2007. p. 183–207.
43. Stedman C. Herbal hepatotoxicity. Semin Liver Dis 2002;22:195–206.
44. Chavez ML, Jordan MA, Chaves PI. Evidence-based drug-herbal interactions. Life Sci 2006;78:2146–57.
45. Koo J, Desai R. Traditional Chinese medicine in dermatology. Dermatol Ther 2003;16:98–105.
46. Xie H. Toxicity of Chinese veterinary herbal medicines. American Journal of Traditional Chinese Veterinary Medicine 2011;6:45–53.
47. Tyler VE. Herbs of choice: the therapeutic use of phytomedicinals. New York: Pharmaceutical Products Press; 1994.
48. Perharic L, Shaw D, Leon C, et al. Possible association of liver damage with the use of Chinese herbal medicine for skin disease. Vet Hum Toxicol 1995;37:562–6.
49. Bukutu C, Deol J, Shamseer L, et al. Complementary, holistic, and integrative medicine: atopic dermatitis. Pediatr Rev 2007;28:87–94.
50. Hektoen L. Review of the current involvement of homeopathy in veterinary practice and research. Vet Rec 2005;157:224–9.
51. Simonart T, Kabagabo C, De Maertelaer V. Homeopathic remedies in dermatology: a systemic review of controlled clinical trials. Br J Dermatol 2011;165: 897–905.

52. Sinha MN, Siddiqui VA, Nayak C, et al. Randomized controlled pilot study to compare homeopathy and conventional therapy in otitis media. Homeopathy 2012;101:5–12.

53. Taylor JA, Jacobs J. Homeopathic ear drops as an adjunct to standard therapy in children with acute otitis media. Homeopathy 2011;100:109–15.

54. Hill PB, Hoare J, Lau-Gillard P, et al. Pilot study of the effect of individualised homeopathy on the pruritus associated with atopic dermatitis in dogs. Vet Rec 2009;164:364–70.

55. Scott DW, Miller WH, Senter DA, et al. Treatment of canine atopic dermatitis with a commercial homeopathic remedy: a single-blinded, placebo-controlled study. Can Vet J 2002;43:601–3.

56. Drosdovech M, Neumann S, Evans D, et al. Not classical homeopathy. Can Vet J 2002;43:908–9.

57. Jouppi R. Studies of homeopathic treatments need to involve both homeopaths and allopaths. Can Vet J 2002;43:910.

58. Kujala C. A poor test of homeopathy. Can Vet J 2002;43:909.

59. Taylor L. Study defies the most basic tenets of homeopathy. Can Vet J 2002;43: 911–2.

60. Van As FM. Homeopathic principles not followed. Can Vet J 2002;43:908.

61. Mathie RT, Hansen L, Elliot MF, et al. Outcomes from homeopathic prescribing in veterinary practice: a prospective, research-targeted, pilot study. Homeopathy 2007;96:27–34.

62. Dantes F, Rampes H. Do homeopathic medicines provoke adverse effects? Br Homeopath J 2000;89:S35–8.

63. Chakraborti D, Mukherjee SC, Saha KC, et al. Arsenic toxicity from homeopathic treatment. J Toxicol Clin Toxicol 2003;41:963–7.

64. Ellis CN, Berberian B, Sulica VI, et al. A double-blind evaluation of topical capsaicin in pruritic psoriasis. J Am Acad Dermatol 1993;29:438–42.

65. Bernstein JE, Parish LC, Rapaport M, et al. Effects of topically applied capsaicin on moderate and severe psoriasis vulgaris. J Am Acad Dermatol 1986;15: 504–7.

66. Fitzgerald M. Capsaicin and sensory neurons: a review. Pain 1983;15:109–30.

67. Lynn B. Capsaicin: actions on C fibre afferents that may be involved in itch. Skin Pharmacol 1992;5:9–13.

68. Wallengren J, Moller H. The effect of capsaicin on some experimental inflammations in human skin. Acta Derm Venereol 1986;66:375–80.

69. Singh S, Natarajan K, Aggarwal BB. Capsaicin is a potent inhibitor of nuclear transcription of factor KB activation by diverse agents. J Immunol 1996;157: 4412–20.

70. Tobin D, Nabarro G, Baart de la Faille H, et al. Increased number of immunoreactive nerve fibers in atopic dermatitis. J Allergy Clin Immunol 1992;90:613–22.

71. Pincelli C, Fantini F, Massimi P, et al. Neuropeptides in skin from patients with atopic dermatitis: an immunohistochemical study. Br J Dermatol 1990;122: 745–50.

72. Heyer G. Abnormal cutaneous neurosensitivity in atopic skin. Acta Derm Venereol Suppl (Stockh) 1992;176:93–4.

73. Thomsen MK. Substance P: a neurogenic mediator of acute cellular inflammation in the dog? J Vet Pharmacol Ther 1991;14:250–6.

74. Marsella R, Nicklin CF, Melloy C. The effects of capsaicin topical therapy in dogs with atopic dermatitis: a randomized, double-blinded, placebo-controlled, cross-over clinical trial. Vet Dermatol 2002;13:131–9.

75. Yosipovitch G. Adverse reactions of topical capsaicin. J Am Acad Dermatol 1998;38:503–4.
76. Park EJ, Park KC, Eo H, et al. Suppression of spontaneous dermatitis in NC/Nga murine model by PG102 isolated from *Actinidia arguta*. J Invest Dermatol 2007; 127:1154–60.
77. Park EJ, Kim B, Eo H, et al. Control of IgE and selective TH1 and TH2 cytokines by PG102 isolated from *Actinidia arguta*. J Allergy Clin Immunol 2005;116: 1151–7.
78. Kim SH, Kim S, Lee SH, et al. The effects of PG 102, a water-soluble extract from *Actinidia arguta*, on serum total IgE levels: a double-blind, randomized, placebo-controlled exploratory clinical study. Eur J Nutr 2011;50:523–9.
79. Marsella R, Messinger L, Zabel S, et al. A randomized, double-blind, placebo-controlled study to evaluate the effect of EFF1001, an *Actinidia arguta* (hardy kiwi) preparation, on CADESI score and pruritus in dogs with mild to moderate atopic dermatitis. Vet Dermatol 2010;21:50–7.
80. Nenoff P, Haustein UF, Brandt W. Antifungal activity of the essential oil *Melaleuca alternifolia* (tea tree oil) against pathogenic fungi in vitro. Skin Pharmacol 1996;9: 388–94.
81. Carson CF, Riley TV. Antimicrobial activity of the major components of the essential oil of *Melaleuca alternifolia*. J Appl Bacteriol 1995;78:364–9.
82. LaPlante KL. In vitro activity of lysostaphin, mupirocin, and tea tree oil against clinical methicillin-resistant *Staphylococcus aureus*. Diagn Microbiol Infect Dis 2007;57:413–8.
83. Mickiene R, Bakutis B, Ballukoniene V. Antimicrobial activity of two essential oils. Ann Agric Environ Med 2011;18:139–44.
84. Weseler A, Geiss HK, Saller R, et al. Antifungal effect of Australian tea tree oil on *Malassezia pachydermatis*. Schweiz Arch Tierheilkd 2002;144:215–21.
85. Reichling J, Fitzi J, Hellmann K, et al. Topical tea tree oil effective in canine localised pruritic dermatitis—a multi-centre randomised double-blind controlled clinical trial in the veterinary practice. Dtsch Tierarztl Wochenschr 2004;111:408–14.
86. Fitzi J, Fürst-Jucker J, Wegener T, et al. Phytotherapy of chronic dermatitis and pruritus of dogs with a topical preparation containing tea tree oil (Bogaskin). Schweiz Arch Tierheilkd 2002;144:223–31.
87. Crawford GH, Sciacca JR, James WD. Tea tree oil: cutaneous effects of the extracted oil of *Melaleuca alternifolia*. Dermatitis 2004;15:59–66.
88. Mozelsio NB, Harris KE, McGrath KG, et al. Immediate systemic hypersensitivity reaction associated with topical application of Australian tea tree oil. Allergy Asthma Proc 2003;24:73–5.
89. Villar D, Knight MJ, Hansen SR, et al. Toxicity of melaleuca oil and related essential oils applied topically on cats and dogs. Vet Hum Toxicol 1994;36:139–42.
90. Bischoff K, Guale F. Australian tea tree (*Melaleuca alternifolia*) oil poisoning in three purebred cats. J Vet Diagn Invest 1998;10:208–10.
91. Della LR. Chamomile extracts exerted anti-inflammatory effects when applied topically in animal models of inflammation. Planta Med 1990;56:657–8.
92. Lee SH, Heo Y, Kim YC. Effect of German chamomile oil application on alleviating atopic dermatitis-like immune alterations in mice. J Vet Sci 2010;11:35–41.
93. Foti C, Nettis E, Panebianco R, et al. Contact urticarial from *Matricaria chamomilla*. Contact Dermatitis 2000;43:360–1.
94. Subiza J, Subiza JL, Hinojosa M, et al. Anaphylactic reaction after the ingestion of chamomile tea: a study of cross-reactivity with other composite pollens. J Allergy Clin Immunol 1989;84:353–8.

95. Brown DJ, Dattner AM. Phytotherapeutic approaches to common dermatologic conditions. Arch Dermatol 1998;134:1401–4.
96. Kumar S, Juresic E, Barton M, et al. Management of skin toxicity during radiation therapy: a review of the evidence. J Med Imaging Radiat Oncol 2010;54: 264–79.
97. Reider N, Komericki P, Hausen BM, et al. The seamy side of natural medicines: contact sensitization to arnica (*Arnica montana* L.) and marigold (*Calendula officinalis* L.). Contact Dermatitis 2001;45:269–72.
98. Baumann LS. Less-known botanical cosmeceuticals. Dermatol Ther 2007;20: 330–42.
99. Pazyar N, Yaghoobi R, Kazerouni A, et al. Oatmeal in dermatology: a brief review. Indian J Dermatol Venereol Leprol 2012;78:142–5.
100. Alexandrescu DT, Vaillant JG, Dasanu CA. Effect of treatment with a colloidal oatmeal lotion on the acneiform eruption induced by epidermal growth factor receptor and multiple tyrosine-kinase inhibitors. Clin Exp Dermatol 2007;32: 71–4.
101. Cerio R, Dohil M, Jeanine D, et al. Mechanism of action and clinical benefits of colloidal oatmeal for dermatologic practice. J Drugs Dermatol 2010;9:1116–20.
102. Eichenfield LF, Fowler JF Jr, Rigel DS, et al. Natural advances in eczema care. Cutis 2007;80:S2–16.
103. Das S, Mishra B, Gill K, et al. Isolation and characterization of novel protein with anti-fungal and anti-inflammatory properties from aloe vera leaf gel. Int J Biol Macromol 2011;48:38–43.
104. Fulton JE. The stimulation of postdermabrasion wound healing with stabilizing aloe vera gel-polyethylene oxide dressing. J Dermatol Surg Oncol 1990;16: 460–7.
105. Syed TA, Ahmad SA, Holt AH, et al. Management of psoriasis with aloe vera extract in a hydrophilic cream: a placebo-controlled double-blind study. Trop Med Int Health 1996;1:505–9.
106. Choonhakarn C, Busaracome P, Sripanikulchai B, et al. A prospective, randomized clinical trial comparing topical aloe vera with 0.1% triamcinolone acetonide in mild to moderate plaque psoriasis. J Eur Acad Dermatol Venereol 2010;24: 168–72.
107. Dat AD, Poon F, Pham KB, et al. Aloe vera for treating acute and chronic wounds. Cochrane Database Syst Rev 2012;(2):CD008762.

Index

Note: Page numbers of article titles are in **boldface** type.

Vet Clin Small Anim 43 (2013) 205–219
http://dx.doi.org/10.1016/S0195-5616(12)00198-2
0195-5616/13/$ – see front matter © 2013 Elsevier Inc. All rights reserved.

Moving?

Make sure your subscription moves with you!

To notify us of your new address, find your **Clinics Account Number** (located on your mailing label above your name), and contact customer service at:

Email: **journalscustomerservice-usa@elsevier.com**

800-654-2452 (subscribers in the U.S. & Canada)
314-447-8871 (subscribers outside of the U.S. & Canada)

Fax number: 314-447-8029

Elsevier Health Sciences Division
Subscription Customer Service
3251 Riverport Lane
Maryland Heights, MO 63043

*To ensure uninterrupted delivery of your subscription, please notify us at least 4 weeks in advance of move.